Pocket Companion
to Guyton and Hall Textbook
of Medical Physiology

TWELFTH EDITION

Pocket Companion
to Guyton and Hall Textbook
of Medical Physiology

John E. Hall PhD

Arthur C. Guyton Professor and Chair
Department of Physiology and Biophysics
Associate Vice Chancellor for Research
University of Mississippi Medical Center
Jackson, Mississippi

ELSEVIER
SAUNDERS

ELSEVIER
SAUNDERS

1600 John F. Kennedy Blvd.
Ste. 1800
Philadelphia, PA 19103-2899

POCKET COMPANION TO GUYTON AND HALL   ISBN: 978-1-4160-5451-1
TEXTBOOK OF MEDICAL PHYSIOLOGY, TWELFTH EDITION

Copyright © 2012, 2006, 2001, 1998 by Saunders, Inc., an imprint of Elsevier Inc.

Notices

Knowledge and best practice in this field are constantly changing. As new research and experience broaden our understanding, changes in research methods, professional practices, or medical treatment may become necessary.

Practitioners and researchers must always rely on their own experience and knowledge in evaluating and using any information, methods, compounds, or experiments described herein. In using such information or methods they should be mindful of their own safety and the safety of others, including parties for whom they have a professional responsibility.

With respect to any drug or pharmaceutical products identified, readers are advised to check the most current information provided (i) on procedures featured or (ii) by the manufacturer of each product to be administered, to verify the recommended dose or formula, the method and duration of administration, and contraindications. It is the responsibility of practitioners, relying on their own experience and knowledge of their patients, to make diagnoses, to determine dosages and the best treatment for each individual patient, and to take all appropriate safety precautions.

To the fullest extent of the law, neither the Publisher nor the authors, contributors, or editors, assume any liability for any injury and/or damage to persons or property as a matter of products liability, negligence or otherwise, or from any use or operation of any methods, products, instructions, or ideas contained in the material herein.

Illustrations by Michael Schenk and Walter Cunningham

International Standard Book Number
978-1-4160-5451-1

Executive Editor: William Schmitt   *Senior Project Manager:* Claire Kramer
Managing Editor: Rebecca Gruliow   *Designer:* Louis Forgione
Publishing Services Manager: Patricia Tannian

Printed in the United States of America

Last digit is the print number: 9   8   7   6   5   4   3   2   1

Thomas H. Adair, PhD
Professor of Physiology and Biophysics
University of Mississippi Medical Center
Jackson, Mississippi
    Membrane Physiology, Nerve, and Muscle
      (Chapters 4–8)
    Respiration (Chapters 37–42)
    Aviation, Space, and Deep-Sea Diving Physiology
      (Chapters 43–44)
    Gastrointestinal Physiology (Chapters 62–66)

David J. Dzielak, PhD
Professor of Surgery
Professor of Health Sciences
Associate Professor of Physiology and Biophysics
University of Mississippi Medical Center
Jackson, Mississippi
    Blood Cells, Immunity, and Blood Coagulation
      (Chapters 32–36)
    The Nervous System. A. General Principles and
      Sensory Physiology (Chapters 45–48)
    The Nervous System: B. The Special Senses
      (Chapters 49–53)
    The Nervous System: C. Motor and Integrative
      Neurophysiology (Chapters 54–59)

John E. Hall, PhD
Arthur C. Guyton Professor and Chair
Department of Physiology and Biophysics
Associate Vice Chancellor for Research
University of Mississippi Medical Center
Jackson, Mississippi
    Introduction to Physiology: The Cell and General
      Physiology (Chapters 1–3)
    The Circulation (Chapters 14–19)
    The Body Fluids and Kidneys (Chapters 25–31)
    The Nervous System: C. Motor and Integrative
      Neurophysiology (Chapters 60–61)

Metabolism and Temperature Regulation
    (Chapters 67–73)
Endocrinology and Reproduction (Chapters 79–83)

Thomas E. Lohmeier, PhD
Professor of Physiology and Biophysics
University of Mississippi Medical Center
Jackson, Mississippi
    Endocrinology and Reproduction (Chapters 74–78)

R. Davis Manning, PhD
Professor of Physiology and Biophysics
University of Mississippi Medical Center
Jackson, Mississippi
    The Heart (Chapters 9–13)
    The Circulation (Chapters 20–24)
    Sports Physiology (Chapter 84)

Human physiology is the discipline that links basic sciences with clinical medicine. It is integrative and encompasses everything from the study of molecules and subcellular components to the study of organ systems and their interactions that allow us to function as living beings. Because human physiology is a rapidly expanding discipline and covers a broad scope, the vast amount of information potentially applicable to the practice of medicine can be overwhelming. Therefore, one of our goals for writing this "Pocket Companion" was to distill this enormous amount of information into a book that would be small enough to be carried in a coat pocket and used often but still contain the basic physiologic principles necessary for the study of medicine.

The pocket companion was designed to accompany Guyton and Hall's *Textbook of Medical Physiology*, 12th Edition, and it cannot serve as a substitute for the parent text. Rather, it is intended to serve as a concise overview of the most important facts and concepts from the parent text, presented in a manner that facilitates rapid comprehension of basic physiologic principles. Some of the most important features of the pocket companion are as follows:

- It has been designed to serve as a guide for students who wish to review a large volume of material from the parent text rapidly and efficiently. The headings of the sections state succinctly the primary concepts in the accompanying paragraphs. Thus the student can quickly review many of the main concepts in the textbook by first studying the paragraph headings.
- The table of contents matches that of the parent text, and each topic has been cross-referenced with specific page numbers from the parent text. The pocket companion has been updated in parallel with the *Textbook of Medical Physiology.*
- The size of the book has been restricted so it can fit conveniently in a coat pocket as an immediate source of information when needed.

Although the pocket companion contains the most important facts necessary for studying physiology, it does not contain the details that enrich the physiologic concepts or the clinical examples of abnormal physiology that are contained in the parent book. We therefore recommend that the pocket companion be used in conjunction with the *Textbook of Medical Physiology*, 12th Edition.

I am grateful to each of the contributors for their careful work on this book. Contributing authors were selected for their knowledge of physiology and their ability to present information effectively to students.

We have strived to make this book as accurate as possible and hope that it will be valuable for your study of physiology. Your comments and suggestions for ways to improve the *Pocket Companion* are always greatly appreciated.

John E. Hall, PhD
Jackson, Mississippi

Contents

UNIT III

The Heart

UNIT IV

The Circulation

UNIT V

The Body Fluids and Kidneys

UNIT VI

Blood Cells, Immunity, and Blood Coagulation

UNIT VII

Respiration

UNIT VIII

Aviation, Space, and Deep-Sea Diving Physiology

UNIT IX

The Nervous System: A. General Principles and Sensory Physiology

UNIT XII

Gastrointestinal Physiology

UNIT XIII

Metabolism and Temperature Regulation

UNIT XIV

Endocrinology and Reproduction

UNIT XV

Sports Physiology

I

Introduction to Physiology: The Cell and General Physiology

Functional Organization of the Human Body and Control of the "Internal Environment"

The goal of physiology is to understand the *function* of living organisms and their parts. In human physiology, we are concerned with the characteristics of the human body that allow us to sense our environment, move about, think and communicate, reproduce, and perform all of the functions that enable us to survive and thrive as living beings.

Human physiology is a broad subject that includes the functions of molecules and subcellular components; tissues; organs; organ systems, such as the cardiovascular system; and the interaction and communication among these components. A distinguishing feature of physiology is that it seeks to integrate the functions of all of the parts of the body to understand the function of the entire human body. Life in the human being relies on this total function, which is considerably more complex than the sum of the functions of the individual cells, tissues, and organs.

Cells Are the Living Units of the Body. Each organ is an aggregate of many cells held together by intercellular supporting structures. The entire body contains about 75 to 100 trillion cells, each of which is adapted to perform special functions. These individual cell functions are coordinated by multiple regulatory systems operating in cells, tissues, organs, and organ systems.

Although the many cells of the body differ from each other in their special functions, all of them have certain basic characteristics. For example, (1) oxygen combines with breakdown products of fat, carbohydrates, or protein to release energy that is required for normal function of the cells; (2) most cells have the ability to reproduce, and whenever cells are destroyed the remaining cells often regenerate new cells until the appropriate number is restored; and (3) cells are bathed in extracellular fluid, the constituents of which are precisely controlled.

"Homeostatic" Mechanisms of the Major Functional Systems (p. 4)

Essentially all of the organs and tissues of the body perform functions that help maintain the constituents of the extracellular fluid relatively constant, a condition called *homeostasis*. Much of our discussion of physiology focuses on the mechanisms by which the cells, tissues, and organs contribute to homeostasis.

Extracellular Fluid Transport and Mixing System— The Blood Circulatory System

Extracellular fluid is transported throughout the body in two stages. The first stage is movement of blood around the *circulatory system,* and the second stage is movement of fluid between the blood capillaries and cells. The circulatory system keeps the fluids of the internal environment continuously mixed by pumping blood through the vascular system. As blood passes through the capillaries, a large portion of its fluid diffuses back and forth into the interstitial fluid that lies between the cells, allowing continuous exchange of substances between the cells and the interstitial fluid and between the interstitial fluid and the blood.

Origin of Nutrients in the Extracellular Fluid

- The *respiratory system* provides oxygen for the body and removes carbon dioxide.
- The *gastrointestinal system* digests food and absorbs various nutrients, including carbohydrates, fatty acids, and amino acids, into the extracellular fluid.
- The *liver* changes the chemical composition of many of the absorbed substances to more usable forms, and other tissues of the body (e.g., fat cells, kidneys, endocrine glands) help modify the absorbed substances or store them until they are needed.
- The *musculoskeletal system* consists of skeletal muscles, bones, tendons, joints, cartilage, and ligaments. Without this system, the body could not move to the appropriate place to obtain the foods required for nutrition. This system also provides protection of internal organs and support of the body.

Removal of Metabolic End Products (p. 5)

- The *respiratory system* not only provides oxygen to the extracellular fluid but also removes carbon dioxide, which is produced by the cells, released from the blood into the alveoli, and then released to the external environment.
- The *kidneys* excrete most of the waste products other than carbon dioxide. The kidneys play a major role in regulating the extracellular fluid composition by controlling the excretion of salts, water, and waste

products of the chemical reactions of the cells. By controlling body fluid volumes and compositions, the kidneys also regulate blood volume and blood pressure.

- The *liver* eliminates certain waste products produced in the body as well as toxic substances that are ingested.

Regulation of Body Functions

- The *nervous system* directs the activity of the muscular system, thereby providing locomotion. It also controls the function of many internal organs through the autonomic nervous system, and it allows us to sense our external and internal environment and to be intelligent beings so we can obtain the most advantageous conditions for survival.
- The *hormone systems* control many of the metabolic functions of the cells, such as growth, rate of metabolism, and special activities associated with reproduction. Hormones are secreted into the bloodstream and are carried to tissues throughout the body to help regulate cell function.

Protection of the Body

- The *immune system* provides the body with a defense mechanism that protects against foreign invaders, such as bacteria and viruses, to which the body is exposed daily.
- The *integumentary system,* which is composed mainly of skin, provides protection against injury and defense against foreign invaders as well as protection of underlying tissues against dehydration. The skin also serves to regulate body temperature.

Reproduction

The *reproductive system* provides for formation of new beings like ourselves. Even this can be considered a homeostatic function because it generates new bodies in which trillions of additional cells can exist in a well-regulated internal environment.

Control Systems of the Body *(p. 6)*

The human body has thousands of control systems that are essential for homeostasis. For example, genetic systems operate in all cells to control intracellular as well as extracellular functions. Other control systems operate within the organs or throughout the entire body to control interactions among the organs.

Regulation of oxygen and carbon dioxide concentrations in the extracellular fluid is a good example of multiple control systems that operate together. In this instance, the respiratory system operates in association with the nervous system. When the carbon dioxide concentration in the blood increases above normal, the respiratory center is excited, causing the person to breathe rapidly and deeply. This increases the expiration of carbon dioxide and therefore removes it from the blood and the extracellular fluid until the concentration returns to normal.

Normal Ranges of Important Extracellular Fluid Constituents

Table 1–1 shows some of the important constituents of extracellular fluid along with their normal values, normal ranges, and maximum limits that can be endured for short periods of time without the occurrence of death. Note the narrowness of the ranges; levels outside these ranges are usually the cause or the result of illnesses.

Characteristics of Control Systems

Most Control Systems of the Body Operate by *Negative Feedback*. For regulation of carbon dioxide concentration as discussed, a high concentration of carbon dioxide in the extracellular fluid increases pulmonary ventilation, which decreases the carbon dioxide concentration toward normal levels. This is an example of *negative feedback;* any stimulus that attempts to change the carbon dioxide concentration is counteracted by a response that is *negative* to the initiating stimulus.

The degree of effectiveness with which a control system maintains constant conditions is determined by the *gain* of the negative feedback. The gain is calculated according to the following formula.

$$\text{Gain} = \text{Correction}/\text{Error}$$

Some control systems, such as those that regulate body temperature, have feedback gains as high as −33, which simply means that the degree of correction is 33 times greater than the remaining error.

Feed-Forward Control Systems Anticipate Changes. Because of the many interconnections between control systems, the total control of a particular body function may be more complex than can be accounted for by

Table 1–1. Some Important Constituents and Physical Characteristics of the Extracellular Fluid, Normal Range of Control, and Approximate Nonlethal Limits for Short Periods

Parameter	Units	Average Normal Values	Normal Ranges	Approximate Nonlethal Limits
Oxygen	mm Hg	40	35–45	10–1000
Carbon dioxide	mm Hg	40	35–45	5–80
Sodium ion	mmol/L	142	138–146	115–175
Potassium ion	mmol/L	4.2	3.8–5.0	1.5–9.0
Calcium ion	mmol/L	1.2	1.0–1.4	0.5–2.0
Chloride ion	mmol/L	108	103–112	70–130
Bicarbonate ion	mmol/L	28	24–32	8–45
Glucose	mg/dL	85	75–95	20–1500
Body temperature	°F (°C)	98.4 (37.0)	98–98.8 (37.0)	65–110 (18.3–43.3)
Acid-base	pH	7.4	7.3–7.5	6.9–8.0

simple negative feedback. For example, some movements of the body occur so rapidly that there is not sufficient time for nerve signals to travel from some of the peripheral body parts to the brain and then back to the periphery in time to control the movements. Therefore, the brain uses feed-forward control to cause the required muscle contractions. Sensory nerve signals from the moving parts apprise the brain in retrospect of whether the appropriate movement, as envisaged by the brain, has been performed correctly. If it has not, the brain corrects the feed-forward signals it sends to the muscles the next time the movement is required. This is also called *adaptive control*, which is, in a sense, delayed negative feedback.

Positive Feedback Can Sometimes Cause Vicious Cycles and Death, and Other Times Can Be Useful. A system that exhibits positive feedback responds to a perturbation with changes that amplify the perturbation and therefore leads to instability rather than stability. For example, severe hemorrhage may lower blood pressure to such a low level that blood flow to the heart is insufficient to maintain normal cardiac pumping; as a result, blood pressure falls even lower, further diminishing blood flow to the heart and causing still more weakness of the heart. Each cycle of this feedback leads to more of the same, which is a *positive feedback* or a *vicious cycle.*

In some cases the body uses positive feedback to its advantage. An example is the generation of nerve signals. When the nerve fiber membrane is stimulated the slight leakage of sodium ions into the cell causes opening of more channels, more sodium entry, more change in membrane potential, and so forth. Therefore, a slight leak of sodium into the cell becomes an explosion of sodium entering the interior of the nerve fiber, which creates the nerve action potential.

Summary—Automaticity of the Body (p. 9)

The body is a social order of about 75 to 100 trillion cells organized into various functional structures, the largest of which are called *organs*. Each functional structure, or organ, has a role in maintaining a constant internal environment. So long as homeostasis is maintained, the cells of the body continue to live and function properly. Thus, each cell benefits from homeostasis and, in turn, each cell contributes its share toward the maintenance of homeostasis. This reciprocal interplay provides continuous *automaticity* of the body until one or more functional systems lose their ability to contribute their share of function. When this loss happens, all cells of the body suffer. Extreme dysfunction leads to death, whereas moderate dysfunction leads to sickness.

CHAPTER 2

The Cell and Its Functions

Organization of the Cell (p. 11)

Figure 2–1 shows a typical cell, including the *nucleus* and *cytoplasm*, which are separated by the *nuclear membrane*. The cytoplasm is separated from *interstitial fluid*, which surrounds the cell, by a *cell membrane*. The substances that make up the cell are collectively called *protoplasm*, which is composed mainly of the following.

- *Water* comprises 70% to 85% of most cells.
- *Electrolytes* provide inorganic chemicals for cellular reactions. Some of the most important electrolytes in the cell are *potassium, magnesium, phosphate, sulfate, bicarbonate,* and small quantities of *sodium, chloride,* and *calcium.*
- *Proteins* normally constitute 10% to 20% of the cell mass. They can be divided into two types: *structural proteins* and *globular (functional) proteins* (which are mainly *enzymes*).
- *Lipids* constitute about 2% of the total cell mass. Among the most important lipids in the cells are *phospholipids, cholesterol, triglycerides,* and *neutral fats.* In *adipocytes* (fat cells), triglycerides may account for as much as 95% of the cell mass.
- *Carbohydrates* play a major role in nutrition of the cell. Most human cells do not store large amounts of carbohydrates, which usually average about 1% of the total cell mass but may be as high as 3% in muscle cells and 6% in liver cells. The small amount of carbohydrates in the cells is usually stored in the form of *glycogen,* an insoluble polymer of glucose.

Physical Structure of the Cell (p. 12)

The cell (Fig. 2–1) is not merely a bag of fluid and chemicals; it also contains highly organized physical structures called *organelles.* Some of the principal organelles of the cell are the *cell membrane, nuclear membrane, endoplasmic reticulum* (ER), *Golgi apparatus, mitochondria, lysosomes,* and *centrioles.*

The Cell and Its Organelles Are Surrounded by Membranes Composed of Lipids and Proteins. These membranes include the *cell membrane, nuclear membrane,* and *membranes of the ER, mitochondria, lysosomes,* and *Golgi apparatus.* They provide barriers that prevent free movement of water and water-soluble substances from one cell compartment to another. Protein

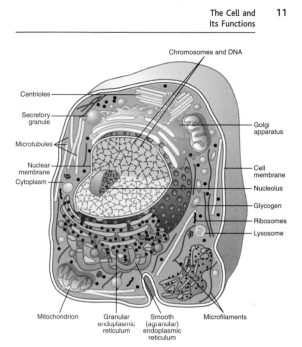

Chromosomes and DNA

Centrioles

Secretory granule

Microtubules

Nuclear membrane

Cytoplasm

Golgi apparatus

Cell membrane

Nucleolus

Glycogen

Ribosomes

Lysosome

Mitochondrion

Granular endoplasmic reticulum

Smooth (agranular) endoplasmic reticulum

Microfilaments

Figure 2–1. Reconstruction of a typical cell, showing the internal organelles of the cytoplasm and nucleus.

molecules in the membrane often penetrate the membrane, providing pathways (channels) to allow movement of specific substances through the membranes.

The Cell Membrane Is a Lipid Bilayer with Inserted Proteins. The lipid bilayer is composed almost entirely of *phospholipids* and *cholesterol.* Phospholipids have a water-soluble portion *(hydrophilic)* and a portion that is soluble only in fats *(hydrophobic).* The hydrophobic portions of the phospholipids face each other, whereas the hydrophilic parts face the two surfaces of the membrane in contact with the surrounding interstitial fluid and the cell cytoplasm.

This lipid bilayer membrane is highly permeable to lipid-soluble substances, such as oxygen, carbon dioxide, and alcohol, but it acts as a major barrier to water-soluble substances, such as ions and glucose. Floating in the lipid bilayer are proteins, most of which are *glycoproteins* (proteins combined with carbohydrates).

There are two types of membrane protein: the *integral proteins*, which protrude through the membrane, and the *peripheral proteins,* which are attached to the inner surface of the membrane and do not penetrate. Many of the integral proteins provide *structural channels* (pores) through which water-soluble substances, especially ions, can diffuse. Other integral proteins act as *carrier proteins* for the transport of substances, sometimes against their gradients for diffusion.

Integral proteins can also serve as *receptors* for substances, such as peptide hormones, that do not easily penetrate the cell membrane.

The peripheral proteins are normally attached to one of the integral proteins and usually function as *enzymes* that catalyze chemical reactions of the cell.

The membrane carbohydrates occur mainly in combination with proteins and lipids in the form of *glycoproteins* and *glycolipids.* The "glyco" portions of these molecules usually protrude to the outside of the cell. Many other carbohydrate compounds, called *proteoglycans,* which are mainly carbohydrate substances bound together by small protein cores, are loosely attached to the outer surface; thus the entire outer surface of the cell often has a loose carbohydrate coat called the *glycocalyx.*

The carbohydrates on the outer surface of the cell have multiple functions: (1) they are often negatively charged and therefore repel other molecules negatively charged; (2) the glycocalyx of cells may attach to other cells (thus the cells attach to each other); (3) some of the carbohydrates act as *receptors* for binding hormones; and (4) some carbohydrate moieties enter into immune reactions, as discussed in Chapter 34.

The *ER* Synthesizes Multiple Substances in the Cell. A large network of tubules and vesicles, called the *ER,* penetrates almost all parts of the cytoplasm. The membrane of the ER provides an extensive surface area for the manufacture of many substances used inside the cells and released from some cells. They include proteins; carbohydrates; lipids; and other structures such as lysosomes, peroxisomes, and secretory granules.

Lipids are made within the ER wall. For the synthesis of proteins, *ribosomes* attach to the outer surface of the *granular ER.* These function in association with *messenger RNA* to synthesize many proteins that then enter the Golgi apparatus, where the molecules are further modified before they are released or used in the cell. Part of the ER has no attached ribosomes and is called the *agranular,* or *smooth, ER.* The agranular ER functions for the synthesis of lipid substances and for other processes of the cells promoted by intrareticular enzymes.

The *Golgi Apparatus* Functions in Association with the ER. The Golgi apparatus has membranes similar to those of the agranular ER, is prominent in secretory cells, and is located on the side of the cell from which the secretory substances are extruded. Small *transport vesicles*, also called ER vesicles, continually pinch off from the ER and then fuse with the Golgi apparatus. In this way, substances entrapped in the ER vesicles are transported from the ER to the Golgi apparatus. The substances are then processed in the Golgi apparatus to form lysosomes, secretory vesicles, and other cytoplasmic components.

Lysosomes Provide an Intracellular Digestive System. Lysosomes, found in great numbers in many cells, are small spherical vesicles surrounded by a membrane that contains digestive enzymes; these enzymes allow lysosomes to break down intracellular substances in structures, especially damaged cell structures, food particles that have been ingested by the cell, and unwanted materials such as bacteria.

The membranes surrounding the lysosomes usually prevent the enclosed enzymes from coming in contact with other substances in the cell and therefore prevent their digestive action. When these membranes are damaged, however, the enzymes are released and split the organic substances with which they come in contact into highly diffusible substances such as amino acids and glucose.

Mitochondria Release Energy in the Cell. An adequate supply of energy must be available to fuel the chemical reactions of the cell. This is provided mainly by the chemical reaction of oxygen with the three types of foods: glucose derived from carbohydrates, fatty acid derived from fats, and amino acid derived from proteins. After entering the cell, the foods are split into smaller molecules that, in turn, enter the mitochondria, where other enzymes remove carbon dioxide and hydrogen ions in a process called the *citric acid cycle*. An oxidative enzyme system, which is also in the mitochondria, causes progressive oxidation of the hydrogen atoms. The end products of the reactions of the mitochondria are water and carbon dioxide. The energy liberated is used by the mitochondria to synthesize another substance, *adenosine triphosphate* (ATP), which is a highly reactive chemical that can diffuse throughout the cell to release its energy whenever it is needed for the performance of cell functions.

Mitochondria are also self-replicative, which means that one mitochondrion can form a second one, a third one, and so on whenever there is a need in the cell for increased amounts of ATP.

There Are Many Cytoplasmic Structures and Organelles. There are hundreds of types of cells in the body, and each has a special structure. Some cells, for example, are rigid and have large numbers of *filamentous* or *tubular structures,* which are composed of *fibrillar proteins.* A major function of these tubular structures is to act as a *cytoskeleton,* providing rigid physical structures for certain parts of cells. Some of the tubular structures, called *microtubules,* can transport substances from one area of the cell to another.

One of the important functions of many cells is to secrete special substances, such as digestive enzymes. Almost all of the substances are formed by the ER-Golgi apparatus system and are released into the cytoplasm inside storage vesicles called *secretory vesicles.* After a period of storage in the cell, they are expelled through the cell membrane to be used elsewhere in the body.

The *Nucleus* Is the Control Center of the Cell and Contains Large Amounts of DNA, Also Called *Genes* (p. 17). The genes determine the characteristics of the proteins of the cell, including the enzymes of the cytoplasm. They also control reproduction. They first reproduce themselves through a process of *mitosis* in which two daughter cells are formed, each of which receives one of the two sets of genes.

The *nuclear membrane,* also called the *nuclear envelope,* separates the nucleus from the cytoplasm. This structure is composed of two membranes; the outer membrane is continuous with the ER, and the space between the two nuclear membranes is also continuous with the compartment inside the ER. Both layers of the membrane are penetrated by several thousand *nuclear pores,* which are almost 100 nanometers in diameter.

The nuclei in most cells contain one or more structures called *nucleoli,* which unlike many of the organelles do not have a surrounding membrane. The nucleoli contain large amounts of RNA and proteins of the type found in ribosomes. A nucleolus becomes enlarged when the cell is actively synthesizing proteins. Ribosomal RNA is stored in the nucleolus and transported through the nuclear membrane pores to the cytoplasm, where it is used to produce mature ribosomes, which play an important role in the formation of proteins.

Functional Systems of the Cell (p. 18)

Ingestion by the Cell—Endocytosis

The cell obtains nutrients and other substances from the surrounding fluid through the cell membrane via *diffusion* and *active transport*. Very large particles enter the cell via *endocytosis,* the principal forms of which are *pinocytosis* and *phagocytosis*.

- *Pinocytosis is the ingestion of small globules of extra-cellular fluid, forming minute vesicles in the cell cyto-plasm.* This is the only method by which large molecules, such as proteins, can enter the cells. These molecules usually attach to specialized recep-tors on the outer surface of the membrane that are concentrated in small pits called *coated pits.* On the inside of the cell membrane underneath these pits is a latticework of a fibrillar protein called *clathrin* and a contractile filament of *actin* and *myosin.* After the protein molecules bind with the receptors, the membrane invaginates and contractile proteins sur-round the pit, causing its borders to close over the attached proteins and form a *pinocytotic vesicle.*

- *Phagocytosis is the ingestion of large particles, such as bacteria, cells, and portions of degenerating tissue.* This ingestion occurs much in the same way as pinocytosis except that it involves large particles instead of mole-cules. Only certain cells have the ability to perform phagocytosis, notably tissue *macrophages* and some *white blood cells.* Phagocytosis is initiated when proteins or large polysaccharides on the surface of the particle bind with receptors on the surface of the phagocyte. In the case of bacteria, these usually are attached to specific antibodies, and the antibodies in turn attach to the phagocyte receptors, dragging the bacteria along with them. This intermediation of antibodies is called *opsonization* and is discussed further in Chapters 33 and 34.

Pinocytic and Phagocytic Foreign Substances Are Digested in the Cell by the Lysosomes. Almost as soon as pinocytic or phagocytic vesicles appear inside a cell, lysosomes become attached to the vesicles and empty their digestive enzymes into the vesicle. Thus, a *digestive vesicle* is formed in which the enzymes begin hydrolyzing the proteins, carbohydrates, lipids, and other substances in the vesicle. The products of digestion are small molecules of amino acids, glucose, phosphate, and so on that can diffuse through the membrane of the vesicle into the cytoplasm. The undigested substances, called the *residual body*, are excreted through the cell membrane via the process of *exocytosis*, which is basically the opposite of endocytosis.

Synthesis of Cellular Structures by ER and Golgi Apparatus *(p. 20)*

The Synthesis of Most Cell Structures Begins in the ER. Many of the products formed in the ER are then passed onto the Golgi apparatus, where they are further processed before release into the cytoplasm. The *granular ER*, characterized by large numbers of ribosomes attached to the outer surface, is the site of protein formation. Ribosomes synthesize the proteins and extrude many of them through the wall of the ER to the interior of the endoplasmic vesicles and tubules, called the *endoplasmic matrix.*

When protein molecules enter the ER, enzymes in the ER wall cause rapid changes, including congregation of carbohydrates to form *glycoproteins.* In addition, the proteins are often cross-linked, folded, and shortened to form more compact molecules.

The ER also synthesizes lipids, especially phospholipid and cholesterol, which are incorporated into the lipid bilayer of the ER. Small ER vesicles, or *transport vesicles,* continually break off from the smooth reticulum. Most of these migrate rapidly to the Golgi apparatus.

The *Golgi Apparatus* Processes Substances Formed in the ER. As substances are formed in the ER, especially proteins, they are transported through the reticulum tubules toward the portions of the smooth ER that lie nearest the Golgi apparatus. Small transport vesicles, composed of small envelopes of smooth ER, continually break away and diffuse to the deepest layer of the Golgi apparatus. The transport vesicles instantly fuse with the Golgi apparatus and empty their contents into the vesicular spaces of the Golgi apparatus. Here, more carbohydrates are added to the secretions, and the ER secretions are compacted. As the secretions pass toward the outermost layers of the Golgi apparatus, the compaction and processing continue; finally, small and large vesicles break away from the Golgi apparatus, carrying with them the compacted secretory substances. These substances can then diffuse throughout the cell.

In a highly secretory cell, the vesicles formed by the Golgi apparatus are mainly *secretory vesicles,* which diffuse to the cell membrane, fuse with it, and eventually empty their substances to the exterior via a mechanism called *exocytosis.* Some of the vesicles made in the Golgi apparatus, however, are destined for intracellular use. For example, specialized portions of the Golgi apparatus form lysosomes.

Extraction of Energy from Nutrients by the Mitochondria *(p. 21)*

The principal substances from which the cells extract energy are oxygen and one or more of the foodstuffs—carbohydrates, fats, proteins—that react with oxygen. In the human body, almost all carbohydrates are converted to *glucose* by the digestive tract and liver before they reach the cell; similarly, proteins are converted to *amino acids,* and fats are converted to *fatty acids.* Inside the cell, these substances react chemically with oxygen under the influence of enzymes that control the rates of reaction and channel the released energy in the proper direction.

Oxidative Reactions Occur inside the Mitochondria, and the Energy Released Is Used to Form Mainly ATP. ATP is a nucleotide composed of the nitrogenous base *adenine,* the pentose sugar *ribose,* and *three phosphate radicals.* The last two phosphate radicals are connected with the remainder of the molecule by *high-energy phosphate bonds,* each of which contains about 12,000 calories of energy per mole of ATP under the usual conditions of the body. The high-energy phosphate bonds are labile so they can be split instantly whenever energy is required to promote other cellular reactions.

When ATP releases its energy, a phosphoric acid radical is split away, and *adenosine diphosphate* (ADP) is formed. Energy derived from cell nutrients causes the ADP and phosphoric acid to recombine to form new ATP, with the entire process continuing over and over again.

Most of the ATP Produced in the Cell Is Formed in the Mitochondria. After entry into the cells, glucose is subjected to enzymes in the cytoplasm that convert it to *pyruvic acid,* a process called *glycolysis.* Less than 5% of the ATP formed in the cell occurs via glycolysis.

The pyruvic acid derived from carbohydrates, the fatty acids derived from lipids, and the amino acids derived from proteins are all eventually converted to the compound *acetyl-coenzyme A* (acetyl-CoA) in the matrix of mitochondria. This substance is then acted on by another series of enzymes in a sequence of chemical reactions called the *citric acid cycle,* or *Krebs cycle.*

In the citric acid cycle, acetyl-CoA is split into *hydrogen ions* and *carbon dioxide.* The hydrogen ions are highly reactive and eventually combine with oxygen that has diffused into the mitochondria. This reaction releases a tremendous amount of energy, which is used to convert large amounts of ADP to ATP. This requires large numbers of protein enzymes that are integral parts of the mitochondria.

The initial event in the formation of ATP is removal of an electron from the hydrogen atom, thereby converting it to a hydrogen ion. The terminal event is movement of the hydrogen ion through large globular proteins called *ATP synthetase,* which protrude through the membranes of the mitochondrial *membranous shelves,* which themselves protrude into the mitochondrial matrix. ATP synthetase is an enzyme that uses the energy and movement of the hydrogen ions to effect the conversion of ADP to ATP, and hydrogen ions combine with oxygen to form water. The newly formed ATP is transported out of the mitochondria to all parts of the cell cytoplasm and nucleoplasm, where it is used to energize the functions of the cell. This overall process is called the *chemosmotic mechanism* of ATP formation.

ATP Is Used for Many Cellular Functions. ATP promotes three types of cell function: (1) *membrane transport,* as occurs with the sodium-potassium pump, which transports sodium out of the cell and potassium into the cell; (2) *synthesis of chemical compounds throughout the cell*; and (3) *mechanical work,* as occurs with the contraction of muscle fibers or with ciliary and ameboid motion.

Locomotion and Ciliary Movements of Cells *(p. 23)*

The most important type of movement that occurs in the body is that of the specialized muscle cells in skeletal, cardiac, and smooth muscle, which constitute almost 50% of the entire body mass. Two other types of movement occur in other cells: *ameboid locomotion* and *ciliary movement.*

Ameboid Locomotion Is the Movement of an Entire Cell in Relation to Its Surroundings. An example of ameboid locomotion is the movement of white blood cells through tissues. Typically, ameboid locomotion begins with protrusion of a *pseudopodium* from one end of the cell. This results from continual exocytosis, which forms a new cell membrane at the leading edge of the pseudopodium, and continual endocytosis of the membrane in the mid and rear portions of the cell.

Two other effects are also essential to the forward movement of the cell. The first effect is attachment of the pseudopodium to the surrounding tissues so it becomes fixed in its leading position while the remainder of the cell body is pulled forward toward the point of attachment. This attachment is effected by receptor proteins that line the insides of the exocytotic vesicles.

The second requirement for locomotion is the presence of the energy needed to pull the cell body in the direction of the pseudopodium. In the cytoplasm of all cells are molecules of the protein *actin*. When these molecules polymerize to form a filamentous network the network contracts when it binds with another protein, an actin-binding protein such as *myosin*. The entire process, which is energized by ATP, takes place in the pseudopodium of a moving cell, in which such a network of actin filaments forms inside the growing pseudopodium.

The most important factor that usually initiates ameboid movement is the process called *chemotaxis*, which results from the appearance of certain chemical substances in the tissue called *chemotactic substances*.

Ciliary Movement Is a Whiplike Movement of Cilia on the Surfaces of Cells. Ciliary movement occurs in only two places in the body: on the inside surfaces of the *respiratory airways* and on the inside surfaces of the *uterine tubes* (fallopian tubes of the reproductive tract). In the nasal cavity and lower respiratory airways, the whiplike motion of the cilia causes a layer of mucus to move toward the pharynx at a rate of about 1 cm/min; in this way, passageways with mucus or particles that become entrapped in the mucus are continually cleared. In the uterine tubes, the cilia cause slow movement of fluid from the ostium of the uterine tube toward the uterine cavity; it is mainly this movement of fluid that transports the ovum from the ovary to the uterus.

The mechanism of the ciliary movement is not fully understood, but there are at least two necessary factors: (1) the presence of ATP and (2) the appropriate ionic conditions, including appropriate concentrations of magnesium and calcium.

CHAPTER 3

Genetic Control of Protein Synthesis, Cell Function, and Cell Reproduction

Genes in Cell Nucleus Control Protein Synthesis *(p. 27)*. The genes control protein synthesis in the cell and in this way control cell function. Proteins play a key role in almost all functions of the cell by serving as enzymes that catalyze the reactions of the cell and as major components of the physical structures of the cell.

Each gene is a double-stranded, helical molecule of *deoxyribonucleic acid* (DNA) that controls the formation of *ribonucleic acid* (RNA). The RNA, in turn, spreads throughout the cells to control the formation of a specific protein. The entire process, from *transcription* of the genetic code in the nucleus to *translation* of the RNA code and formation or proteins in the cell cytoplasm, is often referred to as *gene expression* and is shown in Figure 3–1. Because there are about 30,000 genes in each cell, it is possible to form large numbers of different cellular proteins.

Nucleotides Are Organized to Form Two Strands of DNA Loosely Bound to Each Other. Genes are attached in an end-on-end manner in long, double-stranded, helical molecules of DNA that are composed of three basic building blocks: (1) *phosphoric acid,* (2) *deoxyribose* (a sugar), and (3) four *nitrogenous bases:* two purines (adenine and guanine) and two pyrimidines (thymine and cytosine).

The first stage in the formation of DNA is the combination of one molecule of phosphoric acid, one molecule of deoxyribose, and one of the four bases to form a *nucleotide.* Four nucleotides can therefore be formed, one from each of the four bases. Multiple nucleotides are bound together to form two strands of DNA, and the two strands are loosely bound to each other.

The backbone of each DNA strand is composed of alternating phosphoric acid and deoxyribose molecules. The purine and pyrimidine bases are attached to the side of the deoxyribose molecules, and loose bonds between the purine and pyrimidine bases of the two DNA strands hold them together. *The purine base adenine of one strand always bonds with the pyrimidine base thymine of the other strand, whereas guanine always bonds with cytosine.*

The Genetic Code Consists of Triplets of Bases. Each group of three successive bases in the DNA strand is called a *code word,* and these code words control the

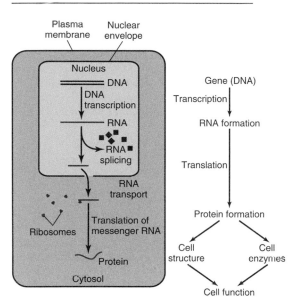

Figure 3–1. General schema by which the genes control cell function.

sequence of amino acids in the protein to be formed in the cytoplasm. One code word, for example, might be composed of a sequence of adenine, thymine, and guanine, whereas the next code word might have a sequence of cytosine, guanine, and thymine. These two code words have entirely different meanings because their bases are different. The sequence of successive code words of the DNA strand is known as the *genetic code.*

DNA Code in the Cell Nucleus Is Transferred to RNA Code in the Cell Cytoplasm—The Process of Transcription *(p. 30)*

Because DNA is located in the nucleus and many of the functions of the cell are carried out in the cytoplasm, there must be some method by which the genes of the nucleus control the chemical reactions of the cytoplasm. This is achieved through RNA, the formation of which is controlled by DNA. During this process the code of DNA is transferred to RNA, a process called *transcription.* The RNA diffuses from the nucleus to the nuclear pores into the cytoplasm, where it controls protein synthesis.

RNA Is Synthesized in the Nucleus from a DNA Template. During the synthesis of RNA the two strands of the DNA molecule separate, and one of the two strands is used as a template for the synthesis of RNA. The code triplets in the DNA cause the formation of *complementary code triplets* (called *codons*) in the RNA; these codons then control the sequence of amino acids in a protein to be synthesized later in the cytoplasm. Each DNA strand in each chromosome carries the code for perhaps as many as 2000 to 4000 genes.

The basic building blocks of RNA are almost the same as those of DNA except that in RNA, the sugar *ribose* replaces the sugar deoxyribose and the pyrimidine *uracil* replaces thymine. The basic building blocks of RNA combine to form four nucleotides, exactly as described for the synthesis of DNA. These nucleotides contain the bases *adenine, guanine, cytosine,* and *uracil.*

The next step in the synthesis of RNA is *activation of the nucleotides.* This occurs through the addition of two phosphate radicals to each nucleotide to form triphosphates. These last two phosphates are combined with the nucleotide by *high-energy phosphate bonds,* which are derived from the adenosine triphosphate (ATP) of the cell. This activation process makes available large quantities of energy, which is used for promoting the chemical reactions that add each new RNA nucleotide to the end of the RNA chain.

The DNA Strand Is Used as a Template to Assemble the RNA Molecule from Activated Nucleotides. The assembly of the RNA molecule occurs under the influence of the enzyme RNA *polymerase* as follows:

1. In the DNA strand immediately ahead of the gene that is to be transcribed is a sequence of nucleotides called the *promoter.* An RNA polymerase recognizes this promoter and attaches to it.
2. The polymerase causes unwinding of two turns of the DNA helix and separation of the unwound portions.
3. The polymerase moves along the DNA strand and begins forming the RNA molecules by binding complementary RNA nucleotides to the DNA strand.
4. The successive RNA nucleotides then bind to each other to form an RNA strand.

5. When the RNA polymerase reaches the end of the DNA gene, it encounters a sequence of DNA molecules called the *chain-terminating sequence*; this causes the polymerase to break away from the DNA strand. The RNA strand is then released into the nucleoplasm.

The code present in the DNA strand is transmitted in complementary form to the RNA molecule as follows:

DNA Base	RNA Base
Guanine	Cytosine
Cytosine	Guanine
Adenine	Uracil
Thymine	Adenine

There Are Four Types of RNA. Each of the four types of RNA plays a different role in protein formation: (1) *messenger RNA* (mRNA) carries the genetic code to the cytoplasm to control the formation of proteins; (2) *ribosomal RNA*, along with proteins, forms the ribosomes, the structures in which protein molecules are assembled; (3) *transfer RNA* (tRNA) transports activated amino acids to the ribosomes to be used in the assembly of the proteins; and (4) *MicroRNA (miRNA)*, which are single-stranded RNA molecules of 21 to 23 nucleotides that can regulate gene transcription and translation.

There are 20 types of tRNA, each of which combines specifically with one of the 20 amino acids and carries this amino acid to the ribosomes, where it is incorporated in the protein molecule. The code in the tRNA that allows it to recognize a specific codon is a triplet of nucleotide bases called an *anticodon*. During formation of the protein molecule, the three anticodon bases combine loosely by hydrogen bonding with the codon bases of the mRNA. In this way, the various amino acids are lined up along the mRNA chain, thus establishing the proper sequence of amino acids in the protein molecule.

Translation Is Synthesis of Polypeptides on the Ribosomes from the Genetic Code Contained in mRNA *(p. 33)*

To manufacture proteins, one end of the mRNA strand enters the ribosome, and then the entire strand threads its way through the ribosome in just over a minute. As it passes through, the ribosome "reads" the genetic code and causes the proper succession of amino acids to bind together to form chemical bonds called *peptide linkages.* The mRNA does not recognize the different types of amino acid but, instead, recognizes the different types of tRNA. Each type of tRNA molecule carries only one specific type of amino acid that is incorporated into the protein.

Thus as the strand of mRNA passes through the ribosome, each of its codons attracts to it a specific tRNA that, in turn, delivers a specific amino acid. This amino acid then combines with the preceding amino acids to form a peptide linkage, and this sequence continues to build until an entire protein molecule is formed. At this point, a *chain-terminating codon* appears and indicates completion of the process, and the protein is released into the cytoplasm or through the membrane of the endoplasmic reticulum to the interior.

Control of Gene Function and Biochemical Activity in Cells *(p. 35)*

The genes control the function of each cell by determining the relative proportion of the various types of enzymes and structural proteins that are formed. Regulation of gene expression covers the entire process from transcription of the genetic code in the nucleus to the formation or proteins in the cytoplasm.

The Promoter Controls Gene Expression. Cellular protein synthesis starts with transcription of DNA into RNA, a process controlled by regulatory elements in the *promoter* of a gene. In eukaryotes, including mammals, the basal promoter consists of a sequence of 7 bases (TATAAAA) called the *TATA box,* the binding site for the *TATA-binding protein* (*TBP*) and several other important *transcription factors* that are collectively referred to as the *transcription factor IID complex.* In addition to the transcription factor IID complex, this region is where transcription factor IIB binds to both the DNA as well as RNA polymerase 2 to facilitate transcription of the DNA into RNA. This basal promoter is found in all protein coding genes and the polymerase must bind with this basal promoter before it can begin traveling along the DNA strand to synthesize RNA. The *upstream promoter* is located further upstream from the transcription start site and contains several binding sites for positive or negative transcription factors that can effect transcription through interactions with proteins bound to the basal promoter. The structure and transcription factor binding sites in the upstream promoter vary from gene to gene to give rise to the different expression patterns of genes in different tissues.

Transcription of genes in eukaryotes is also influenced by *enhancers*, which are regions of DNA that can bind transcription factors. Enhancers can be located a great distance from the gene they act on or even on a different chromosome. However, although enhancers may be located a great distance away from their target gene, they may be relatively close when DNA is coiled in the nucleus. It is estimated that there are 110,000 gene enhancer sequences in the human genome.

Control of the Promoter through Negative Feedback by the Cell Product. When the cell produces a critical amount of substance, it causes negative feedback inhibition of the promoter that is responsible for its synthesis. This inhibition can be accomplished by causing a regulatory repressor protein to bind at the repressor operator or a regulatory activator protein to break this bond. In either case, the promoter becomes inhibited.

There are other mechanisms available for control of transcription by the promoter, including the following:

1. A promoter may be controlled by transcription factors located elsewhere in the genome.
2. In some instances, the same regulatory protein functions as an activator for one promoter and as a repressor for another, allowing different promoters to be controlled at the same time by the same regulatory protein.
3. The nuclear DNA is packaged in specific structural units, the *chromosomes*. Within each chromosome, the DNA is wound around small proteins called *histones*, which are held together tightly in a compacted state with other proteins. So long as the DNA is in this compacted state, it cannot function to form RNA. Multiple mechanisms exist, however, that can cause selected areas of the chromosomes to become decompacted, allowing RNA transcription. Even then, specific transcriptor factors control the actual rate of transcription by the promoter in the chromosome.

The DNA-Genetic System Also Controls Cell Reproduction *(p. 37)*

The genes and their regulatory mechanisms determine not only the growth characteristics of cells but also when and whether these cells divide to form new cells.

In this way, the genetic system controls each stage of the development of the human from the single-cell fertilized ovum to the whole functioning body.

Most cells of the body, with the exception of mature red blood cells, striated muscle cells, and neurons, are capable of reproducing other cells of their own type. Ordinarily, as sufficient nutrients are available, each cell increases in size until it automatically divides via *mitosis* to form two new cells. Different cells of the body have different life cycle periods that vary from as short as 10 hours for highly stimulated bone marrow cells to the entire lifetime of the human body for nerve cells.

Cell Reproduction Begins with Replication of DNA. Only after all of the DNA in the chromosomes has been replicated can mitosis take place. The DNA is duplicated only once, so the net result is two exact replicates of all DNA. These replicates then become the DNA of the two daughter cells that will be formed at mitosis. The replication of DNA is similar to the way RNA is transcribed from DNA, except for a few important differences:

1. Both strands of the DNA are replicated, not just one of them.
2. Both strands of the DNA helix are replicated from end to end rather than small portions of them, as occurs during the transcription of RNA by genes.
3. The principal enzymes for replication of DNA are a complex of several enzymes called *DNA polymerase,* which is comparable to RNA polymerase.
4. Each newly formed strand of DNA remains attached by loose hydrogen bonding to the original DNA strand that is used as its template. Two DNA helixes are formed, therefore, that are duplicates of each other and are still coiled together.
5. The two new helixes become uncoiled by the action of enzymes that periodically cut each helix along its entire length, rotate each segment sufficiently to cause separation, and then resplice the helix.

DNA Strands are "Repaired" and "Proofread." During the time between the replication of DNA and the beginning of mitosis, there is a period of "proofreading" and "repair" of the DNA strands. Whenever inappropriate DNA nucleotides have been matched up with the nucleotides of the original template strand, special enzymes cut out the defective areas and replace them with the appropriate complementary nucleotides. Because of proofreading and repair, the transcription process rarely makes a mistake. When a mistake is made, however, it is called a *mutation*.

Entire Chromosomes Are Replicated. The DNA helixes of the nucleus are each packaged as a single chromosome. The human cell contains 46 chromosomes arranged in 23 pairs. In addition to the DNA in the chromosome, there is a large amount of protein composed mainly of *histones*, around which small segments of each DNA helix are coiled. During mitosis, the successive coils are packed against each other, allowing the long DNA molecule to be packaged in a coiled and folded arrangement. Replication of the chromosomes in their entirety occurs soon after replication of the DNA helixes. The two newly formed chromosomes remain temporarily attached to each other at a point called the *centromere*, which is located near their center. These duplicated but still-attached chromosomes are called *chromatids.*

Mitosis Is the Process by which the Cell Splits into Two New Daughter Cells. Two pairs of *centrioles*, which are small structures that lie close to one pole of the nucleus, begin to move apart from each other. This movement is caused by successive polymerization of protein microtubules growing outward from each pair of centrioles. As the tubules grow, they push one pair of centrioles toward one pole of the cell and the other toward the opposite pole. At the same time, other microtubules grow radially away from each of the centriole pairs, forming a spiny star called the *aster* at each end of the cell. The complex of microtubules extending between the centriole pairs is called the *spindle*, and the entire set of microtubules plus the pairs of centrioles is called the *mitotic apparatus.* Mitosis then proceeds through several phases.

- *Prophase* is the beginning of mitosis. While the spindle is forming, the chromosomes of the nucleus become condensed into well-defined chromosomes.
- *Prometaphase* is the stage at which the growing microtubular spines of the aster puncture and fragment the nuclear envelope. At the same time, the microtubules from the aster become attached to the chromatids at the centromere, where the paired chromatids are still bound to each other.
- *Metaphase* is the stage at which the two asters of the mitotic apparatus are pushed farther and farther apart by additional growth of the mitotic spindle.

Simultaneously, the chromatids are pulled tightly by the attached microtubules to the center of the cell, lining up to form the *equatorial plate* of the mitotic spindle.

- *Anaphase* is the stage at which the two chromatids of each chromosome are pulled apart at the centromere. Thus all 46 pairs of chromosomes are separated, forming two sets of 46 daughter chromosomes.

- *Telophase* is the stage at which the two sets of daughter chromosomes are pulled completely apart. Then the mitotic apparatus dissolves, and a new nuclear membrane develops around each set of chromosomes.

Cell Differentiation Allows Different Cells of the Body to Perform Different Functions. As a human develops from a fertilized ovum, the ovum divides repeatedly until trillions of cells are formed. Gradually, however, the new cells differentiate from each other, with certain cells having different genetic characteristics from other cells. This differentiation process occurs as a result of inactivation of certain genes and activation of others during successive stages of cell division. This process of differentiation leads to the ability of different cells in the body to perform different functions.

II

Membrane Physiology, Nerve, and Muscle

CHAPTER 4

Transport of Substances through Cell Membranes

Differences between the composition of intracellular and extracellular fluids are caused by transport mechanisms of cell membranes. These differences include the following:

- Extracellular fluid has a high sodium concentration, high chloride concentration, and low potassium concentration. The opposite is true of intracellular fluid.
- The concentrations of phosphates and proteins in intracellular fluid are greater than those in extracellular fluid.

The Cell Membrane Consists of a Lipid Bilayer with "Floating" Protein Molecules. The lipid bilayer constitutes a barrier for the movement of most water-soluble substances. However, most lipid-soluble substances can pass directly through the lipid bilayer. Protein molecules in the lipid bilayer constitute an alternate transport pathway.

- *Channel proteins* provide a watery pathway for molecules to move through the membrane.
- *Carrier proteins* bind with specific molecules and then undergo conformational changes that move molecules through the membrane.

Transport through the Cell Membrane Occurs through Diffusion or Active Transport

- *Diffusion* means random movement of molecules either through intermolecular spaces in the cell membrane or in combination with a carrier protein. The energy that causes diffusion is the energy of the normal kinetic motion of matter.
- *Active transport* means movement of substances across the membrane in combination with a carrier protein but also against an electrochemical gradient. This process requires a source of energy in addition to kinetic energy.

Diffusion (p. 46)

Diffusion Is the Continual Movement of Molecules in Liquids or Gases. Diffusion through the cell membrane is divided into the following two subtypes:

- *Simple diffusion* means that molecules move through a membrane without binding with carrier proteins. Simple diffusion can occur by way of two pathways:

(1) through the interstices of the lipid bilayer and (2) through watery channels in transport proteins that span the cell membrane.

• *Facilitated diffusion* requires a carrier protein. The carrier protein aids in passage of molecules through the membrane, probably by binding chemically with them and shuttling them through the membrane in this form.

The Rate of Diffusion of a Substance through the Cell Membrane Is Directly Proportional to Its Lipid Solubility. The lipid solubilities of oxygen, nitrogen, carbon dioxide, anesthetic gases, and most alcohols are so high they can dissolve directly in the lipid bilayer and diffuse through the cell membrane.

Water and Other Lipid-Insoluble Molecules Diffuse through Protein Channels in the Cell Membrane. Water readily penetrates the cell membrane and can also pass through transmembrane protein channels. Other lipid-insoluble molecules (mainly ions) can pass through the water-filled protein channels in the same way as water molecules if they are sufficiently small.

Protein Channels Have Selective Permeability for Transport of One or More Specific Molecules. This permeability results from the characteristics of the channel itself, such as its diameter, its shape, and the nature of the electrical charges along its inside surfaces.

Gating of Protein Channels Provides a Means for Controlling Their Permeability. The gates are thought to be gatelike extensions of the transport protein molecule, which can close over the channel opening or be lifted from the opening by a conformational change in the protein molecule itself. The opening and closing of gates are controlled in two principal ways:

• *Voltage gating.* In this instance, the molecular conformation of the gate responds to the electrical potential across the cell membrane. For example, the normal negative charge on the inside of the cell membrane causes the sodium gates to remain tightly closed. When the inside of the membrane loses its negative charge (becomes less negative), these gates open allowing sodium ions to pass inward through the sodium channels. The opening of sodium channel gates is the basic cause of action potentials in nerves.

• *Chemical gating.* Some protein channel gates are opened by the binding of another molecule with the protein; this causes a conformational change in the protein molecule that opens or closes the gate. This is called chemical (or ligand) gating. One of the most important instances of chemical gating is the effect of acetylcholine on the "acetylcholine channel" of the neuromuscular junction.

Facilitated Diffusion Is Also Called Carrier-Mediated Diffusion. A substance transported in this manner usually cannot pass through the cell membrane without the assistance of a specific carrier protein.

- Facilitated diffusion involves the following two steps: (1) the molecule to be transported enters a blind-ended channel and binds to a specific receptor and (2) a conformational change occurs in the carrier protein, so the channel now opens to the opposite side of the membrane.
- Facilitated diffusion differs from simple diffusion in the following important way. The rate of simple diffusion increases proportionately with the concentration of the diffusing substance. With facilitated diffusion, the rate of diffusion approaches a maximum as the concentration of the substance increases. This maximum rate is dictated by the rate at which the carrier protein molecule can undergo the conformational change.
- Among the most important substances that cross cell membranes through facilitated diffusion are glucose and most of the amino acids.

Factors That Affect the Net Rate of Diffusion
(p. 50)

Substances Can Diffuse in Both Directions through the Cell Membrane. Therefore, what is usually important is the net rate of diffusion of a substance in the desired direction. This net rate is determined by the following factors:

- *Permeability.* The permeability of a membrane for a given substance is expressed as the net rate of diffusion of the substance through each unit area of the membrane for a unit concentration difference between the two sides of the membrane (when there are no electrical or pressure differences).
- *Concentration difference.* The rate of net diffusion through a cell membrane is proportional to the difference in concentration of the diffusing substance on the two sides of the membrane.

- *Electrical potential.* If an electrical potential is applied across a membrane, the ions move through the membrane because of their electrical charges. When large amounts of ions have moved through the membrane, a concentration difference of the same ions develops in the direction opposite to the electrical potential difference. When the concentration difference rises to a sufficiently high level, the two effects balance each other creating a state of *electrochemical equilibrium.* The electrical difference that balances a given concentration difference can be determined with the Nernst equation.

Osmosis across Selectively Permeable Membranes— "Net Diffusion of Water" *(p. 51)*

Osmosis Is the Process of Net Movement of Water Caused by a Concentration Difference of Water. Water is the most abundant substance to diffuse through the cell membrane. However, the amount that diffuses in each direction is so precisely balanced under normal conditions that not even the slightest net movement of water occurs. Therefore, the volume of a cell remains constant. However, a concentration difference for water can develop across a cell membrane. When this happens, net movement of water occurs across the cell membrane, causing the cell to either swell or shrink, depending on the direction of the net movement. The pressure difference required to stop osmosis is the *osmotic pressure.*

The Osmotic Pressure Exerted by Particles in a Solution Is Determined by the Number of Particles per Unit Volume of Fluid and Not by the Mass of the Particles. On average, the kinetic energy of each molecule or ion that strikes a membrane is about the same regardless of its molecular size. Consequently, the factor that determines the osmotic pressure of a solution is the concentration of the solution in terms of number of particles per unit volume but not in terms of mass of the solute.

The Osmole Expresses Concentration in Terms of Number of Particles. One osmole is 1 g molecular weight of undissociated solute. Thus 180 g of glucose, which is 1 g molecular weight of glucose, is equal to 1 osmole of glucose because glucose does not dissociate. A solution that has 1 osmole of solute dissolved in each kilogram of water is said to have an osmolality of 1 osmole per kilogram, and a solution that has

1/1000 osmole dissolved per kilogram has an osmolality of 1 milliosmole per kilogram. The normal osmolality of the extracellular and intracellular fluids is about 300 milliosmoles per kilogram, and the osmotic pressure of these fluids is about 5500 mm Hg.

"Active Transport" of Substances through Membranes (p. 52)

Active Transport Can Move a Substance against an Electrochemical Gradient. An electrochemical gradient is the sum of all the diffusion forces acting at the membrane—the forces caused by a concentration difference, an electrical difference, and a pressure difference. That is, substances cannot diffuse "uphill." When a cell membrane moves a substance uphill against a concentration gradient (or uphill against an electrical or pressure gradient), the process is called *active transport.*

Active Transport Is Divided into Two Types According to the Source of the Energy Used to Effect the Transport. In both instances, transport depends on carrier proteins that penetrate the membrane, which is also true for facilitated diffusion.

• *Primary active transport.* The energy is derived directly from the breakdown of adenosine triphosphate (ATP) or some other high-energy phosphate compound.
• *Secondary active transport.* The energy is derived secondarily from energy that has been stored in the form of ionic concentration differences between the two sides of a membrane, originally created by primary active transport. The sodium electrochemical gradient drives most secondary active transport processes.

Primary Active Transport (p. 53)

The Sodium-Potassium (Na^+-K^+) Pump Transports Sodium Ions out of Cells and Potassium Ions into Cells. This pump is present in all cells of the body, and it is responsible for maintaining the sodium and potassium concentration differences across the cell membrane as well as for establishing a negative electrical potential inside the cells. The pump operates in the following manner. Three sodium ions bind to a carrier protein on the inside of the cell, and two potassium ions bind to the carrier protein on the outside of the cell. The carrier protein has ATPase activity, and the simultaneous binding of sodium and potassium ions causes the ATPase function of the protein to become activated. This then cleaves one molecule of ATP, splitting it to form adenosine diphosphate (ADP) and liberating a high-energy phosphate bond of energy. This energy is then believed to cause a conformational change in the protein carrier molecule, extruding the sodium ions to the outside and the potassium ions to the inside.

The Na^+-K^+ Pump Controls Cell Volume. The Na^+-K^+ pump transports three molecules of sodium to the outside of the cell for every two molecules of potassium pumped to the inside. This continual net loss of ions from the cell interior initiates an osmotic force to move water out of the cell. Furthermore, when the cell begins to swell, this automatically activates the Na^+-K^+ pump, moving to the exterior still more ions that are carrying water with them. Therefore, the Na^+-K^+ pump performs a continual surveillance role in maintaining normal cell volume.

Active Transport Saturates in the Same Way That Facilitated Diffusion Saturates. When the difference in concentration of the substance to be transported is small, the rate of transport rises approximately in proportion to increases in its concentration. At high concentrations, the rate of transport is limited by the rates at which the chemical reactions of binding, release, and carrier conformational changes can occur.

Co-Transport and Counter-Transport Are Two Forms of Secondary Active Transport. When sodium ions are transported out of cells by primary active transport, a large concentration gradient of sodium normally develops. This gradient represents a storehouse of energy because the excess sodium outside the cell membrane is always attempting to diffuse to the cell interior.

- *Co-transport.* The diffusion energy of sodium can pull other substances along with the sodium (in the same direction) through the cell membrane using a special carrier protein.
- *Counter-transport.* The sodium ion and substance to be counter-transported move to opposite sides of the membrane, with sodium always moving to the cell interior. Here again, a protein carrier is required.

Glucose and Amino Acids Can Be Transported into Most Cells through Sodium Co-Transport. The transport carrier protein has two binding sites on its exterior side—one for sodium and one for glucose or amino acids. Again, the concentration of sodium ions is very high on the outside and very low on the inside, providing the energy for the transport. A special property of the transport protein is that the conformational change to allow sodium movement to the cell interior does not occur until a glucose or amino acid molecule also attaches.

Calcium and Hydrogen Ions Can Be Transported out of Cells through the Sodium Counter-Transport Mechanism

- *Calcium counter-transport* occurs in most cell membranes, with sodium ions moving to the cell interior and calcium ions moving to the exterior, both bound to the same transport protein in a counter-transport mode.
- *Hydrogen counter-transport* occurs especially in the proximal tubules of the kidneys, where sodium ions move from the lumen of the tubule to the interior of the tubular cells, and hydrogen ions are counter-transported into the lumen.

CHAPTER 5

Membrane Potentials and Action Potentials

Electrical potentials exist across the membranes of essentially all cells of the body. In addition, nerve and muscle cells are "excitable" (i.e., capable of self-generating electrical impulses at their membranes). The present discussion is concerned with membrane potentials that are generated both at rest and during action potentials by nerve and muscle cells.

Basic Physics of Membrane Potentials
(p. 57)

A Concentration Difference of Ions across a Selectively Permeable Membrane Can Produce a Membrane Potential

- *Potassium diffusion potential.* Suppose a cell membrane is permeable to potassium ions but not to any other ions. Potassium ions tend to diffuse outward because of the high potassium concentration inside the cell. Because potassium ions are positively charged, the loss of potassium ions from the cell creates a negative potential inside the cell. Within a few milliseconds, the potential change becomes sufficiently great to block further net diffusion of potassium despite the high potassium ion concentration gradient. In the normal large mammalian nerve fiber, the potential difference required to stop further net diffusion is about −94 millivolts.

- *Sodium diffusion potential.* Now suppose a cell membrane is permeable to sodium ions but not to any other ions. Sodium ions tend to diffuse into the cell because of the high sodium concentration outside the cell. Diffusion of sodium ions into the cell creates a positive potential inside the cell. Again, the membrane potential rises sufficiently high within milliseconds to block further net diffusion of sodium ions into the cell; however, this time, for the large mammalian nerve fiber, the potential is about +61 millivolts.

The Nernst Equation Describes the Relation of Diffusion Potential to Concentration Difference. The membrane potential that prevents net diffusion of an ion in either direction through the membrane is called the

Nernst potential for that ion. The following is the Nernst equation:

$$\text{EMF(millivolts)} = \pm 61 \log\left(\frac{\text{concentration inside}}{\text{concentration outside}}\right)$$

where EMF is the electromotive force. The sign of the potential is positive (+) if the ion under consideration is a negative ion and negative (−) if it is a positive ion.

The Goldman Equation Is Used to Calculate the Diffusion Potential When the Membrane Is Permeable to Several Different Ions. In this case, the diffusion potential that develops depends on three factors: (1) the polarity of the electrical charge of each ion, (2) the permeability of the membrane (P) to each ion, and (3) the concentrations (C) of the respective ions on the inside (i) and outside (o) of the membrane. The following is the Goldman equation:

$$\text{EMF(millivolts)} =$$
$$- 61 \log\left(\frac{C_{Na^+i}P_{Na^+} + C_{K^+i}P_{K^+} + C_{Cl^-o}P_{Cl^-}}{C_{Na^+o}P_{Na^+} + C_{K^+o}P_{K^+} + C_{Cl^-i}P_{Cl^-}}\right)$$

Note the following features and implications of the Goldman equation:

• Sodium, potassium, and chloride ions are most importantly involved in the development of membrane potentials in neurons and muscle fibers as well as in the neuronal cells in the central nervous system.
• The degree of importance of each ion in determining the voltage is proportional to the membrane permeability for that particular ion.
• A positive ion concentration gradient from inside the membrane to the outside causes electronegativity inside the membrane.

Resting Membrane Potential of Nerves (p. 59)

The Resting Membrane Potential Is Established by the Diffusion Potentials, Membrane Permeability, and Electrogenic Nature of the Na⁺-K⁺ Pump

• *Potassium diffusion potential.* A high ratio of potassium ions from inside to outside the cell, 35:1, produces a Nernst potential of −94 millivolts according to the Nernst equation.

- *Sodium diffusion potential.* The ratio of sodium ions from inside to outside the membrane is 0.1, which gives a calculated Nernst potential of +61 millivolts.
- *Membrane permeability.* The permeability of the nerve fiber membrane to potassium is about 100 times as great as that to sodium, so the diffusion of potassium contributes far more to the membrane potential. The use of this high value of permeability in the Goldman equation gives an internal membrane potential of −86 millivolts, which is near the potassium diffusion potential of −94 millivolts.
- *Electrogenic nature of the Na^+-K^+ pump.* The Na^+-K^+ pump transports three sodium ions to the outside of the cell for each two potassium ions pumped to the inside, which causes a continual loss of positive charges from inside the membrane. Therefore the Na^+-K^+ pump is electrogenic because it produces a net deficit of positive ions inside the cell; this causes a negative charge of about −4 millivolts inside the cell membrane.

Nerve Action Potential *(p. 60)*

Nerve signals are transmitted by action potentials, which are rapid changes in the membrane potential. Each action potential begins with a sudden change from the normal resting negative potential to a positive membrane potential and then ends with an almost equally rapid change back to the resting negative potential.

The successive stages of the action potential are as follows:

- *Resting stage.* This is the resting membrane potential before the action potential occurs.
- *Depolarization stage.* At this time, the membrane suddenly becomes permeable to sodium ions, allowing tremendous numbers of positively charged sodium ions to flow to the interior of the axon, and the potential rises rapidly in the positive direction.
- *Repolarization stage.* Within a few 10,000ths of a second after the membrane becomes highly permeable to sodium ions the sodium channels begin to close and the potassium channels open more than they normally do. Then rapid diffusion of potassium ions to the exterior re-establishes the normal negative resting membrane potential.

Voltage-Gated Sodium and Potassium Channels Are Activated and Inactivated during the Course of an Action Potential. The necessary factor for both depolarization and repolarization of the nerve membrane during the action potential is the *voltage-gated sodium channel.* The voltage-gated potassium channel also plays an important role in increasing the rapidity of repolarization of the membrane. *These two voltage-gated channels are present in addition to the Na^+-K^+ pump and the Na^+-K^+ leak channels that establish the resting permeability of the membrane.*

The Events That Cause the Action Potential Can Be Summarized as Follows

- *During the resting state,* before the action potential begins, the conductance for potassium ions about 100 times as great as the conductance for sodium ions. This is caused by much greater leakage of potassium ions than sodium ions through the leak channels.

- *At the onset of the action potential,* the sodium channels instantaneously become activated and allow up to a 5000-fold increase in sodium permeability (also called sodium conductance). Then the inactivation process closes the sodium channels within a few fractions of a millisecond. The onset of the action potential also causes voltage gating of the potassium channels, causing them to begin opening more slowly.

- *At the end of the action potential,* the return of the membrane potential to the negative state causes the potassium channels to close back to their original status but, again, only after a delay.

A Positive-Feedback, Vicious Circle Opens the Sodium Channels. If any event causes the membrane potential to rise from −90 millivolts toward the zero level, the rising voltage itself causes many voltage-gated sodium channels to begin opening. This allows rapid inflow of sodium ions, which causes still further rise of the membrane potential, thus opening still more voltage-gated sodium channels. This process is a positive-feedback vicious circle that continues until all of the voltage-gated sodium channels have become activated (opened).

An Action Potential Does Not Occur until the Threshold Potential Has Been Reached. This happens when the number of sodium ions entering the nerve fiber becomes greater than the number of potassium ions leaving the fiber. A sudden increase in the membrane potential in a large nerve fiber from −90 millivolts to about −65 millivolts usually causes explosive development of the action potential. This level of −65 millivolts is said to be the threshold of the membrane for stimulation.

A New Action Potential Cannot Occur When the Membrane Is Still Depolarized from the Preceding Action Potential. Shortly after the action potential is initiated, the sodium channels become inactivated, and any amount of excitatory signal applied to these channels at this point does not open the inactivation gates. The only condition that can reopen them is when the membrane potential returns either to or almost to the original resting membrane potential level. Then, within another small fraction of a second, the inactivation gates of the channels open, and a new action potential can then be initiated.

- *Absolute refractory period.* An action potential cannot be elicited during the absolute refractory period, even with a strong stimulus. This period for large myelinated nerve fibers is about 1/2500 second, which means that a maximum of about 2500 impulses can be transmitted per second.

- *Relative refractory period.* This period follows the absolute refractory period. During this time, stronger than normal stimuli can excite the nerve fiber, and an action potential can be initiated.

Propagation of the Action Potential *(p. 64)*

An action potential elicited at any one point on a membrane usually excites adjacent portions of the membrane, resulting in propagation of the action potential. Thus the depolarization process travels along the entire extent of the fiber. Transmission of the depolarization process along a nerve or muscle fiber is called a nerve or muscle impulse.

- *Direction of propagation.* An excitable membrane has no single direction of propagation, instead the action potential travels in both directions away from the stimulus.

- *All-or-nothing principle.* Once an action potential has been elicited at any point on the membrane of a normal fiber, the depolarization process travels over the entire membrane if conditions are right, or it might not travel at all if conditions are not right.

Re-establishing Sodium and Potassium Ionic Gradients after Action Potentials Are Completed—Importance of Energy Metabolism (p. 65)

Transmission of each impulse along the nerve fiber reduces infinitesimally the concentration differences of sodium and potassium between the inside and outside of the membrane. From 100,000 to 50 million impulses can be transmitted by nerve fibers before the ion concentration differences have decreased to the point that action potential conduction ceases. Even so, with time it becomes necessary to re-establish the sodium and potassium membrane concentration differences. This is achieved by the action of the Na^+-K^+ pump.

Special Characteristics of Signal Transmission in Nerve Trunks (p. 67)

Large Nerve Fibers Are Myelinated, and the Small Ones Are Unmyelinated. The central core of the fiber is the axon, and the membrane of the axon is used for conducting the action potential. Surrounding the larger axons is a thick myelin sheath deposited by Schwann cells. The sheath consists of multiple layers of cellular membrane containing the lipid substance sphingomyelin, which is an excellent insulator. At the juncture between two successive Schwann cells, a small noninsulated area only 2 to 3 µm in length remains where ions can still flow with ease between the extracellular fluid and the axon. This area is the *node of Ranvier.*

"Saltatory" Conduction Occurs in Myelinated Fibers. Even though ions cannot flow significantly through the thick sheaths of myelinated nerves, they can flow with considerable ease through the nodes of Ranvier. Thus the nerve impulse jumps from node to node along the fiber, which is the origin of the term "saltatory." Saltatory conduction is of value for two reasons:

• *Increased velocity.* First, by causing the depolarization process to jump long intervals along the axis of the nerve fiber, this mechanism increases the velocity of nerve transmission in myelinated fibers as much as 5- to 50-fold.

• *Energy conservation.* Second, saltatory conduction conserves energy for the axon because only the nodes depolarize, allowing perhaps a hundred times smaller loss of ions than would otherwise be necessary and therefore requiring little energy for re-establishing the sodium and potassium concentration differences across the membrane after a series of nerve impulses.

Conduction Velocity Is Greatest in Large, Myelinated Nerve Fibers. The velocity of action potential conduction in nerve fibers varies from as low as 0.25 m/sec in very small unmyelinated fibers to as high as 100 m/sec in very large myelinated fibers. The velocity increases approximately with the fiber diameter in myelinated nerve fibers and approximately with the square root of the fiber diameter in unmyelinated fibers.

Contraction of Skeletal Muscle

About 40% of the body mass is skeletal muscle, and perhaps another 10% is smooth muscle and cardiac muscle. Many of the principles of contraction apply to all three types of muscle. In this chapter, the function of skeletal muscle is considered. The functions of smooth muscle are discussed in Chapter 8, and the functions of cardiac muscle are discussed in Chapter 9.

Physiologic Anatomy of Skeletal Muscle (p. 71)

Skeletal Muscle Fiber

Figure 6–1 shows the organization of skeletal muscle. In most muscles the fibers extend the entire length of the muscle. Each fiber is innervated by only one nerve ending.

Myofibrils Are Composed of Actin and Myosin Filaments. Each muscle fiber contains hundreds to thousands of myofibrils, and, in turn, each myofibril (see Fig. 6–1*D*) is composed of about 1500 myosin filaments and 3000 actin filaments lying side by side. These filaments are large polymerized protein molecules that are responsible for muscle contraction. In Figure 6–1 the thick filaments are myosin, and the thin filaments are actin; note the following features:

- *Light and dark bands.* The myosin and actin filaments partially interdigitate and thus cause the myofibrils to have alternate light and dark bands. The light bands contain only actin filaments and are called I bands. The dark bands called A bands contain myosin filaments as well as the ends of the actin filaments. The length of the A band is the length of the myosin filament.

- *Cross-bridges.* The small projections from the sides of the myosin filaments are cross-bridges. They protrude from the surfaces of the myosin filament along its entire length except in the center. Myosin cross-bridges interact with actin filaments causing contraction.

- *Z disc.* The ends of the actin filaments are attached to Z discs (see Fig. 6–1*E*). The Z disc passes across the myofibril and from one to another, attaching and aligning the myofibrils across the muscle fiber.

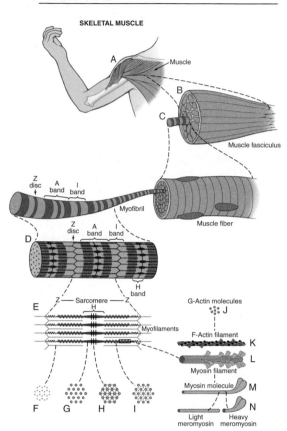

Figure 6–1. Organization of skeletal muscle, from the gross to the molecular level. *F, G, H,* and *I* are cross sections at the levels indicated.

The entire muscle fiber therefore has light and dark bands, giving skeletal and cardiac muscle a striated appearance.

- *Sarcomere.* The portion of a myofibril that lies between two successive Z discs is called a sarcomere. During rest, the actin filaments overlap the myosin filaments with an optimal amount of interdigitation in skeletal muscle and slightly shorter than optimal interdigitation in cardiac muscle.

General Mechanism of Muscle Contraction (p. 73)

The initiation and execution of muscle contraction occur in the following sequential steps:

1. An action potential travels along a motor nerve to its endings on muscle fibers, and each nerve ending secretes a small amount of the neurotransmitter substance acetylcholine.
2. The acetylcholine acts on a local area of the muscle membrane to open acetylcholine-gated cation channels, which allows mainly sodium ions but also calcium ions to flow into the muscle fiber causing a local depolarization. The local depolarization in turn leads to opening of voltage-gated sodium channels resulting in an action potential.
3. The action potential travels along the muscle fiber membrane, causing the sarcoplasmic reticulum to release calcium ions into the myofibrils that have been stored in the sarcoplasmic reticulum.
4. The calcium ions initiate attractive forces between the actin and myosin filaments, causing them to slide together; this is the contractile process.
5. The calcium ions are continually pumped back into the sarcoplasmic reticulum, where they remain stored until a muscle action potential arrives; this removal of the calcium ions from the myofibrils causes muscle contraction to cease.

Molecular Mechanism of Muscle Contraction (p. 74)

Muscle Contraction Occurs by a Sliding Filament Mechanism. Mechanical forces generated by the interaction of myosin cross-bridges with actin filaments cause the actin filaments to slide inward among the myosin filaments. Under resting conditions, these forces are inhibited, but when an action potential travels over the muscle fiber membrane, the sarcoplasmic reticulum releases large quantities of calcium ions, which activate the forces between the myosin and actin filaments, and contraction begins.

The Myosin Filament Is Composed of Multiple Myosin Molecules. The tails of myosin molecules bundle together to form the body of the filament, whereas the myosin heads and part of each myosin molecule hang outward to the sides of the body, providing an arm that extends the head outward from the body. The protruding arms and heads together are called cross-bridges. An important feature of the myosin head is that it functions as an adenosine triphosphatase (ATPase) enzyme, which allows it to cleave adenosine triphosphate (ATP) and thus energize the contraction process.

The Actin Filament Is Composed of Actin, Tropomyosin, and Troponin. Each actin filament is about 1 μm long. The bases of the actin filaments are inserted strongly into the Z discs, whereas the other ends protrude in both directions into the adjacent sarcomeres where they lie in the spaces between the myosin molecules.

Interaction of One Myosin Filament, Two Actin Filaments, and Calcium Ions to Cause Contraction *(p. 75)*

The actin filament is inhibited by the troponin-tropomyosin complex: activation is stimulated by calcium ions.

• *Inhibition by the troponin-tropomyosin complex.* The active sites on the normal actin filament of the relaxed muscle are inhibited or physically covered by the troponin-tropomyosin complex. Consequently, the sites cannot attach to the heads of the myosin filaments to cause contraction until the inhibitory effect of the troponin-tropomyosin complex is itself inhibited.

• *Activation by calcium ions.* The inhibitory effect of the troponin-tropomyosin complex on the actin filaments is inhibited in the presence of calcium ions. Calcium ions combine with troponin C, causing the troponin complex to tug on the tropomyosin molecule. This "uncovers" the active sites of the actin, allowing contraction to proceed.

A "Walk Along" Theory Can Explain How the Activated Actin Filament and the Myosin Cross-Bridges Interact to Cause Contraction. When a myosin head attaches to an active site, the head tilts automatically toward the arm that is dragging along the actin filament. This tilt of the head is called the power stroke. Immediately after tilting, the head automatically breaks away from the active site. The head then returns to its normal perpendicular direction. In this position, it combines with a new active site farther along the actin filament. Thus, the heads of the cross-bridges bend back and forth and, step by step, walk along the actin filament, pulling the ends of the actin filaments toward the center of the myosin filament.

The Amount of Actin and Myosin Filament Overlap Dictates Tension Development by the Contracting Muscle *(p. 77)*

The Strength of Contraction Is Maximal When There Is Maximal Overlap between Actin Filaments and the Cross-Bridges of the Myosin Filaments. A muscle cannot develop tension at very long sarcomere lengths because there is no overlap between actin and myosin filaments. As the sarcomere shortens and actin and myosin filaments begin to overlap, the tension increases progressively. Full tension is maintained at a sarcomere length of about 2.0 µm because the actin filament has overlapped all of the cross-bridges of the myosin filament. On further shortening, the ends of the two actin filaments begin to overlap (in addition to overlapping the myosin filaments), causing muscle tension to decrease. When the sarcomere length decreases to about 1.65 µm, the two Z discs of the sarcomere abut the ends of the myosin filaments, and the strength of contraction decreases precipitously.

Energetics of Muscle Contraction *(p. 78)*

Muscle Contraction Requires ATP to Perform Three Main Functions

- Most of the ATP is used to activate the walk-along mechanism of muscle contraction.
- Calcium is pumped back into the sarcoplasmic reticulum causing the contraction to terminate.
- Sodium and potassium ions are pumped through the muscle fiber membrane to maintain an appropriate ionic environment for the propagation of action potentials.

There Are Three Main Sources of Energy for Muscle Contraction. The concentration of ATP in the muscle fiber is sufficient to maintain full contraction for only 1 to 2 seconds. After the ATP is split into adenosine diphosphate (ADP), the ADP is rephosphorylated to form a new ATP. There are several sources of energy for this rephosphorylation.

- *Phosphocreatine* carries a high-energy bond similar to that of ATP but has more free energy. The energy released from this bond causes bonding of a new phosphate ion to ADP to reconstitute the ATP. The combined energy of ATP and phosphocreatine is capable of causing maximal muscle contraction for only 5 to 8 seconds.
- The *breakdown of glycogen* to pyruvic acid and lactic acid liberates energy that is used to convert ADP to ATP. The glycolytic reactions can occur in the absence of oxygen. The rate of formation of ATP by the glycolytic process is about 2.5 times as rapid as ATP formation when the cellular foodstuffs react with oxygen. Glycolysis alone can sustain maximum muscle contraction for only about 1 minute.
- *Oxidative metabolism* occurs when oxygen is combined with the various cellular foodstuffs to liberate ATP. More than 95% of all energy used by the muscles for sustained, long-term contraction is derived from this source. The foodstuffs consumed are carbohydrates, fats, and proteins.

Characteristics of Whole Muscle Contraction (p. 79)

Isometric Contractions Do Not Shorten Muscle, Whereas Isotonic Contractions Do Shorten Muscle

- *Isometric contraction* occurs when the muscle does not shorten during contraction. True isometric contractions cannot be generated in the intact body because the so-called *series elastic components* stretch during the contraction, allowing some shortening of the muscle. These elastic elements include the tendons, sarcolemmal ends of muscle fibers, and perhaps the hinged arms of the myosin cross-bridges.
- *Isotonic contraction* occurs when the muscle shortens and the tension on the muscle remains constant. The characteristics of the isotonic contraction depend on the load against which the muscle contracts as well as on the inertia of the load.

Fast Fibers Are Adapted for Powerful Muscle Contractions, Whereas Slow Fibers Are Adapted for Prolonged Muscle Activity. Each muscle is composed of a mixture of so-called fast and slow muscle fibers, with still other fibers that are between these two extremes. However, a given muscle may have predominantly fast muscle fibers (e.g., anterior tibialis), whereas other muscles may have predominantly slow muscle fibers (e.g., soleus).

- *Slow fibers (type I, red muscle)* (1) are smaller muscle fibers, (2) have high capillarity and large numbers of mitochondria to support high levels of oxidative metabolism, and (3) contain large amounts of myoglobin, which gives the slow muscle a reddish appearance and the name "red muscle." The deficit of red myoglobin in fast muscle provides the name white muscle.

- *Fast fibers (type II, white muscle)* (1) are larger for greater strength of contraction, (2) have extensive sarcoplasmic reticulum for rapid release of calcium ions, (3) have large amounts of glycolytic enzymes for rapid release of energy, and (4) have lower capillarity and fewer mitochondria because oxidative metabolism is of secondary importance.

Mechanics of Skeletal Muscle Contraction *(p. 80)*

Force Summation Is the Adding Together of Individual Twitch Contractions to Increase the Intensity of Overall Muscle Contraction. Summation occurs in two ways:

- *Multiple motor unit summation.* When the central nervous system sends a weak signal to contract a muscle, the motor units in the muscle that contain the smallest and fewest muscle fibers are stimulated in preference to the larger motor units. Then, as the strength of the signal increases, larger motor units also begin to be excited, with the largest motor units often having up to 50 times as much contractile force as the smallest units.

- *Frequency summation and tetanization.* As the frequency of muscle contraction increases, there comes a point at which each new contraction occurs before the preceding one ends. As a result, the second contraction is added partially to the first, so the total strength of contraction rises progressively with increasing frequency. When the frequency reaches a critical level, the successive contractions fuse, and the action appears to be completely smooth; this is called tetanization.

Muscle Hypertrophy Is an Increase in the Total Mass of a Muscle; Muscle Atrophy Is a Decrease in the Mass

- *Muscle hypertrophy* results from an increase in the number of actin and myosin filaments in each muscle fiber. When the number of contractile proteins increases sufficiently, the myofibrils split within each muscle fiber to form new myofibrils. It is mainly this great increase in the number of additional myofibrils that causes muscle fibers to hypertrophy; however, under special conditions, the total number of muscle fibers can also increase.

- *Muscle atrophy.* When a muscle remains unused for a long period, the rate of decay of the contractile proteins occurs more rapidly than the rate of replacement; therefore muscle atrophy occurs. Atrophy begins almost immediately when a muscle loses its nerve supply because it no longer receives the contractile signals that are required to maintain normal muscle size.

CHAPTER 7

Excitation of Skeletal Muscle: Neuromuscular Transmission and Excitation-Contraction Coupling

Transmission of Impulses from Neurons to Skeletal Muscle Fibers: The Neuromuscular Junction (p. 83)

Skeletal muscle fibers are innervated by large, myelinated nerve fibers that originate in motoneurons of the spinal cord. Each nerve fiber normally stimulates three fibers to several hundred skeletal muscle fibers. The nerve ending makes a junction, called the *neuromuscular junction,* and the action potential in the muscle fiber travels in both directions toward the muscle fiber ends.

Secretion of Acetylcholine by the Nerve Terminals (p. 83)

When a Nerve Impulse Reaches the Neuromuscular Junction, Vesicles Containing Acetylcholine Are Released into the Synaptic Space. On the inside surface of the neural membrane are linear dense bars. To the side of each dense bar are voltage-gated calcium channels. When the action potential spreads over the nerve terminal, these channels open allowing calcium ions to diffuse into the terminal. The calcium ions are believed to exert an attractive influence on the acetylcholine vesicles, drawing them adjacent to the dense bars. Some of the vesicles fuse with the neural membrane and empty their acetylcholine into the synaptic space via the process of exocytosis.

Acetylcholine Opens Acetylcholine-Gated Ion Channels on the Postsynaptic Membrane. Acetylcholine-gated cation channels are located on the muscle membrane immediately below the dense bar areas. When two acetylcholine molecules attach to the channel receptors, a conformational change opens the channel. The principal effect of opening the acetylcholine-gated channels is to allow large numbers of sodium ions to pour into the inside of the muscle fiber, carrying with them large numbers of positive charges. This effect creates a local potential change at the muscle fiber membrane called the end-plate potential. In turn, this end-plate potential normally leads to opening of voltage-gated sodium channels, which initiate an action potential at the muscle membrane and thus causes muscle contraction.

Acetylcholine Released into the Synaptic Space Is Destroyed by Acetylcholinesterase or Simply Diffuses Away. The acetylcholine, once released into the synaptic space, continues to activate the acetylcholine receptors for as long as it remains in the space. Most of the acetylcholine is destroyed by the enzyme acetylcholinesterase. A small amount diffuses out of the synaptic space. The short period during which the acetylcholine remains in the synaptic space—a few milliseconds at most—is always sufficient to excite the muscle fiber under normal conditions.

Acetylcholine Produces an End-Plate Potential That Excites the Skeletal Muscle Fiber. The movement of sodium ions into the muscle fiber causes the internal membrane potential in the local area of the end-plate to increase in the positive direction as much as 50 to 75 millivolts, creating a local potential called the *end-plate potential*. The end-plate potential created by acetylcholine stimulation is normally far greater than that necessary to initiate an action potential in the muscle fiber.

Drugs That Enhance or Block Transmission at the Neuromuscular Junction *(p. 86)*

Drugs Can Affect the Neuromuscular Junction by Having Acetylcholine-Like Actions, Blocking Neuromuscular Transmission, and Inactivating Acetylcholinesterase

- *Drugs that have acetylcholine-like actions.* Many compounds, including methacholine, carbachol, and nicotine, have the same effect on the muscle fiber as does acetylcholine. The difference between these drugs and acetylcholine is that they are not destroyed by cholinesterase, or they are destroyed slowly.

- *Drugs that block neuromuscular transmission.* A group of drugs known as the curariform drugs can prevent passage of impulses from the end-plate into the muscle. Thus d-tubocurarine competes with acetylcholine for the acetylcholine receptor sites, so the acetylcholine generated by the end-plate cannot increase the permeability of the muscle membrane acetylcholine channels sufficiently to initiate an action potential.

- *Drugs that inactivate acetylcholinesterase.* Three particularly well-known drugs—neostigmine, physostigmine, and diisopropyl fluorophosphate—inactivate acetylcholinesterase. As a result, acetylcholine levels increase with successive nerve impulses, causing large amounts of acetylcholine to accumulate and then repetitively stimulate the muscle fiber.

Neostigmine and physostigmine last up to several hours. Diisopropyl fluorophosphate, which has potential military use as a powerful "nerve" gas poison, inactivates acetylcholinesterase for weeks.

Myasthenia Gravis Causes Muscle Paralysis

Paralysis Occurs Because of the Inability of the Neuromuscular Junctions to Transmit Signals from the Nerve Fibers to the Muscle Fibers. Pathologically, myasthenia gravis is thought to be an autoimmune disease in which patients have developed antibodies against their own acetylcholine-gated ion channels. The end-plate potentials that occur in the muscle fibers are too weak to initiate opening of voltage-gated sodium channels so that muscle fiber depolarization does not occur. If the disease is sufficiently intense, the patient dies of paralysis—in particular, paralysis of the respiratory muscles. The disease usually can be ameliorated by administration of neostigmine or another anticholinesterase drug. This treatment allows acetylcholine to accumulate in the synaptic cleft.

Muscle Action Potential *(p. 87)*

The Conduction of Action Potentials in Nerve Fibers is *Qualitatively* Similar to That in Skeletal Muscle Fibers. Some of the *quantitative* differences and similarities include the following:

- *The resting membrane potential* is about −80 to −90 millivolts in skeletal muscle fibers, which is similar to that of large myelinated nerve fibers.
- *The duration of the action potential* is 1 to 5 milliseconds in skeletal muscle, which is about five times as long as that in large myelinated nerves.
- *The velocity of conduction* is 3 to 5 m/sec in skeletal muscle, which is about 1/18 the velocity of conduction in the large myelinated nerve fibers that excite skeletal muscle.

Excitation-Contraction Coupling *(p. 88)*

Transverse Tubules Are Internal Extensions of the Cell Membrane. The transverse tubules (T tubules) run transverse to the myofibrils. They begin at the cell membrane and penetrate from one side of the muscle fiber to the opposite side. At the point at which the

T tubules originate from the cell membrane, they are open to the exterior and thus contain extracellular fluid in their lumens. Because the T tubules are internal extensions of the cell membrane, when an action potential spreads over a muscle fiber membrane it also spreads along the T tubules to the interior of the muscle fiber.

The Sarcoplasmic Reticulum Is Composed of Longitudinal Tubules and Terminal Cisternae. The longitudinal tubules run parallel to the myofibrils and terminate in large chambers called terminal cisternae. The cisternae abut the T tubules. In cardiac muscle, a single T tubule network for each sarcomere is located at the level of the Z disc. In mammalian skeletal muscle, there are two T tubule networks for each sarcomere located near the two ends of the myosin filaments, which are the points at which the mechanical forces of muscle contraction are created. Thus mammalian skeletal muscle is optimally organized for rapid excitation of muscle contraction.

Calcium Ions Are Released from the Terminal Cisternae of the Sarcoplasmic Reticulum. Calcium ions located in the sarcoplasmic reticulum are released when an action potential occurs in the adjacent T tubule. The action potential itself is thought to cause rapid opening of calcium channels through the membranes of the terminal cisternae of the sarcoplasmic reticulum. These channels remain open for a few milliseconds; during this time the calcium ions responsible for muscle contraction are released into the sarcoplasm surrounding the myofibrils.

Calcium Pump Removes Calcium Ions from the Sarcoplasmic Fluid. A continually active calcium pump located in the walls of the sarcoplasmic reticulum pumps calcium ions away from the myofibrils back into the sarcoplasmic tubules. This pump can concentrate the calcium ions about 10,000-fold inside the tubules. In addition, inside the reticulum is a calcium-binding protein called *calsequestrin* that can provide another 40-fold increase in the storage of calcium. This transfer of calcium into the sarcoplasmic reticulum depletes calcium ions in the myofibrillar fluid, thereby terminating the muscle contraction.

CHAPTER 8

Excitation and Contraction of Smooth Muscle

Contraction of Smooth Muscle

Many of the principles of contraction that apply to skeletal muscle also apply to smooth muscle. Most important, essentially the same attractive forces that occur between myosin and actin filaments in skeletal muscle also cause contraction in smooth muscle, but the internal physical arrangement of actin and myosin filaments in smooth muscle fibers is entirely different from that of skeletal muscle.

Types of Smooth Muscle (p. 91)

In general, smooth muscle can be divided into two major types:

- *Multi-unit smooth muscle.* The most important characteristics of multi-unit smooth muscle fibers are that each fiber can contract independently of the others and the control is exerted mainly by nerve signals. Examples include the smooth muscle fibers of the ciliary muscle of the eye, the iris of the eye, and the piloerector muscles that cause erection of the hairs when stimulated by the sympathetic nervous system.

- *Single-unit smooth muscle.* This type is also called *unitary smooth muscle, syncytial smooth muscle,* and *visceral smooth muscle.* A mass of hundreds to millions of muscle fibers contract together as a single unit. The cell membranes are joined by gap junctions so action potentials can travel from one fiber to the next and cause the muscle fibers to contract together. This type of muscle is found in the walls of the gastrointestinal tract, bile ducts, ureters, uterus, oviducts, and blood vessels.

Physical Basis for Smooth Muscle Contraction (p. 92)

Smooth Muscle Does Not Have the Same Striated Arrangement of Actin and Myosin Filaments As Is Found in Skeletal Muscle

- *Actin filaments attach to dense bodies.* Some of the dense bodies are dispersed inside the cell and held in place by a scaffold of structural proteins linking one dense body to another. Others are attached to the cell membrane and form bonds with dense bodies of adjacent cells, allowing the force of contraction to be transmitted from one cell to the next.

- *Myosin filaments are interspersed among the actin filaments.* The myosin filaments have a diameter that is more than twice as large as that of the actin filaments.
- *Contractile units.* The individual contractile units consist of actin filaments radiating from two dense bodies; these filaments overlap a single myosin filament that is located midway between the dense bodies.

Comparison of Smooth Muscle Contraction and Skeletal Muscle Contraction *(p. 92)*

Unlike Skeletal Muscle Contractions, Most Smooth Muscle Contractions Are Prolonged Tonic Ones That Sometimes Last Hours or Even Days. Both the physical and chemical characteristics of smooth muscle are different than those of skeletal muscle. The following are some of the differences:

- *Slow cycling of the cross-bridges.* The rapidity of cross-bridge cycling in smooth muscle (i.e., the rate of myosin cross-bridge attachment and release with actin) is much slower in smooth muscle than in skeletal muscle.
- *Low energy requirement.* Only 1/10 to 1/300 as much energy is required to sustain a contraction in smooth muscle compared with that of skeletal muscle.
- *Slow onset of contraction and relaxation.* A typical smooth muscle tissue begins to contract 50 to 100 milliseconds after it is excited and has a total contraction time of 1 to 3 seconds, which is 30 times as long as that of an average skeletal muscle.
- *Increased maximum force of contraction.* The maximum force of contraction of smooth muscle is often greater than that of skeletal muscle. This increased force of attraction is postulated to result from the prolonged period of attachment of the myosin cross-bridges to the actin filaments.

Smooth Muscle Can Shorten by a Higher Percentage of Its Length Than Can Skeletal Muscle. Skeletal muscle has a useful distance of contraction of only about one fourth to one third of its stretched length, whereas smooth muscle can often contract more than two thirds of its stretched length.

The "Latch Mechanism" Facilitates Prolonged Holding Contractions. Once smooth muscle has developed full contraction, the degree of activation of the muscle can usually be reduced to far less than the initial level, yet the muscle can maintain its full force of contraction. This is called the "latch mechanism." The importance of the latch mechanism is that it can maintain prolonged tonic contraction in smooth muscle for hours with little use of energy.

Regulation of Contraction by Calcium Ions
(p. 93)

Calcium Ions Combine with Calmodulin to Cause Activation of Myosin Kinase and Phosphorylation of the Myosin Head. Smooth muscle does not contain troponin but, instead, has *calmodulin,* another regulatory protein. Although this protein reacts with calcium ions, it is different from troponin in the manner in which it initiates the contraction; calmodulin does this by activating the myosin cross-bridges. Regulation of contraction is thus myosin based in smooth muscle, rather than actin based as it is in skeletal muscle. This activation and subsequent contraction occur in the following sequence:

1. The calcium ions bind with calmodulin; the calmodulin-calcium complex then joins with and activates *myosin kinase,* a phosphorylating enzyme.
2. One of the light chains of each myosin head, called the *regulatory chain,* becomes phosphorylated in response to the myosin kinase.
3. When the regulatory chain is phosphorylated, the head has the capability of binding with the actin filament, causing muscle contraction. When this myosin light chain is not phosphorylated, the attachment–detachment cycling of the head with the actin filament does not occur.

Myosin Phosphatase Is Important for Cessation of Contraction. When the calcium ion concentration falls below a critical level, the aforementioned processes automatically reverse except for phosphorylation of the myosin head. Reversal of this step requires another enzyme, myosin phosphatase, which splits the phosphate from the regulatory light chain; the cycling then stops, and the contraction ceases.

Nervous and Hormonal Control of Smooth Muscle Contraction *(p. 94)*

Neuromuscular Junctions of Smooth Muscle

Neuromuscular Junctions of the Highly Structured Type Found on Skeletal Muscle Fibers Are Not Present in Smooth Muscle

- *Diffuse junctions.* These are the sites of transmitter release. In most instances, the autonomic nerve fibers form so-called diffuse junctions that secrete their transmitter substance into the matrix coating of the smooth muscle; the transmitter substance then diffuses to the cells.

- *Varicosities on the axons.* The axons that innervate smooth muscle fibers do not have typical branching end feet of the type found in the motor end-plate on skeletal muscle fibers. Instead, most of the fine terminal axons have multiple varicosities that are distributed along their axes. The varicosities contain vesicles loaded with transmitter substance.

- *Contact junctions.* In the multi-unit type of smooth muscle, the varicosities lie directly on the muscle fiber membrane. These so-called contact junctions have a function similar to that of the skeletal muscle neuromuscular junctions.

Acetylcholine and Norepinephrine Can Have Excitatory or Inhibitory Effects at the Smooth Muscle Neuromuscular Junction. These transmitter substances are secreted by the autonomic nerves innervating smooth muscle, but they are never both secreted by the same nerve fibers. Acetylcholine is an excitatory transmitter substance for smooth muscle fibers in some organs but an inhibitory substance for smooth muscle in others. When acetylcholine excites a muscle fiber, norepinephrine ordinarily inhibits it—and vice versa.

Membrane Potentials and Action Potentials in Smooth Muscle *(p. 95)*

The resting membrane potential depends on the type of smooth muscle and the momentary condition of the muscle. It is usually about −50 to −60 millivolts, or about 30 millivolts less negative than in skeletal muscle.

Action Potentials Occur in Single-Unit Smooth Muscle, Such as Visceral Smooth Muscle, in a Manner Similar to That of Skeletal Muscle. They do not occur in most multi-unit types of smooth muscle. The action potentials of visceral smooth muscle occur in two forms:

- *Spike potentials.* Typical spike action potentials occur in most types of single-unit smooth muscle. They can be elicited by electrical stimulation, stretch, or the action of hormones and transmitter substances, or they may be the result of spontaneous generation in the muscle fiber itself.

- *Action potentials with plateaus.* The onset of this type of action potential is similar to that of the typical spike potential. However, repolarization is delayed for several hundred milliseconds. The plateau accounts for the prolonged periods of contraction that occur in the ureter, the uterus under some conditions, and some types of vascular smooth muscle.

Calcium Ions Are Important for Generating Smooth Muscle Action Potentials. Sodium participates little in generation of the action potential in most smooth muscle. Instead, the flow of calcium ions to the interior of the fiber is mainly responsible for the action potential.

Slow-Wave Potentials in Single-Unit Smooth Muscle Can Lead to Generation of Action Potentials. Slow waves are slow oscillations in membrane potential. The slow wave itself is not an action potential.

- *Cause of slow waves.* Two possible causes of slow waves are (1) oscillations in sodium pump activity, which cause the membrane potential to become more negative when sodium is pumped rapidly and less negative when sodium is pumped slowly and (2) the conductance of the ion channels, which may increase and decrease rhythmically.

- *Importance of slow waves.* Action potentials can be initiated when the potential of the slow wave rises above threshold (about −35 millivolts). The action potential spreads over the muscle mass, and contraction occurs.

Spontaneous Action Potentials Are Often Generated When Visceral (Single-Unit) Smooth Muscle Is Stretched. Spontaneous action potentials result from a combination of the normal slow wave potentials in addition to a decrease in the negativity of the membrane potential caused by the stretch itself. This response to stretch allows the gut wall, when excessively stretched, to contract automatically thereby resisting the stretch.

Effect of Local Tissue Factors and Hormones on Smooth Muscle Contraction without Action Potentials *(p. 97)*

Smooth Muscle Relaxation in Blood Vessels Occurs in Response to Local Tissue Factors. This vasodilatory response is extremely important for local control of blood flow.

Most of the Circulating Hormones in the Body Affect Smooth Muscle Contraction to Some Degree. A hormone causes contraction when the muscle cell membrane contains excitatory receptors for the respective hormone. Conversely, the hormone causes inhibition if the membrane contains inhibitory receptors.

Source of Calcium Ions That Cause Contraction *(p. 97)*

Most of the Calcium Ions That Cause Contraction Enter the Muscle Cell from the Extracellular Fluid. Because smooth muscle fibers are relatively small compared with skeletal muscle fibers, the calcium ions can diffuse to all parts of a smooth muscle fiber and elicit the contractile process. Therefore, the force of contraction of smooth muscle is highly dependent on the extracellular fluid calcium ion concentration. The sarcoplasmic reticulum is only rudimentary in most smooth muscle.

Calcium Pumps Remove Calcium Ions from the Intracellular Fluids and Thereby Terminate Contraction. Calcium is removed by calcium pumps. These pumps move the calcium ions out of the smooth muscle fiber and back into the extracellular fluid, or they pump the calcium ions into the sarcoplasmic reticulum.

III

The Heart

CHAPTER 9

Cardiac Muscle; The Heart as a Pump and Function of the Heart Valves

The human heart is composed of two pumps: the *right heart*, which receives blood from the peripheral organs and pumps it through the lungs, and the *left heart*, which receives oxygenated blood from the lungs and pumps it back to the peripheral organs. Each pump is composed of an *atrium* and a *ventricle*. The atria function as primer pumps that fill the ventricles with blood. The ventricles contract and impart high pressure to the blood, which is responsible for propelling it through the circulation. The heart has a special conduction system that maintains its own rhythmicity and transmits action potentials throughout the heart muscles.

Distinguishing Features of Cardiac Muscle Compared with Skeletal Muscle (p. 101)

The similarities and differences in cardiac and skeletal muscle include the following:

- *Both cardiac and skeletal muscle are striated and have actin and myosin filaments* that interdigitate and slide along each other during contraction.
- *Cardiac muscle has intercalated discs between cardiac muscle cells,* which is one of the differences from skeletal muscle. These discs have very low electrical resistance allowing an action potential to travel freely between cardiac muscle cells.
- The *cardiac muscle is a syncytium* of many heart muscle cells in which the action potential spreads rapidly from cell to cell.
- *The atrioventricular (A-V) bundle slowly conducts impulses from the atria to the ventricles.* This is an exclusive pathway because the atrial syncytium and ventricular syncytium are normally insulated from one another by fibrous tissue.

Action Potentials in Cardiac Muscle (p. 102)

The resting membrane potential of cardiac muscle is about -85 to -95 millivolts, and the action potential is 105 millivolts. The membranes remain depolarized for 0.2 second in the atria and for 0.3 second in the ventricles.

Slow Entry of Sodium and Calcium Ions into the Cardiac Muscle Cells Is One of the Causes of the Action Potential Plateau. The action potential of skeletal muscle is caused by entry of sodium through *fast sodium* *channels,* which remain open for only a few 10,000ths of a second. In cardiac muscle, the fast sodium channels also open at the initiation of the action potential, but cardiac muscle has unique *slow calcium channels,* or *calcium-sodium channels.* Calcium and sodium ions flow through the slow channels into the cell after the initial spike of the action potential, and they maintain the plateau. Calcium that enters the cell through these channels also promotes cardiac muscle contraction.

Another Cause of the Plateau of the Action Potential Is a Decrease in the Permeability of Cardiac Muscle Cells to Potassium Ions. The decrease in cardiac potassium permeability also prevents return of the membrane potential in cardiac muscle; this mechanism is not present in skeletal muscle. When the slow calcium-sodium channels close after 0.2 to 0.3 second, the potassium permeability increases rapidly and thus returns the membrane potential to its resting level.

Diffusion of Calcium Into the Myofibrils Promotes Muscle Contraction. The action potential spreads into each cardiac muscle fiber along the *transverse (T) tubules,* causing the longitudinal sarcoplasmic tubules to release calcium ions into the sarcoplasmic reticulum. These calcium ions catalyze the chemical reactions that promote the sliding of the actin and myosin filaments along one another to cause muscle contraction. This mechanism is also present in skeletal muscle.

Another means of calcium entry into the sarcoplasm, however, is unique to cardiac muscle. The T tubules of cardiac muscles have 25 times as great a volume as those in skeletal muscle volume. These T tubules contain large amounts of calcium that are released during the action potential. In addition, the T tubules open directly into the extracellular fluid in cardiac muscle, so their calcium content highly depends on the extracellular calcium concentration. At the end of the plateau of the action potential, the influx of calcium ions into the muscle fiber abruptly stops, and calcium is pumped back into the sarcoplasmic reticulum and T tubules. Thus, the contraction ends.

The Cardiac Cycle *(p. 105)*

The events that occur at the beginning of a heartbeat and last until the beginning of the next heartbeat are called the *cardiac cycle.*

- Each beat of the heart begins with a spontaneous action potential that is initiated in the *sinus node* of the right atrium near the opening of the superior vena cava.

- The action potential travels through both atria and the *A-V node and bundle* into the ventricles.
- A delay of more than 1/10 of a second occurs in the A-V node and bundle, which allows the atria to contract before the ventricles contract.

Figure 9–1 shows the events of the cardiac cycle. The ventricles fill with blood during *diastole* and contract during *systole.* The top three curves in Figure 9–1 show the aortic pressure, left ventricular pressure, and left atrial pressure. The curves below them are the changes in ventricular volume, the electrocardiogram, and the phonocardiogram (a recording of heart sounds).

The Spread of the Action Potential in the Heart Initiates Each Heartbeat. The electrocardiogram is a recording of the voltage generated by the heart from the surface of the body during each heartbeat (see Fig. 9–1).

- The *P wave is caused by spread of depolarization across the atria,* which causes atrial contraction. Atrial pressure increases just after the P wave.

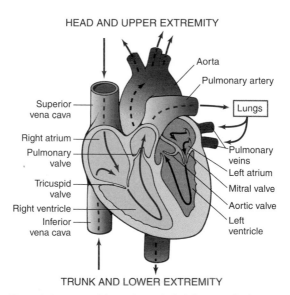

HEAD AND UPPER EXTREMITY

Aorta

Pulmonary artery

Lungs

Superior vena cava

Right atrium

Pulmonary valve

Tricuspid valve

Right ventricle

Inferior vena cava

Pulmonary veins

Left atrium

Mitral valve

Aortic valve

Left ventricle

TRUNK AND LOWER EXTREMITY

Figure 9–1. Events of the cardiac cycle for left ventricular function showing changes in left atrial pressure, left ventricular pressure, aortic pressure, ventricular volume, the electrocardiogram, and the phonocardiogram.

- The *QRS waves appear as a result of ventricular depolarization* about 0.16 second after the onset of the P wave, and this initiates ventricular contraction; then the ventricular pressure begins to increase.
- The *ventricular T wave is caused by repolarization of the ventricle.*

The Atria Function as Primer Pumps for the Ventricles. About 75% of ventricular filling occurs during diastole before contraction of the atria, which causes the remaining 25% of ventricular filling. When the atria fail to function properly, such as during atrial fibrillation, little difficulty is encountered unless a person exercises, and then shortness of breath and other symptoms of heart failure occur. The atrial pressure waves (see Fig. 9–1) include the following:

- The *a wave, which is caused by atrial contraction*
- The *c wave, which occurs during ventricular contraction* because of slight backflow of blood and bulging of the A-V valves toward the atria
- The *v wave, which is caused by in-filling of the atria* from the venous return

The Ventricles Fill with Blood During Diastole. The following events occur just before and during diastole:

- During *systole, the A-V valves are closed,* and the atria fill with blood.
- At the beginning of *diastole* is the period of *isovolumic relaxation,* caused by ventricular relaxation. When ventricular pressure decreases below that of the atria, *the A-V valves open.*
- The higher pressure in the atria pushes blood into the ventricles during diastole.
- The *period of rapid filling of the ventricles* occurs during the first third of diastole and provides most of the ventricular filling.
- *Atrial contraction* occurs during the last third of diastole and contributes about 25% of the filling of the ventricle. This contraction is commonly known as the "atrial kick."

Outflow of Blood from the Ventricles Occurs during Systole. The following events occur during systole:

- *At the beginning of systole, ventricular contraction occurs,* the A-V valves close, and pressure begins to build up in the ventricle. No outflow of blood occurs during the first 0.2 to 0.3 second of ventricular contraction *(period of isovolumic contraction).* Note that isovolumic means "the same volume" and refers to the ventricular volume.

- When the left ventricular pressure exceeds the aortic pressure of about 80 mm Hg and the right ventricular pressure exceeds the pulmonary artery pressure of 8 mm Hg, the aortic and pulmonary valves open. Ventricular outflow occurs, and this is called the *period of ejection.*
- Most ejection occurs during the first part of this period *(period of rapid ejection).*
- This is followed by the *period of slow ejection.* During this period, aortic pressure may slightly exceed the ventricular pressure because the kinetic energy of the blood leaving the ventricle is converted to the pressure in the aorta, which slightly increases its pressure.
- During the last period of systole the ventricular pressures fall below the aortic and pulmonary artery pressures. Thus the aortic and pulmonary valves close at this time.

The Fraction of the End-Diastolic Volume That Is Ejected Is Called the Ejection Fraction

- At the end of diastole, the volume of each ventricle is 110 to 120 mL; this volume is called the *end-diastolic volume.*
- The *stroke volume,* which has a value of about 70 mL, is the amount of blood ejected with each beat.
- The *end-systolic volume* is the remaining volume in the ventricle at the end of systole and measures about 40 to 50 mL.
- The *ejection fraction* is calculated by dividing the stroke volume by the end-diastolic volume; it has a value of about 60%. The stroke volume of the heart can be doubled by increasing the end-diastolic volume and decreasing the end-systolic volume.

Ventricular Ejection Increases Pressure in the Aorta to 120 mm Hg (Systolic Pressure). When the ventricular pressure exceeds the diastolic pressure in the aorta, the aortic valve opens and blood is ejected into the aorta. Pressure in the aorta increases to about 120 mm Hg and distends the elastic aorta and other arteries.

When the aortic valve closes at the end of ventricular ejection, there is a slight backflow of blood followed by a sudden cessation of flow, which causes an *incisura,* or a slight increase in aortic pressure. During diastole, blood continues to flow into the peripheral circulation, and the arterial pressure decreases to 80 mm Hg (diastolic pressure).

The Heart Valves Prevent Backflow of Blood. The A-V valves (*tricuspid* and *mitral* valves) prevent backflow of blood from the ventricles to the atria during systole. In a similar fashion, the *semilunar valves* (*aortic* and *pulmonary* valves) prevent backflow of blood from the aorta and pulmonary artery into the ventricle during diastole. The A-V valves have papillary muscles attached to them by the *chordae tendineae*. During systole, the papillary muscles contract to help prevent the valves from bulging back too far into the atria. The aorta and pulmonary valves are thicker than the A-V valves and do not have any papillary muscles attached.

Work Output of the Heart *(p. 108)*

The *stroke work output* of the ventricles is the output of energy by the heart during each heartbeat. The heart performs two types of work:

- *The volume-pressure work of the heart* is the work done to increase the pressure of the blood; in the left heart, it equals stroke volume multiplied by the difference between the left ventricular mean ejection pressure and the left ventricular mean input pressure. The volume-pressure work of the right ventricle is only about one sixth that of the left ventricle because the ejection pressure of the right ventricle is much lower.
- *The work to be done to supply kinetic energy to the blood* equals $MV^2/2$, where M is the mass of blood ejected, and V is the velocity.

Usually, only about 1% of the work of the heart creates kinetic energy. However, with a condition such as aortic stenosis the opening of the aortic valve is very small, and the velocity of blood is very high. Supplying kinetic energy therefore can consume as much as 50% of the total work output of the heart.

The Volume-Pressure Diagram of the Left Ventricle Determines the Cardiac Work Output. The cardiac cycle can be depicted in a *volume-pressure diagram* that plots intraventricular pressure as a function of left ventricular volume. The phases of the cardiac cycle include the following:

- ***Phase I:*** *Period of filling* during which the left ventricular volume increases from the *end-systolic* volume to the *end-diastolic* volume, or from 45 mL to 115 mL, an increase of 70 mL.

- **Phase II:** *Period of isovolumic contraction* during which the volume of the ventricle remains at the end-diastolic volume but the intraventricular pressure increases to the level of the aortic diastolic pressure, or 80 mm Hg.
- **Phase III:** *Period of ejection* during which the systolic pressure increases further because of additional ventricular contraction, and the ventricular volume decreases by 70 mL, which is the *stroke volume.*
- **Phase IV:** *Period of isovolumic relaxation during which the ventricular volume remains at 45 mL, but the intraventricular pressure decreases to its diastolic pressure level.*

The area inside the volume-pressure diagram represents the volume-pressure work (or external work output) of the ventricle during each cardiac cycle. This diagram and cardiac work are affected by the *preload* and *afterload* on the heart. Preload is usually considered to be the end-diastolic pressure, and the afterload is considered to be the pressure in the artery exiting the ventricle (aorta or pulmonary artery).

Oxygen Consumption by the Heart Depends on Cardiac Work. Cardiac oxygen consumption mainly depends on the volume-pressure type of work. This oxygen consumption has also been found to be proportional to the tension of the heart multiplied by the time the tension is maintained. Wall tension in the heart is proportional to the pressure times the diameter of the ventricle. Ventricular wall tension therefore increases at high systolic pressures or when the heart is dilated.

Regulation of Heart Pumping *(p. 110)*

The Frank-Starling Mechanism Intrinsically Regulates Cardiac Pumping Ability. When *venous return* of blood increases, the heart muscle stretches more, which makes it pump with a greater force of contraction. The *Frank-Starling* mechanism of the heart can be stated in another way: *Within physiological limits, the heart pumps all the blood that comes to it without allowing excess accumulation of blood in the veins.* The extra stretch of the cardiac muscle during increased venous return, within limits, causes the actin and myosin filaments to interdigitate at a more optimal length for force generation. In addition, more stretch of the right atrial wall causes a reflex increase in the heart rate of 10% to 20%, which helps the heart pump more blood.

The ability of the heart to pump blood can be illustrated graphically in several ways. First, stroke work output can be plotted for each ventricle as a function of its corresponding atrial pressure. Ventricular output (or *cardiac output*) can also be plotted as a function of atrial pressure (see Fig. 20–1).

The Autonomic Nervous System Affects Cardiac Pumping. Under strong sympathetic stimulation, the heart rate of an adult increases from a resting value of 72 beats per minute up to 180 to 200 beats per minute, and the force of contraction of the heart muscles increases dramatically. Sympathetic stimulation therefore can increase cardiac output two- to threefold. The heart has a resting sympathetic tone; therefore inhibition of the sympathetic system decreases the heart rate and the force of contraction of the heart, and thus cardiac output decreases. This is explained further in Chapter 20.

Parasympathetic stimulation mainly affects the atria and can decrease the heart rate dramatically and the force of contraction of the ventricles slightly. The combined effect decreases cardiac output by 50% or more.

Cardiac Contractility Is Affected by Several Factors. Among the factors that affect cardiac contractility are the *extracellular electrolyte concentrations.* Excess potassium in extracellular fluid causes the heart to become flaccid and reduces the heart rate, thereby causing a large decrease in contractility. Excess calcium in the extracellular fluid causes the heart to go into spastic contraction. In contrast, a decrease in calcium ions causes the heart to become flaccid.

Assessment of cardiac contractility has proven to be difficult. The *rate of change of ventricular pressure,* or dP/dt, has been used as an index of contractility, especially the peak dP/dt. This index, however, is affected by both preload and afterload; another index that is more reliable is (dP/dt)/P.

CHAPTER 10

Rhythmical Excitation of the Heart

The heart has a special system for self-excitation of rhythmical impulses to cause repetitive contraction of the heart. This system conducts impulses throughout the heart and causes the atria to contract one-sixth of a second before the ventricles contract, which allows extra filling of the ventricles with blood before contraction.

Specialized Excitatory and Conductive System of the Heart (p. 115)

The parts of the rhythmical conduction system and their function are as follows:

- *Sinus node* (or the *sinoatrial node*), which initiates the cardiac impulse
- *Internodal pathway*, which conducts impulses from the sinus node to the atrioventricular (A-V) node
- *A-V node*, which delays impulses from the atria to the ventricles
- *A-V bundle*, which delays impulses and conducts impulses from the A-V node to the ventricles
- Right and left bundles of *Purkinje fibers*, which conduct impulses to all parts of the ventricles

The Sinus Node Controls the Rate of Beat of the Entire Heart. The membrane potential of a sinus node fiber is −55 to −60 millivolts compared with −85 to −90 millivolts in a ventricular muscle fiber.

The action potential in the sinus node is caused by the following:

- The *fast sodium channels* are inactivated at the normal resting membrane potential, but there is slow leakage of sodium into the fiber.
- Between action potentials the resting potential gradually increases because of this *slow leakage of sodium* until the potential reaches −40 millivolts.
- At this time, the *calcium-sodium channels* become activated, allowing rapid entry of calcium and sodium, but especially calcium, thus causing the action potential.
- Greatly increased numbers of *potassium channels open* within about 100 to 150 milliseconds after the calcium-sodium channels open, allowing potassium to escape from the cells. This returns the membrane potential to its resting potential, and the self-excitation cycle starts again, with sodium leaking slowly into the sinus nodal fibers.

Internodal and Interatrial Pathways Transmit Impulses in the Atrium. The parts of the *internodal pathway* are the *anterior internodal pathway, middle internodal pathway,* and *posterior internodal pathway,* all of which carry impulses from the sinoatrial node to the A-V node. Small bundles of atrial muscle fibers transmit impulses more rapidly than the normal atrial muscle; and one of these, the *anterior interatrial band,* conducts impulses from the right atrium to the anterior part of the left atrium.

The A-V Node Delays Impulses from the Atria to the Ventricles. This delay time allows the atria to empty their contents into the ventricles before ventricular contraction occurs. Table 10–1 shows the time of the arrival of impulses at parts of the conduction system from an impulse initiated at the sinus node.

Note that a delay of 0.09 second occurs between the A-V node and the A-V bundle. The velocity of conduction of this system is only 0.02 to 0.05 m/sec, or one-twelfth that of normal cardiac muscle. The reason for this slow conduction in the A-V node and bundle is that (1) the membrane potential is much less negative in the A-V node and bundle than in normal cardiac muscle and (2) few gap junctions exist between the cells in the A-V node and bundle, so the resistance to ion flow is great.

Transmission of Impulses through the Purkinje System and Cardiac Muscle Is Rapid. The *Purkinje fibers* lead from the A-V node, through the A-V bundle, and into the ventricles. The A-V bundle lies just under the endocardium and receives the cardiac impulse first. The A-V bundle then divides into the *left* and *right bundles.* The following are characteristics of the Purkinje system:

• The action potentials travel at a velocity of 1.5 to 4.0 m/sec, which is six times the velocity in cardiac muscle.

Table 10–1. Time of Arrival of Impulse

Sinus node	0.00 sec
A-V node	0.03 sec
A-V bundle	0.12 sec
Ventricular septum	0.16 sec

A-V, atrioventricular.

- The high permeability of the gap junctions at the intercalated discs between the Purkinje fiber cells likely causes the high velocity of transmission.

The Atrial and Ventricular Syncytia Are Separate and Insulated from One Another. The methods of this separation are the following: *The atria and ventricles are separated by a fibrous barrier that acts as an insulator,* forcing the atrial impulses to enter the ventricles through the A-V bundle.

The Transmission of Impulses through Cardiac Muscles Travels at a Velocity of 0.3 to 0.5 m/sec. Because the Purkinje fibers lie just under the endocardium, the action potential spreads into the rest of the ventricular muscle from this area. Then the cardiac impulses travel up the spirals of the cardiac muscle and finally reach the epicardial surface. The endocardium-to-epicardium transit time is 0.03 second. The transmission time from the initial bundle branches to the epicardial surface of the last part of the heart to be stimulated and is therefore 0.06 second.

Control of Excitation and Conduction in the Heart *(p. 118)*

The Sinus Node Is the Normal Pacemaker of the Heart. The intrinsic rhythmical rates of the different areas of the heart are shown in Table 10–2.

The reason the sinus node is the normal pacemaker is that it discharges faster than the other tissues in the cardiac conduction system. When the sinus node discharges, it sends impulses to the A-V node and Purkinje fibers and thereby discharges them before they can discharge intrinsically. The tissues and sinus node then repolarize at the same time, but the sinus node loses its hyperpolarization faster and discharges again—before the A-V node and Purkinje fibers can undergo self-excitation. Occasionally, some cardiac tissue develops a rhythmical rate faster than that of the sinus node; this

Table 10–2. Intrinsic Discharge Rate

Origin of Discharge	Times/Minute
Sinus node	70–80
A-V node	40–60
Purkinje system	15–40

is called an *ectopic pacemaker*. The most common location of this new pacemaker is the A-V node or the penetrating portion of the A-V bundle.

A-V Block Occurs When Impulses Fail to Pass from the Atria to the Ventricles. During *A-V block* the atria continue to beat normally, but the ventricular pacemaker lies in the Purkinje system, which normally discharges at a rate of 15 to 40 beats per minute. After a sudden block, the Purkinje system does not emit its rhythmical impulses for 5 to 30 seconds because it has been overdriven by the sinus rhythm. During this time, therefore, the ventricles fail to contract, and the person may faint because of the lack of cerebral blood flow. This condition is called the *Stokes-Adams syndrome.*

Control of Heart Rhythmicity and Conduction by the Cardiac Nerves: Sympathetic and Parasympathetic Nerves *(p. 119)*

Parasympathetic (Vagal) Stimulation Slows the Cardiac Rhythm. Stimulation of parasympathetic nerves to the heart releases the neurotransmitter *acetylcholine* from the vagal nerve endings. Acetylcholine causes the following effects:

• The rate of sinus node discharge decreases.
• The excitability of the fibers between the atrial muscle and the A-V node decreases.

The heart rate decreases to one-half normal under mild or moderate vagal stimulation, but strong stimulation can temporarily stop the heartbeat, resulting in a lack of impulses traversing the ventricles. Under these conditions, the Purkinje fibers develop their own rhythm at 15 to 40 beats per minute. This phenomenon is called *ventricular escape.*

The mechanisms of vagal effects on the heart rate are as follows:

1. Acetylcholine increases the permeability of the sinus node and A-V junctional fibers to potassium, which causes *hyperpolarization* of these tissues and makes them less excitable.
2. The membrane potential of the sinus nodal fibers decreases from -55 to -60 millivolts to -65 to -75 millivolts.

The normal upward drift in membrane potential that is caused by sodium leakage in these tissues requires a much longer time to reach the threshold for self-excitation.

Sympathetic Stimulation Increases the Cardiac Rhythm. Stimulation of the sympathetic nerves to the heart has the following three basic effects:

- *The rate of sinus node discharge increases.*
- *The cardiac impulse conduction rate increases* in all parts of the heart.
- *The force of contraction increases* in both atrial and ventricular muscle.

Sympathetic stimulation releases *norepinephrine* at the sympathetic nerve endings. The mechanisms of norepinephrine effects on the heart are not clear, but they are believed to involve two basic effects. First, norepinephrine is believed to increase the permeability of cardiac muscle fibers to sodium and calcium, which increases the resting membrane potential and makes the heart more excitable; therefore the heart rate increases. Second, the greater calcium permeability increases the force of contraction of cardiac muscle.

CHAPTER 11

The Normal Electrocardiogram

As the depolarization wave passes through the heart, electrical currents pass into surrounding tissue, and a small part of the current reaches the surface of the body. The electrical potential generated by these currents can be recorded from electrodes placed on the skin on the opposite sides of the heart; this recording is called an *electrocardiogram.*

The normal electrocardiogram (see Fig. 9–1) is composed of the following:

- A *P wave* caused by the electrical potential generated from depolarization of the atria before their contraction
- A *QRS complex* caused by the electrical potential generated from the ventricles before their contraction
- A *T wave* caused by the potential generated from repolarization of the ventricles

Atrial and Ventricular Contractions Are Related to the Electrocardiogram Waves. In Figure 9–1, the relationships between the electrocardiogram and atrial and ventricular contractions can be seen and indicate the following:

- *The P wave immediately precedes atrial contraction.*
- *The QRS complex immediately precedes ventricular contraction.*
- *The ventricles remain contracted until a few milliseconds after the end of the T repolarization wave.*
- *The atria remain contracted until they are repolarized,* but an atrial repolarization wave cannot be seen on the electrocardiogram because it is obscured by the QRS wave.
- *The P-Q or P-R interval on the electrocardiogram has a normal value of 0.16 second* and is the duration of time between the first deflection of the P wave and the beginning of the QRS wave; this represents the time between the beginning of atrial contraction and the beginning of ventricular contraction.
- *The Q-T interval has a normal value of 0.35 second,* which is the duration of time from the beginning of the Q wave to the end of the T wave. This approximates the time of ventricular contraction.
- *The heart rate can be determined with the reciprocal of the time interval between each heartbeat.*

During the Depolarization Process, the Average Electrical Current Flows from the Base of the Heart toward the Apex. The heart is suspended in a highly conductive medium, so when one area of the heart depolarizes current flows from this area toward a polarized area. The first area that depolarizes is the ventricular septum, and current flows quickly from this area to the other endocardial surfaces of the ventricle. Then current flows from the electronegative inner surfaces of the heart to the electropositive outer surfaces, with the average current flowing from the base of the heart to the apex in an elliptical pattern. An electrode placed near the base of the heart is electronegative, and one placed near the apex is electropositive.

Electrocardiographic Leads (p. 124)

Bipolar Limb Leads Involve an Electrocardiogram Recorded from Electrodes on Two Different Limbs. There Are Three Bipolar Limb Leads

- To record from *lead I, the negative terminal of the electrocardiogram is connected to the right arm, and the positive terminal is connected to the left arm.* During the depolarization cycle, the point at which the right arm connects to the chest is electronegative compared with the point at which the left arm connects, so the electrocardiogram records positively when this lead is used.

- To record from *lead II, the negative terminal of the electrocardiogram is connected to the right arm, and the positive terminal is connected to the left leg.* During most of the depolarization cycle, the left leg is electropositive compared with the right arm, so the electrocardiogram records positively when this lead is used.

- To record from *lead III, the negative terminal is connected to the left arm, and the positive terminal is connected to the left leg.* During most of the depolarization cycle, the left leg is electropositive compared with the left arm, so the electrocardiogram records positively when this lead is used.

Einthoven's Law States That the Electrical Potential of Any Limb Lead Equals the Sum of the Potentials of the Other Two Limb Leads. The positive and negative signs of the various leads must be observed when using this law. The following example illustrates *Einthoven's law.* We first assume that the right arm is 0.2 millivolt negative with respect to the average potential in the body, the left arm is 0.3 millivolt positive, and the left leg is 1.0 millivolt positive. Therefore, lead I has a potential of 0.5 millivolt because this is the difference between

−0.2 millivolt in the right arm and 0.3 millivolt in the left arm. Similarly, lead II has a potential of 1.2 millivolts, and lead III has a potential of 0.7 millivolt.

Chest Leads (Precordial Leads) Can Be Used to Detect Minor Electrical Abnormalities in the Ventricles. Chest leads, known as leads V_1, V_2, V_3, V_4, V_5, and V_6 are connected to the positive terminal of the electrocardiograph, and the *indifferent electrode,* or the negative electrode, is simultaneously connected to the left arm, left leg, and right arm. The QRS recordings from the V_1 and V_2 lead, which are placed over the heart near the base, usually read negatively; and the QRS recording from leads V_4, V_5, and V_6 which are closer to the apex, usually read positively. Because these leads can record the electrical potential immediately underneath the electrode, small changes in electrical potential of the cardiac musculature can be detected, such as that generated by a small myocardial infarction.

Augmented Unipolar Leads Are Also Used to Record Electrocardiograms. Another system of leads in wide use is the augmented unipolar limb lead. With this type of recording, two of the limbs are connected through electrical resistances to the negative terminal of the electrocardiograph, and the third limb is connected to the positive terminal. When the positive terminal is on the right arm, the lead is known as the aVR lead; when it is on the left arm, it is known as the aVL lead; and when it is on the left leg (or foot), it is known as the aVF lead.

CHAPTER 12

Electrocardiographic Interpretation of Cardiac Muscle and Coronary Blood Flow Abnormalities: Vectorial Analysis

Any change in the transmission of impulses through the heart alters the electrical potentials around the heart, which causes changes in the electrocardiogram waves. Therefore most abnormalities in the cardiac muscle can be detected by analyzing the electrocardiogram.

Principles of Vectorial Analysis of Electrocardiograms *(p. 129)*

Vectors Can Be Used to Represent Electrical Potentials Several principles are used in the vectorial analysis of electrical potentials:

- The current in the heart flows from the area of depolarization to the polarized areas, and the electrical potential generated can be represented by a vector, with the *arrowhead pointing in the positive direction.*
- The length of the vector is *proportional to the voltage of the potential.*
- The generated potential at any instance can be represented by an *instantaneous mean vector.*
- When a vector is horizontal and points toward the subject's left side, the axis is defined as zero degrees.
- The scale of the vectors rotates clockwise from the zero-degree reference point.
- If a vector points directly downward, the axis has a direction of +90 degrees.
- If a vector points horizontally to the subject's right side, the axis has a direction of +180 degrees.
- If a vector points directly upward, the axis has a direction of −90 or +270 degrees.
- *The axis of lead I is zero degrees* because the electrodes lie in the horizontal direction on each of the arms.
- *The axis of lead II is +60 degrees* because the right arm connects to the torso in the top right corner, and the left leg connects to the torso in the bottom left corner.
- *The axis of lead III is 120 degrees.*
- When the vector representing the mean direct current flow in the heart is perpendicular to the axis of one of the bipolar limb leads, the voltage recorded in the electrocardiogram in this lead is very low.

- When the vector has approximately the same direction as the axis of one of the bipolar limb leads, nearly the entire voltage is recorded in this lead.

The Normal Electrocardiogram Represents the Vectors That Occur During Electrical Potential Changes in the Cardiac Cycle

- *The QRS complex represents ventricular depolarization* that begins at the ventricular septum and proceeds toward the apex of the heart with an average direction of 59 degrees.
- *The ventricular T wave represents repolarization of the ventricle* that begins near the apex of the heart and proceeds toward the base. Because the cardiac muscle near the apex becomes electropositive after it repolarizes and the muscle near the base is still electronegative, the T wave vector has a direction similar to that of the QRS wave.
- *The atrial P wave represents depolarization of the atria* that begins at the sinus node and spreads in all directions, but the average vector points toward the atrioventricular (A-V) node.

Several Factors Shift the Mean Electrical Axis of the Ventricles to the Left (Counterclockwise)

- *Changes in the position of the heart,* such as occur during expiration or when a person is *recumbent* and the abdominal contents press upward against the diaphragm
- *Accumulation of abdominal fat,* which also presses upward on the heart
- *Left bundle branch block,* which is when the cardiac impulse spreads through the right ventricle two to three times as fast as in the left ventricle. Consequently, the left ventricle remains polarized much longer than the right, and a strong electrical vector points from the right ventricle to the left
- *Hypertrophy of the left ventricle,* which is caused by hypertension, aortic valvular stenosis, or aortic valvular regurgitation

An example of left axis deviation caused by hypertension and the resulting effects on left ventricular hypertrophy of the electrocardiogram is shown in Figure 12–1. *Note that the lead I and III vectors are plotted in this figure and that a vertical dotted line is extended from the ends of these vectors. The resultant vector is drawn from the origin to the intersection of*

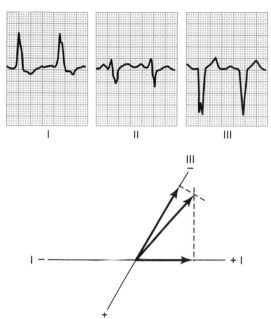

Figure 12–1. Left axis deviation in hypertensive heart disease. Note the slightly prolonged QRS complex.

the two dotted lines and represents the mean electrical axis in this condition.

Several Factors Shift the Mean Electrical Axis of the Ventricles to the Right (Clockwise)

- *Inspiration*
- *Standing up*
- *Lack of abdominal fat,* which allows the heart to rotate clockwise compared with the normal individual
- *Right bundle branch block*
- *Right ventricular hypertrophy*

Conditions That Cause Abnormal Voltage of the QRS Complex *(p. 137)*

Hypertrophy of the Heart Increases the Voltage of the QRS Complex. When the sum of the voltages of the QRS waves from the three standard limb leads is greater than 4 millivolts, a high-voltage electrocardiogram is considered to exist. The most common cause of high-voltage QRS complexes is right or left ventricular hypertrophy.

The Following Conditions Decrease Voltage of the QRS Complex

• *Hearts with old myocardial infarctions* and the resultant decreased cardiac muscle mass. This condition also slows the conduction wave through the heart and decreases the amount of muscle that is depolarized at one time. Therefore, decreased QRS voltage and prolongation of the QRS complex result.

• *Conditions surrounding the heart that effectively "short-circuit" the cardiac electrical potential. Fluid in the pericardium* and *pleural effusion* both conduct currents from around the heart and prevent much of the voltage from reaching the surface of the body. *Pulmonary emphysema* also decreases conduction of the cardiac potentials because the excess volume of air in the lungs insulates the heart.

The Following Conditions Cause a Prolonged QRS Complex

• The most common cause of an extended QRS complex is *prolonged conduction* through the ventricles. This occurs in both hypertrophied and dilated hearts and increases the duration of the QRS waves by about 0.02 to 0.05 second. A prolonged QRS wave caused by left ventricular hypertrophy is shown in Figure 12–1.

• *Blockade of the impulses in the Purkinje system* prolongs the QRS complex because the duration of ventricular depolarization increases in one or both ventricles.

Current of Injury *(p. 138)*

Several abnormalities cause a portion of the heart to remain *depolarized all of the time,* and the current that flows from the depolarized area to the polarized areas of the heart is called the *current of injury.* Some of the abnormalities that can cause a current of injury are as follows:

• Mechanical trauma
• Infectious processes that damage the cardiac muscle membrane
• Coronary ischemia

The Axis of the Current of Injury Can Be Determined with the Electrocardiogram. When a portion of the heart is injured and emits a current of injury, the only time the heart returns to zero potential is at the end of the QRS wave because all of the heart is depolarized at this time (see Fig. 9–1). The axis of the current of injury is determined in the following way:

1. First, *determine the J point,* which is the point of zero potential at the end of QRS wave.
2. *Determine the level of the T-P segment* with respect to the J point on the three standard leads.
3. *Plot the voltages on the coordinates of the three leads* to determine the axis of the current of injury, and note that the negative end of the vector originates in the *injured* area of the ventricles.

Acute Anterior and Posterior Wall Infarctions Can Be Diagnosed with the Electrocardiogram. The current of injury is also useful for determining whether an infarction is in the anterior or posterior portion of the heart. A negative injury potential found on one of the precordial leads indicates that this electrode is in an area of strong negative potential and that the current of injury originates in the anterior wall of the ventricles. In contrast, a positive T P segment with respect to the J point indicates the existence of a posterior ventricular wall infarction.

Abnormalities in the T Wave *(p. 141)*

Normally, the apex of the ventricle repolarizes before the base, and the resultant T wave has a mean electrical axis similar to that of the QRS wave. Several conditions alter the electrical axis of the T wave:

• *During bundle branch block, one of the ventricles depolarizes before the other.* The first ventricle to depolarize is also the first to repolarize, and this causes an axis deviation in the T wave. Therefore, a left bundle branch block causes a rightward axis deviation of the T wave.

During shortening in the depolarization of the base of the heart, the base repolarizes before the apex, which *inverts the T wave.* The most common cause of shortened depolarization is *mild ischemia* of cardiac muscle in the base of the ventricles.

CHAPTER 13

Cardiac Arrhythmias and Their Electrocardiographic Interpretation

Often the heart malfunctions not because of abnormal heart muscle but because of an abnormal rhythm of the heart. The causes of cardiac arrhythmias include (1) abnormal rhythmicity of the sinus node, (2) shift of the pacemaker function from the sinus node to other parts of the heart, (3) block of impulse transmission in the heart, (4) abnormal pathway of transmission in the heart, and (5) spontaneous generation of abnormal impulses from any part of the heart.

Abnormal Sinus Rhythms (p. 143)

Stimulation of the Pacemaker of the Heart Causes Tachycardia. An increase in heart rate, called *tachycardia,* is usually defined as a heart rate greater than 100 beats per minute. The causes of sinus-initiated tachycardia include the following:

- *Increased body temperature*
- *Sympathetic stimulation of the heart,* which occurs after blood loss that decreases arterial pressure and increases sympathetic stimulation through baroreceptor mechanisms. In this instance, the heart rate may increase up to 150 to 180 beats per minute
- *Toxic conditions of the heart* (e.g., digitalis intoxication)

Vagal Stimulation of the Heart Decreases Heart Rate. A slow heart rate, usually less than 60 beats per minute, is called *bradycardia.* Stimulation of the vagus nerve decreases the heart rate because of release of the parasympathetic transmitter agent acetylcholine, which decreases the membrane potential of the sinus node. With *carotid sinus syndrome,* an atherosclerotic process causes excess sensitivity of the baroreceptors in the arterial wall. As a result, increased external pressure on the neck causes the atherosclerotic plaque in the carotid sinus to stimulate the baroreceptors, which then stimulate the vagus nerve and cause bradycardia.

Abnormal Cardiac Rhythms That Result from Impulse Conduction Block (p. 144)

Rarely, the impulse from the sinoatrial node is blocked before it enters the atrial muscle in a condition known as *sinoatrial block.* With this condition, the atrial

P wave may be obscured by the QRS wave, and the ventricles pick up a rhythm that usually originates from the atrioventricular (A-V) node.

A-V Block Inhibits or Completely Blocks Impulses Originating in the Sinoatrial Node. The conditions that cause A-V block include the following:

- *Ischemia of the A-V node or A-V bundle,* which occurs during coronary ischemia if the region of ischemia includes the A-V node or bundle
- *Compression of the A-V bundle,* which can be caused by scar tissue or calcified portions of the heart
- *Inflammation of the A-V node or bundle,* which can occur during myocarditis, diphtheria, or rheumatic fever
- *Strong vagal stimulation of the heart*

The types of A-V block include the following:

- *First degree block.* With this condition, the *P-R (or P-Q) interval increases* from a normal value of 0.16 second to about 0.20 second in a heart beating at a normal rate.
- *Second degree block.* When conduction through the A-V junction slows sufficiently for the *P-R interval to increase to 0.25 to 0.45 second,* only a portion of the impulses pass through to the ventricle. Therefore, the atria beat faster than the ventricles, and "dropped beats" of the ventricles occur.
- *Third degree block.* This is *complete A-V junction block,* and complete dissociation of the P waves and QRS waves occurs. Therefore, the ventricles "escape" from the influence of the sinoatrial pacemaker. A condition in which A-V block comes and goes is called *Stokes-Adams syndrome.*

Premature Contractions (p. 146)

Most premature contractions *(extrasystoles)* result from *ectopic foci* that generate abnormal cardiac impulses. The causes of ectopic foci include the following:

- Local ischemia
- Irritation of cardiac muscle as a result of pressure from calcified plaque
- Toxic irritation of the A-V node, Purkinje system, or myocardium by drugs, nicotine, or caffeine

Ectopic Foci Can Cause Premature Contractions That Originate in the Atria, A-V Junction, or Ventricle. The consequences of premature contractions are as follows:

- *Premature atrial contraction.* The P-R interval decreases in this condition, with the amount dependent on how far the origin of the ectopic foci is from the A-V junction. Premature atrial contraction causes premature ventricular beats that may have a *pulse deficit* if the ventricles do not have sufficient time to fill with blood.
- *A-V nodal or A-V bundle premature contractions.* The P wave is often missing from the electrocardiogram because it is superimposed on the QRS wave.
- *Premature ventricular contractions (PVCs).* The ectopic foci originate in the ventricle, and the QRS complex is often prolonged because the impulses must pass through cardiac muscle, which conducts at a much lower rate than the Purkinje system. The QRS voltage increases because one side of the heart depolarizes ahead of the other, causing a large electrical potential between the depolarized and polarized muscle.

Paroxysmal Tachycardia (p. 148)

The cause of paroxysmal tachycardia is believed to be re-entrant pathways that set up local repeated self–re-excitation. The rapid rhythm of the area causes it to become the new pacemaker of the heart. *Paroxysmal tachycardia* means that the heart rate increases in rapid bursts and then, after a few seconds, minutes, or hours, returns to normal. Treatment is administration of pharmacological agents that decrease the sodium or potassium permeability of cardiac muscle and thus inhibits the fast rhythmical discharge of the irritable area.

Two basic types of paroxysmal tachycardia occur:

- *Atrial paroxysmal tachycardia.* When the origin of the tachycardia is in the atrium but is not close to the sinoatrial node, an inverted P wave appears caused by atrial depolarization in the direction opposite from normal. When the abnormal rhythm originates in the A-V node, P waves are obscured or inverted; this condition is called *supraventricular tachycardia.*
- *Ventricular paroxysmal tachycardia.* This type of tachycardia usually does not occur unless significant ischemic damage is present in the ventricles. This abnormality often initiates lethal fibrillation.

Ventricular Fibrillation (p. 149)

Ventricular fibrillation is the most serious of all cardiac arrhythmias. It occurs when an impulse stimulates first one portion of the ventricular muscles and then another and finally stimulates itself. This stimulation causes many portions of the ventricles to contract at the same time while other portions relax. Therefore, impulses travel around the heart muscle; the phenomenon is also referred to as *circus movements*.

Circus Movements

Circus movements are the basis for ventricular fibrillation. When an impulse travels throughout an entire normal ventricle, it dies because all of the ventricular muscle is in a refractory state. However, three conditions allow the impulse to continue around the heart and start circus movements:

- *Increased pathway around the ventricle.* By the time the impulses return to an originally stimulated muscle, it is no longer in a refractory state, and the impulse then continues to travel around the heart. This is especially likely to occur in hearts that are dilated or have valvular disease or other conditions with a long pathway of conduction.
- *Decreased velocity of conduction.* By the time the slower impulse travels around the heart, the muscle is no longer refractory to a new impulse and is stimulated again. This often occurs in the Purkinje system during ischemia of the cardiac muscle or with high blood potassium concentration.
- *Shortened refractory period of the muscles.* This condition allows repeated stimulation as the impulse travels around the heart and occurs after epinephrine administration or repetitive electrical stimulation.

Defibrillation of the heart causes essentially all parts of the ventricles to become refractory. Clinically, the heart can be defibrillated by applying high-voltage direct current through the chest with electrodes placed on either side of the heart.

Atrial Fibrillation (p. 151)

Because the atria and ventricles are insulated from one another, ventricular fibrillation can occur without atrial fibrillation, and atrial fibrillation can occur without ventricular fibrillation. The causes of atrial fibrillation are identical to those of ventricular fibrillation; a frequent cause of atrial fibrillation is an enlarged atrium resulting from heart valve lesions. The atria do not pump if they are fibrillating, and the efficiency of ventricular pumping decreases 20% to 30%. A person can live for years with atrial fibrillation, although there is some cardiac debility.

Atrial flutter is different from atrial fibrillation in that a single large wave front travels around and around the atria. Thus the atria contract 250 to 300 times per minute; because one side of the atrium contracts while the other relaxes, the strength of the atrial contraction is weak.

IV

The Circulation

CHAPTER 14

Overview of the Circulation; Biophysics of Pressure, Flow, and Resistance

The main function of the circulation is to serve the needs of the tissues by transporting nutrients to them, transporting away waste products, carrying hormones from one part of the body to another, and in general maintaining homeostatic conditions in the tissue fluids for optimal survival and function of the cells.

Physical Characteristics of the Circulation (p. 157)

The circulation is divided into the *pulmonary circulation*, which supplies the lungs, and the *systemic circulation*, which supplies tissues in the remainder of the body. The functional parts of the circulation are the following:

- The *arteries*, which transport blood under high pressure to the tissues and have strong vascular walls and rapid blood flow.
- The *arterioles,* which are the last small branches of the arterial system and act as control valves through which blood is released into the capillaries. These vessels have strong muscular walls that can be constricted or dilated, giving them the capability of markedly altering blood flow to the capillaries in response to changing tissue needs.
- The *capillaries*, which exchange fluids, nutrients, and other substances between the blood and the interstitial fluid. They have thin walls and are highly permeable to small molecules.
- The *venules*, which collect blood from the capillaries and gradually coalesce into progressively larger veins.
- The *veins*, which function as conduits to transport blood from the tissues back to the heart; veins also serve as reservoirs for blood. They have thin walls, low pressure, and rapid blood flow.

The Circulation Is a Complete Circuit. Contraction of the left heart propels blood into the systemic circulation through the aorta, which empties into smaller arteries, arterioles, and eventually capillaries. Because the blood vessels are distensible, each contraction of the heart distends the vessels during relaxation of the heart, the vessels recoil, thereby continuing flow to the tissues, even between heartbeats. Blood leaving the tissues enters the venules and then flows into increasingly larger veins, which carry the blood to the right heart.

The right heart then pumps the blood through the pulmonary artery, small arteries, arterioles, and capillaries, where oxygen and carbon dioxide are exchanged between the blood and the tissues. From the pulmonary capillaries, blood flows into venules and large veins and empties into the left atrium and left ventricle before it is again pumped into the systemic circulation.

Because Blood Flows Around the Same Vessels, Any Change in Flow in a Single Part of the Circuit Transiently Alters Flow in Other Parts. For example, strong constriction of the arteries in the systemic circulation can transiently reduce the total cardiac output, in which case blood flow to the lungs decreases equally as much as flow through the systemic circulation.

Another feature of the circulation is that sudden constriction of a blood vessel must always be accompanied by opposite dilation of another part of the circulation because blood volume cannot change rapidly and blood itself is not compressible. For instance, strong constriction of the veins in the systemic circulation displaces blood into the heart, dilating the heart and causing it to pump with increased force. This is one of the mechanisms by which cardiac output is regulated. With prolonged constriction or dilation of a portion of the circulation, changes in total blood volume can occur through exchange with the interstitial fluid or because of changes in fluid excretion by the kidneys.

Most of the Blood Volume Is Distributed in the Veins of the Systemic Circulation. About 84% of the total blood volume is in the systemic circulation, with 64% in the veins, 13% in the arteries, and 7% in the systemic arterioles and capillaries. The heart contains about 7% of the blood volume and the pulmonary vessels 9%.

Velocity of Blood Flow Is Inversely Proportional to the Vascular Cross-Sectional Area. Because approximately the same volume of blood flows through each segment of the circulation, vessels with a large cross-sectional area, such as the capillaries, have slower blood flow velocity. The approximate total cross-sectional areas of the systemic vessels for the average human being are as follows:

Vessel	Cross Sectional Area (cm^2)
Aorta	2.5
Small arteries	20
Arterioles	40
Capillaries	2500
Venules	250
Small veins	80
Venae cavae	8

Thus, under resting conditions, the velocity of blood flow in capillaries is only about 1/1000 the velocity of flow in the aorta.

Pressures Vary in the Different Parts of the Circulation. Because the pumping action of the heart is pulsatile, the aortic arterial pressure rises to its highest point, the *systolic pressure*, during systole and falls to its lowest point, the *diastolic pressure*, at the end of diastole. In the healthy adult, systolic pressure is approximately 120 mm Hg, and diastolic pressure is 80 mm Hg. This is usually written as 120/80 mm Hg. The difference between systolic and diastolic pressure is called the *pulse pressure* (120 − 80 = 40 mm Hg). As blood flows through the systemic circulation, its pressure falls progressively to approximately 0 mm Hg by the time it reaches the termination of the venae cavae in the right atrium of the heart.

Pressure in the systemic capillaries varies from as high as 35 mm Hg near the arteriolar ends to as low as 10 mm Hg near the venous ends, but the average functional capillary pressure is about 17 mm Hg.

Pressures in the Pulmonary Circulation Are Much Lower Than Those in the Systemic Circulation. Pressure in the pulmonary arteries is also pulsatile, but systolic arterial pressure is about 25 mm Hg and diastolic pressure 8 mm Hg, with a mean pulmonary artery pressure of only 16 mm Hg. Pulmonary capillary pressure averages only 8 mm Hg, yet the total blood flow through the lungs is the same as that in the systemic circulation because of the lower vascular resistance of the pulmonary blood vessels.

Basic Principles of Circulatory Function (p. 158)

The details of circulatory function are complex and are described later, but there are three basic principles that underlie the major functions of the circulatory system:

- *The blood flow to each tissue of the body is controlled according to the tissue's needs.* Tissues need more blood flow when they are active than when they are at rest—occasionally as much as 20 times more. The microvessels of each tissue continuously monitor the tissue needs and control the blood flow at the level required for the tissue activity. Nervous and hormonal mechanisms provide additional control of tissue blood flow.

- *The cardiac output is the sum of all the local tissue blood flows.* After blood flows through a tissue, it immediately returns by way of the veins to the heart. The heart responds automatically to the inflow of blood by pumping almost all of it immediately back into the arteries. In this sense, the heart responds to the demands of the tissues, although it often needs help in the form of nervous stimulation to make it pump the required amounts of blood flow.

- *The arterial pressure is usually controlled independently of local blood flow or cardiac output control.* The circulatory system is provided with an extensive system for controlling arterial pressure. If arterial pressure falls below normal, a barrage of nervous reflexes elicits a series of circulatory changes that elevate the pressure back toward normal, including increased force of heart pumping, contraction of large venous reservoirs to provide more blood to the heart, and constriction of most of the arterioles throughout the body. Over more prolonged periods of time, the kidneys play additional roles by secreting pressure-controlling hormones and by regulating blood volume.

Interrelationships of Pressure, Flow, and Resistance *(p. 159)*

Blood Flow through a Vessel Is Determined by the Pressure Gradient and Vascular Resistance. The flow of blood through a vessel can be calculated by the formula $F = \Delta P/R$, where F is blood flow, ΔP is the pressure difference between the two ends of the vessel, and R is the vascular resistance. Note that it is the *difference in pressure* between the two ends of the vessel that provides the driving force for flow, not the absolute pressure in the vessel. For example, if the pressure at both ends of the vessel were 100 mm Hg, there would be no flow despite the presence of high pressure.

Because of the extreme importance of the relationship among pressure, flow, and resistance, the reader should become familiar with the other two algebraic forms of this relationship: $\Delta P = F \times R$ and $R = \Delta P/F$.

Blood pressure is usually expressed in millimeters of mercury (mm Hg), and blood flow is expressed in milliliters per minute (ml/min); vascular resistance is expressed as mm Hg/ml per minute. In the pulmonary circulation, the pressure gradient is much lower than that in the systemic circulation, whereas the blood flow is the same as that in the systemic circulation; *therefore the total pulmonary vascular resistance is much lower than the systemic vascular resistance.*

Vessel Diameter Has a Marked Effect on Resistance to Blood Flow—Poiseuille's Law. According to the *theory of Poiseuille,* vascular resistance is directly proportional to the viscosity of the blood and the length of the blood vessel and inversely proportional to the radius of the vessel raised to the fourth power:

$$\text{Resistance} \, \alpha \, \frac{(\text{Constant} \times \text{Viscosity} \times \text{Length})}{\text{Radius}^4}$$

Decreased Radius of a Blood Vessel Markedly Increases Vascular Resistance. Because vascular resistance is inversely related to the *fourth power* of the radius, even small changes in radius can cause very large changes in resistance. For example, if the radius of a blood vessel increases from one to two (two times normal), resistance decreases to 1/16 of normal ($\frac{1}{2}^4$) and flow increases to 16 times normal if the pressure gradient remains unchanged. Small vessels in the circulation have the greatest amount of resistance, whereas large vessels have little resistance to blood flow.

For a parallel arrangement of blood vessels, as occurs in the systemic circulation in which different organs are each supplied by an artery that branches into multiple vessels, the total resistance can be expressed as

$$\frac{1}{R_{total}} = \frac{1}{R_1} + \frac{1}{R_2} + \ldots \frac{1}{R_n}$$

where R_1, R_2, and R_n, are the resistances of each of the various vascular beds in the circulation. The total resistance is less than the resistance of any of the individual vascular beds.

For a series arrangement of blood vessels, as occurs within a tissue in which blood flows through arteries, arterioles, capillaries, and veins, the total resistance is the sum of the individual resistances, as

$$R_{total} = R_1 + R_2 + \ldots R_n$$

where R_1, R_2, and R_n are the resistances of the various blood vessels in series within the tissues.

Conductance is a measure of the ease of which blood can flow through a vessel and is the reciprocal of resistance.

$$\text{Conductance} = 1/\text{Resistance}$$

Increased Blood Hematocrit and Increased Viscosity Raise Vascular Resistance and Decrease Blood Flow. The greater the viscosity, the less is the flow of blood in a vessel if all other factors remain constant. The normal viscosity of blood is about three times as great as the viscosity of water. The main factor that makes blood so viscous is that it has large numbers of suspended red blood cells, each of which exerts frictional drag against adjacent cells and against the wall of the blood vessel.

The percentage of blood comprising cells, called the *hematocrit,* is normally about 40; this indicates that about 40% of the blood is cells, and the remainder is plasma. The greater the percentage of cells in the blood—that is, the greater the hematocrit—the greater is the viscosity of blood and therefore the greater is the resistance to blood flow.

"Autoregulation" Attenuates the Effect of Arterial Pressure on Tissue Blood Flow. The effect of arterial pressure on blood flow in many tissues is usually far less than one would expect, based on our previous discussion. The reason for this is that an increase in arterial pressure usually initiates compensatory increases in vascular resistance within a few seconds through activation of the local control mechanisms discussed in Chapter 17. Conversely, with reductions in arterial pressure vascular resistance is promptly reduced in most tissues and blood flow is maintained relatively constant. The ability of each tissue to adjust its vascular resistance and to maintain normal blood flow during changes in arterial pressure between approximately 70 and 175 mm Hg is called *blood flow autoregulation.*

Changes in tissue blood flow rarely last for more than a few hours even when increases in arterial pressure or increased levels of vasoconstrictors or vasodilators are sustained. The reason for the relative constancy of blood flow is that each tissue's local autoregulatory mechanisms eventually override most of the effects of vasoconstrictors to provide a blood flow that is appropriate for the needs of the tissue.

CHAPTER 15

Vascular Distensibility and Functions of the Arterial and Venous Systems

Vascular Distensibility (p. 167)

The distensibility of the arteries allows them to accommodate the pulsatile output of the heart and average out the pressure pulsations; this provides smooth, continuous flow of blood through the small blood vessels of the tissues. Veins are even more distensible than arteries, allowing them to store large quantities of blood that can be called into use when needed. On average, veins are about eight times as distensible as arteries in the systemic circulation. In the pulmonary circulation, the distensibility of veins is similar to that of the systemic circulation. The lung's arteries, however, are more distensible than those of the systemic circulation.

Vascular distensibility is normally expressed as follows:

$$\text{Vascular Distensibilty} = \frac{\text{Increase in Volume}}{\text{Increase in Pressure} \times \text{Original Volume}}$$

Vascular compliance (capacitance) is the total quantity of blood that can be stored in a given part of the circulation for each millimeter of mercury of pressure. It is calculated as follows:

The greater the compliance of the vessel, the more easily it can be distended by pressure.

$$\text{Vascular Compliance} = \frac{\text{Increase in Volume}}{\text{Increase in Pressure}}$$

Compliance is related to distensibility as follows:

$$\text{Compliance} = \text{Distensibility} \times \text{Volume}$$

The compliance of a vein in the systemic circulation is about 24 times as great as its corresponding artery because it is about eight times as distensible and has a volume that is three times as great ($8 \times 3 = 24$).

Sympathetic Stimulation Decreases Vascular Capacitance. Sympathetic stimulation increases smooth muscle tone in veins and arteries, causing a shift of blood to the heart, which is an important method the body uses to increase heart pumping. For example, during hemorrhage, enhanced sympathetic tone of the vessels, especially of the veins, reduces vessel size so the circulation can continue to operate almost normally even when as much as 25% of the total blood volume has been lost.

Vessels Exposed to Increased Volume at First Exhibit a Large Increase in Pressure, but Delayed Stretch of the Vessel Wall Allows the Pressure to Return toward Normal. This phenomenon is often referred to as "*delayed compliance*" or "*stress relaxation.*" Delayed compliance is a valuable mechanism by which the circulation can accommodate extra amounts of blood when necessary, such as after a transfusion that was too large. Delayed compliance in the reverse direction permits the circulation to readjust itself over a period of minutes or hours to a diminished blood volume after serious hemorrhage.

Arterial Pressure Pulsations (p. 168)

With each heartbeat a new surge of blood fills the arteries. Were it not for the distensibility of the arterial system, blood flow through the tissues would occur only during cardiac systole, with no blood flowing during diastole. The combination of distensibility of the arteries and their resistance to flow reduces the pressure pulsations to almost none by the time the blood reaches the capillaries, allowing continuous rather than pulsatile flow through the tissues.

In the young adult, the pressure at the height of each pulse, the *systolic pressure,* is normally about 120 mm Hg; and pressure at its lowest point, the *diastolic pressure,* is about 80 mm Hg. The difference between these two pressures, about 40 mm Hg, is called the *pulse pressure.*

The two most important factors that can *increase* pulse pressure are (1) *increased stroke volume* (the amount of blood pumped into the aorta with each heartbeat) and (2) *decreased arterial compliance.* Decreased arterial compliance can result when the arteries "harden" with aging *(arteriosclerosis).*

Abnormal Pressure Pulse Contours. Several other pathophysiologic conditions of the circulation can cause abnormal *contours* of the pressure pulse wave in addition to changing the pulse pressure (Fig. 15–1):

- With *aortic valve stenosis,* the aortic pulse pressure is greatly decreased because of diminished blood flow through the stenotic aortic valve.
- With *patent ductus arteriosus,* some of the blood pumped into the aorta flows immediately through the open ductus arteriosus into the pulmonary artery,

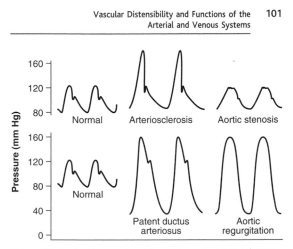

Figure 15–1. Aortic pressure pulse contours in arteriosclerosis, aortic stenosis, patent ductus arteriosus, and aortic regurgitation.

allowing the diastolic pressure to fall very low before the next heartbeat, thereby increasing pulse pressure.

- With *aortic regurgitation,* the aortic valve is absent or functions poorly. After each heartbeat, the blood that flows into the aorta flows immediately back into the left ventricle during diastole, causing the aortic pressure to fall to a very low level between heartbeats, thereby increasing the pulse pressure.

The Pressure Pulses Are Damped in the Smaller Vessels. Pressure pulsations in the aorta are progressively diminished (damped) by (1) the resistance to blood movement in the vessels and (2) the compliance of the vessels. The resistance damps the pulsations because a small amount of blood must flow forward to distend the next segment of the vessel; the greater the resistance, the more difficult it is for this to occur. The compliance damps the pulsation because the more compliant a vessel, the greater is quantity of blood required to cause a rise in pressure. *The degree of damping of arterial pulsations is directly proportional to the product of the resistance and compliance.*

Blood Pressure Can Be Measured Indirectly by the Auscultatory Method. With this method, a stethoscope is placed over a vessel, such as the antecubital artery, and a blood pressure cuff is inflated around the upper arm proximal to the vessel. So long as the cuff inflation is not sufficient to collapse the vessel, no sounds are heard with the stethoscope despite the fact that blood in the artery is pulsing. When the cuff pressure is sufficient to close the artery during part of the arterial pressure cycle, a sound is heard with each pulsation; these sounds are called *Korotkoff sounds*.

When determining blood pressure by the auscultatory method, pressure in the cuff is first inflated well above the arterial systolic pressure. So long as the pressure is higher than the systolic pressure, the brachial artery remains collapsed and no blood jets into the lower artery during the cardiac cycle; therefore, no Korotkoff sounds are heard in the lower artery. As soon as the pressure in the cuff falls below the systolic pressure, blood slips through the artery underneath the cuff during the peak systolic pressure, and one begins to hear *tapping sounds* in the antecubital artery in synchrony with the heartbeat. As soon as these sounds are heard, the pressure level indicated by the manometer connected to the cuff is about equal to the systolic pressure.

As pressure in the cuff is further lowered, the Korotkoff sounds change in quality, having a rhythmical, harsher sound. Finally, when the pressure in the cuff falls to the level of the diastolic pressure (the artery no longer closes during diastole), the sounds suddenly change to a muffled quality and then usually disappear entirely after another 5- to 10-millimeter drop in cuff pressure. When the Korotkoff sounds change to the muffled quality, the manometer pressure is about equal to the diastolic pressure, although this slightly overestimates the diastolic pressure. Many clinicians believe that the pressure at which the Korotkoff sounds completely disappear should be used as the diastolic pressure except in situations in which the disappearance of sounds cannot reliably be determined because sounds are audible even after complete deflation of the cuff. For example, in patients with arteriovenous fistulas for hemodialysis or with aortic insufficiency, Korotkoff sounds may be heard after complete deflation of the cuff.

The mean arterial pressure can be estimated from the systolic and diastolic pressures measured by the auscultatory method as follows:

Mean Arterial Pressure

$$= \frac{2}{3} \text{ Diastolic Pressure} + \frac{1}{3} \text{ Systolic Pressure}$$

For the average young adult, the mean arterial pressure is about ($\frac{2}{3} \times 80$ mm Hg) ($\frac{1}{3} \times 120$ mm Hg), or 93.3 mm Hg.

Veins and Their Function *(p. 171)*

The veins, as discussed previously, are capable of constricting and enlarging and thereby storing either small or large quantities of blood, making this blood available when it is needed by the remainder of the circulation. Veins can also propel blood forward by means of a "venous pump," and they help regulate cardiac output.

Venous Pressure: Relationship to Right Atrial Pressure (Central Venous Pressure) and Peripheral Venous Pressure. Because blood from systemic veins flows into the right atrium, anything that affects the right atrial pressure usually affects venous pressure everywhere in the body. *Right atrial pressure is regulated by a balance between the ability of the heart to pump blood out of the right atrium and a tendency of blood to flow from the peripheral vessels back to the right atrium.*

The normal right atrial pressure is about 0 mm Hg, but it can rise to as high as 20 to 30 mm Hg under abnormal conditions, such as with serious heart failure or after massive transfusion.

Increased Venous Resistance Can Increase the Peripheral Venous Pressure. When large veins are distended, they offer little resistance to blood flow. Many of the large veins entering the thorax are compressed by the surrounding tissues, however, so they are at least partially collapsed or collapsed to an ovoid state. For these reasons, large veins usually offer significant resistance to blood flow, and the pressure in the peripheral veins is usually 4 to 7 mm Hg higher than the right atrial pressure. Partial obstruction of a large vein markedly increases the peripheral venous pressure distal to the obstruction.

Increased Right Atrial Pressure Increases Peripheral Venous Pressure. When the right atrial pressure rises above its normal state of 0 mm Hg, blood begins to back up in large veins and open them up. Pressures in the peripheral veins do not rise until the collapsed points between the peripheral veins and the large central veins have opened, which usually occurs at a right atrial pressure of about 4 to 6 mm Hg. When the right atrial pressure rises still further, as occurs during severe heart failure, it causes a corresponding rise in peripheral venous pressure.

Gravitational Pressure Affects Venous Pressure. The pressure at the surface of a body of water exposed to air is equal to the atmospheric pressure, but the pressure rises 1 mm Hg for each 13.6 mm Hg distance below the surface. This pressure results from the weight of the water and therefore is called *gravitational hydrostatic pressure.*

Gravitational hydrostatic pressure also occurs in the vascular system because of the weight of the blood in the vessels. In an adult who is standing absolutely still, pressure in the veins of the feet is approximately +90 mm Hg because of the hydrostatic weight of the blood in the veins between the heart and feet.

The Venous Valves and "Venous Pump" Influence Venous Pressure.   Were it not for the valves of the veins, the gravitational pressure effect would cause venous pressure in the feet to always be about +90 mm Hg in a standing adult. Each time one tightens the muscles and moves the legs, however, it compresses the veins either in the muscles or adjacent to them and squeezes the blood out of the veins.

The valves in the veins are arranged so the direction of blood flow can only be toward the heart. Consequently, each time a person moves the legs or tenses the muscles, a certain amount of blood is propelled toward the heart, and the pressure in the veins is lowered. This pumping system is known as the "venous pump" or "muscle pump," and it keeps the venous pressure in the feet of a walking adult near 25 mm Hg.

If a person stands perfectly still, however, the venous pump does not work, and venous pressure quickly rises to the full hydrostatic value of 90 mm Hg. If the valves of the venous system become incompetent or are destroyed, the effectiveness of the venous pump is also decreased. When valve incompetence develops, greater pressure in the veins of the legs may further increase the size of the veins and finally destroy the function of the valves entirely. When this occurs, the person develops *varicose veins,* and the venous and capillary pressures increase to high levels, causing leakage of fluid from the capillaries and edema in the legs when standing.

The Veins Function as Blood Reservoirs.   More than 60% of the blood in the circulatory system is usually contained in the veins. For this reason and because the veins are so compliant, the venous system can serve as a blood reservoir for the circulation. For example, when blood is lost from the body, activation of the sympathetic nervous system causes the veins to constrict, which takes up much of the "slack" of the circulatory system caused by the lost blood.

Certain portions of the circulatory system are so compliant they are especially important as blood reservoirs. These areas include (1) the *spleen,* which can sometimes decrease in size to release as much as 100 mL of blood into the reservoir of the circulation; (2) the *liver,* the sinuses of which can release several hundred milliliters of blood into the rest of the circulation; (3) the *large abdominal veins,* which can contribute as much as 300 mL; and (4) the *venous plexus underneath the skin,* which can contribute several hundred milliliters.

CHAPTER 16

The Microcirculation and Lymphatic System: Capillary Fluid Exchange, Interstitial Fluid, and Lymph Flow

A primary function of the circulation—to transport nutrients to the tissues and remove waste products—occurs in the capillaries. The capillaries have only a single layer of highly permeable endothelial cells, permitting rapid interchange of nutrients and cellular waste products between the tissues and circulating blood. About 10 billion capillaries, which have a total surface area of 500 to 700 square meters (about one eighth the size of a football field) provide this function for the body.

Structure of the Microcirculation *(p. 177)*

Blood Enters the Capillaries through an Arteriole and Leaves through a Venule. Blood from the arteriole passes into a series of *metarterioles*, which have structures midway between those of arterioles and capillaries. Arterioles are highly muscular and play a major role in controlling blood flow to the tissues. The metarterioles do not have a continuous smooth muscle coat, but smooth muscle fibers encircle the vessel at intermittent points called *precapillary sphincters.* Contraction of the muscle in these sphincters can open and close the entrance to the capillary.

This arrangement of the microcirculation is not found in all parts of the body, but similar arrangements serve the same purposes. Both the metarterioles and arterioles are in close contact with the tissues they serve, and local conditions, such as changes in the concentration of nutrients or waste products of metabolism, can have direct effects on these vessels in controlling the local blood flow.

The Thin Capillary Wall Consists of a Single Layer of Endothelial Cells. Capillaries are also very porous, with several million slits, or *pores,* between the cells that make up their walls to each square centimeter of capillary surface. Because of the high permeability of the capillaries for most solutes and the high surface area, as blood flows through the capillaries large amounts of dissolved substances diffuse in both directions through these pores. In this way, almost all dissolved substances in the plasma, except the plasma proteins, continually mix with the interstitial fluid.

Blood Flows Intermittently through Capillaries, a Phenomenon Called "Vasomotion." In many tissues, blood flow through capillaries is not continuous but, instead, turns on and off every few seconds. The cause of this intermittence is contraction of the *metarterioles* and *precapillary sphincters*, which are influenced mainly by *oxygen* and *waste products of tissue metabolism.* When oxygen concentrations of the tissue are reduced (e.g., because of increased oxygen utilization), the periods of blood flow occur more often and last longer, thereby allowing the blood to carry increased quantities of oxygen and other nutrients to the tissues.

Exchange of Nutrients and Other Substances between Blood and Interstitial Fluid (p. 179)

Diffusion Is the Most Important Means for Transferring Substances between Plasma and Interstitial Fluid. As blood traverses the capillary, tremendous numbers of water molecules and dissolved substances diffuse back and forth through the capillary wall, providing continual mixture of the interstitial fluid and plasma. Lipid-soluble substances, such as oxygen and carbon dioxide, can diffuse directly through the cell membranes without having to go through the pores. Water-soluble substances, such as glucose and electrolytes, diffuse only through intercellular pores in the capillary membrane. The rate of diffusion for most solutes is so great that cells as far as 50 μm away from the capillaries can receive adequate quantities of nutrients.

The primary factors that affect the rate of diffusion across the capillary walls are as follows:

1. *The pore size in the capillary.* In most capillaries, the pore size is 6 to 7 nanometers. The pores of some capillary membranes, such as the liver capillary sinusoids, are much larger and are therefore much more highly permeable to substances dissolved in plasma.

2. *The molecular size of the diffusing substance.* Water and most electrolytes, such as sodium and chloride, have a molecular size that is smaller than the pore size, allowing rapid diffusion across the capillary wall. Plasma proteins, however, have a molecular size that is slightly greater than the width of the pores, restricting their diffusion.

3. *The concentration difference of the substance between the two sides of the membrane.* The greater the difference between the concentrations of a substance on the two sides of the capillary membrane, the greater is the rate of diffusion in one direction through the membrane. The concentration of oxygen in the blood is normally higher than in the interstitial fluid, allowing large quantities of oxygen to move from the blood toward the tissues. Conversely, the concentrations of the waste products of metabolism are greater in tissues than in blood, allowing them to move into the blood and to be carried away from the tissues.

The Interstitium and Interstitial Fluid (p. 180)

About one sixth of the body consists of spaces between cells, which collectively are called the *interstitium.* The fluid in these spaces is the *interstitial fluid.* The interstitium has two major types of solid structures: (1) *collagen fiber bundles* and (2) *proteoglycan filaments.* The collagen provides most of the tensional strength of the tissues, whereas the proteoglycan filaments, composed mainly of *hyaluronic acid,* are very thin and form a filler of fine reticular filaments, often described as a "brush pile."

"Gel" in the Interstitium Consists of Proteoglycan Filaments and Entrapped Fluid. Fluid in the interstitium is derived by filtration and diffusion from the capillaries and has almost the same constituency as plasma except with lower concentrations of protein. The interstitial fluid is mainly entrapped in the minute spaces among the proteoglycan filaments and has the characteristics of a *gel.*

Because of the large number of proteoglycan filaments, fluid and solutes do not flow easily through the tissue gel. Instead, solutes mainly *diffuse* through the gel. This diffusion occurs about 95% to 99% as rapidly as it does through free fluid.

The Amount of "Free" Fluid in the Interstitium in Most Tissues Is Less Than 1%. Although almost all the fluid in the interstitium is entrapped in the tissue gel, small amounts of *"free" fluid* are also present. When the tissues develop *edema,* these small pockets of free fluid can expand tremendously.

Capillary Fluid Filtration Is Determined by Hydrostatic and Colloid Osmotic Pressures, and Capillary Filtration Coefficient *(p. 181)*

Although the exchange of nutrients, oxygen, and metabolic waste products across the capillaries occurs almost entirely by diffusion, the distribution of fluid across the capillaries is determined by another process—the *bulk flow* or *ultrafiltration* of protein-free plasma. As discussed previously, capillary walls are highly permeable to water and most plasma solutes, except plasma proteins; therefore, hydrostatic pressure differences across the capillary wall push protein-free plasma (ultrafiltrate) through the capillary wall into the interstitium. In contrast, osmotic pressure caused by the plasma proteins (called *colloid osmotic pressure*) tends to produce fluid movement by osmosis from the interstitial spaces into the blood. Interstitial fluid hydrostatic and colloid osmotic pressures also influence fluid filtration across the capillary wall.

The rate at which ultrafiltration occurs across the capillary depends on the difference in hydrostatic and colloid osmotic pressures of the capillary and interstitial fluid. These forces are often called *Starling forces* in honor of Ernest Starling, the physiologist who described their functional significance more than a century ago.

Four Forces Determine Fluid Filtration through the Capillary Membrane. The four primary forces that determine fluid movement across the capillaries are shown in Figure 16–1; the forces are as follows:

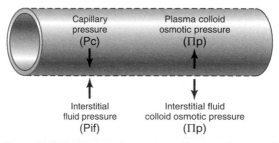

Figure 16–1. Forces operative at the capillary membrane tend to move fluid outward or inward through the membrane pores.

- The *capillary hydrostatic pressure* (Pc), which forces fluid outward through the capillary membrane
- The *interstitial fluid hydrostatic pressure* (Pif), which forces fluid inward through the capillary membrane when the Pif is positive but outward into the interstitium when the Pif is negative
- The *plasma colloid osmotic pressure* (Πp), which tends to cause osmosis of the fluid inward through the capillary membrane
- The *interstitial fluid colloid osmotic pressure* (Πif), which tends to cause osmosis of fluid outward through the capillary membrane

The net rate of filtration out of the capillary is determined by the balance of these forces as well as by the *capillary filtration coefficient* (K_f) as follows:

$$\text{Filtration} = K_f \times (Pc - Pif - \Pi p + \Pi if)$$

Functional Capillary Hydrostatic Pressure Averages about 17 mm Hg in Many Tissues. When blood is flowing through many capillaries, the pressure averages 30 to 40 mm Hg on the arterial ends and 10 to 15 mm Hg on the venous ends, or about 25 mm Hg in the middle. When the capillaries are closed, the pressure in the capillaries beyond the closure is about equal to the pressure at the venous ends of the capillaries (10 mm Hg). When averaged over a period of time, including the periods of opening and closure of the capillaries, the *functional mean capillary pressure* is closer to the pressure in the venous ends of the capillaries than to the pressure in the arteriole ends; it averages about 17 mm Hg in many tissues. In some tissues, such as the kidneys, capillary hydrostatic pressure may be as high as 60 to 65 mm Hg (see Chapter 26).

Interstitial Fluid Hydrostatic Pressure Is Subatmospheric (Negative Pressure) in Loose Subcutaneous Tissue and Positive in Tightly Encased Tissues. Measurements of interstitial fluid hydrostatic pressure have yielded an average value of about −3 mm Hg in loose subcutaneous tissue. One of the basic reasons for this negative pressure is the lymphatic pumping system (discussed later). When fluid enters the lymphatic capillaries, any movement of the tissue propels the fluid forward through the lymphatic system and eventually back into the circulation. In this way, free fluid that accumulates in the tissue is pumped away as a consequence of tissue movement. This pumping action of lymphatic capillaries appears to account for the slight intermittent negative pressure that occurs in the tissues at rest.

In Tissues Surrounded by Tight Encasements, Such as the Brain, Kidneys, and Skeletal Muscle (Surrounded by Fibrous Sheaths), Interstitial Fluid Hydrostatic Pressures Are Usually Positive. For instance, the brain interstitial fluid hydrostatic pressure averages about $+4$ to $+16$ mm Hg. In the kidneys, interstitial fluid hydrostatic pressure averages about $+6$ mm Hg.

Plasma Colloid Osmotic Pressure Averages about 28 mm Hg. The proteins are the only dissolved substances in the plasma that do not readily pass through the capillary membrane. These substances exert an osmotic pressure referred to as the *colloid osmotic pressure.* The normal concentration of plasma protein averages about 7.3 g/dL. About 19 mm Hg of the colloid osmotic pressure is due to the dissolved protein, but an additional 9 mm Hg is due to the positively charged cations, mainly sodium ions, that bind to the negatively charged plasma proteins. This is called the *Donnan equilibrium effect,* which causes the colloid osmotic pressure in the plasma to be about 50% greater than that produced by the proteins alone.

The plasma proteins are mainly a mixture of albumin, globulin, and fibrinogen. About 80% of the total colloid osmotic pressure of the plasma results from the albumin fraction, 20% from the globulin, and only a tiny amount from the fibrinogen.

Interstitial Fluid Colloid Osmotic Pressure Averages about 8 mm Hg. Although the size of the usual capillary pore is smaller than the molecular size of the plasma protein, this is not true of all pores; therefore, small amounts of plasma protein leak through the pores into the interstitial spaces. The average protein concentration of the interstitial fluid is around 40% of that in the plasma, or about 3 g/dL, giving a colloid osmotic pressure of about 8 mm Hg. In some tissues, such as the liver, the interstitial fluid colloid osmotic pressure is much greater because the capillaries are much more permeable to plasma proteins.

Summary of Fluid Volume Exchange through the Capillary Membrane. The average capillary pressure at the arteriolar ends of the capillaries is 15 to 25 mm Hg greater than at the venular ends. Because of this difference, fluid filters out of the capillaries at the arteriolar ends, and fluid is reabsorbed back into the capillaries at their venular ends. A small amount of fluid flows through the tissues from the arteriolar ends of the capillaries to the venular ends.

Under normal conditions, however, a state of near-equilibrium exists between the amount of fluid filtering outward at the arteriolar ends of the capillaries and the amount of fluid returned to the circulation by absorption at the venular ends of the capillaries. There is a slight disequilibrium that occurs, and a small amount of fluid is filtered in excess of that reabsorbed. This fluid is eventually returned to the circulation by way of the lymphatics. Table 16–1 shows the *average* forces that exist across the entire capillaries and illustrates the principles of this equilibrium. The pressures in the arterial and venous capillaries in Table 16–1 are averaged to calculate the mean functional capillary pressure, which is about 17.3 mm Hg.

The small imbalance of forces, 0.3 mm Hg, causes slightly more filtration than reabsorption of fluid into the interstitial spaces.

The Rate of Filtration in the Capillaries Is Also Determined by the *Capillary Filtration Coefficient* (K_f). The filtration coefficient in an average tissue is about 0.01 mL of fluid per minute per millimeter of mercury per 100 g of tissue. For the entire body, the capillary filtration coefficient is about 6.67 mL of fluid per minute

Table 16–1. Equilibrium of Forces across Capillaries

Forces	mm Hg
Mean forces tending to move fluid outward	
Mean capillary hydrostatic pressure	17.3
Negative interstitial free fluid pressure	3.0
Interstitial fluid colloid osmotic pressure	8.0
Total outward force	28.3
Mean force tending to move fluid inward	
Plasma colloid osmotic pressure	28.0
Total inward force	28.0
Summation of mean forces	
Outward	28.3
Inward	−28.0
Net outward force	0.3

per millimeter of mercury. Thus the net rate of capillary filtration for the entire body is expressed as follows:

$$\text{Net Filtration} = K_f \times \text{Net Filtration Pressure}$$
$$= 6.67 \times 0.3$$
$$= 2\,mL/min$$

Because of the extreme differences in the permeabilities and surface areas of the capillary systems in different tissues, the capillary filtration coefficient may vary more than 100-fold among tissues. For example, the capillary filtration coefficient in the kidneys is about 4.2 mL/min per millimeter of mercury per 100 g of kidney weight, a value almost 400 times as great as the K_f of many other tissues. This obviously causes a much greater rate of filtration in the glomerular capillaries of the kidney.

An Abnormal Imbalance of Pressures in the Capillary Can Cause Edema. *If the mean capillary hydrostatic pressure rises* above the normal 17 mm Hg, the net pressure causing filtration of fluid into the tissue spaces also rises. A rise in mean capillary pressure of 20 mm Hg causes an increase in the net filtration pressure from 0.3 mm Hg to 20.3 mm Hg, which results in 68 times as much net filtration of fluid into the interstitial spaces as normally occurs. Prevention of accumulation of excess fluid in the spaces would require 68 times the normal flow of fluid into the lymphatic system, an amount that is too great for the lymphatics to carry away. As a result, large increases in capillary pressure can cause accumulation of fluid in the interstitial spaces, a condition referred to as *edema.*

Similarly, a *decrease in plasma colloid osmotic pressure* increases the net filtration force and therefore the net filtration rate of fluid into the tissues.

The Lymphatic System *(p. 186)*

The lymphatic system carries fluid from tissue spaces into the blood. Importantly, the lymphatics also carry away proteins and large particulate matter from the tissue spaces, neither of which can be removed through absorption directly into the blood capillary.

Almost all tissues of the body have lymphatic channels. Most of the lymph from the lower part of the body flows up the *thoracic duct* and empties into the venous system at the juncture of the left interior jugular vein and subclavian vein. Lymph from the left side of the head, left arm, and parts of the chest region also enters the thoracic duct before it empties into the veins. Lymph from the right side of the neck and head, right arm, and parts of the thorax enter the *right lymph duct,* which then empties into the venous system at the juncture of the right subclavian vein and internal jugular vein.

Lymph Is Derived from Interstitial Fluid. As lymph first flows from the tissue, it has almost the same composition as the interstitial fluid. In many tissues, the protein concentration averages about 2 g/dL, but in other tissues such as the liver the protein concentration may be as high as 6 g/dL.

In addition to carrying fluid and protein from the interstitial spaces to the circulation, the lymphatic system is one of the major routes for absorption of nutrients from the gastrointestinal tract, as discussed in Chapter 65. After a fatty meal, for instance, thoracic duct lymph sometimes contains as much as 1% to 2% fat.

The Rate of Lymph Flow Is Determined by Interstitial Fluid Hydrostatic Pressure and the Lymphatic Pump. The total rate of lymph flow is approximately 120 mL/hr, or 2 to 3 L per day. This rate of formation can change dramatically, however, in certain pathological conditions associated with excessive fluid filtration from the capillaries into the interstitium.

- *Increased interstitial fluid hydrostatic pressure increases the lymph flow rate.* At normal interstitial fluid hydrostatic pressures in the subatmospheric range, lymph flow is very low. As the pressure rises to values slightly higher than 0 mm Hg, the lymph flow increases by more than 20-fold. When interstitial pressure reaches +1 to +2 mm Hg, lymph flow fails to rise further. This results from the fact that rising tissue pressure not only increases the entry of fluid into the lymphatic capillaries but also compresses the larger lymphatics, thereby impeding lymph flow.

- *The lymphatic pump increases lymph flow.* Valves exist in all lymph channels. In addition, each segment of the lymphatic vessel functions as a separate automatic pump; that is, filling of a segment causes it to contract, and the fluid is pumped through the valve into the next lymphatic segment. This fills the lymphatic segment, and within a few seconds it too contracts, with the process continuing along the lymph vessel until the fluid is finally emptied. This pumping action propels the lymph forward toward the circulation. In addition to pumping caused by intrinsic contraction of the vessels, external factors also compress lymph vessels. For example, contraction of muscles surrounding lymph vessels or movement of body parts may increase lymphatic pumping. Under some conditions, such as during exercise, the lymphatic pump may increase lymph flow by as much as 10- to 30-fold.

The Lymphatic System Is Important as an "Overflow Mechanism" That Returns to the Circulation Excess Proteins and Fluid Volume That Enter the Tissue Spaces. When the lymphatic system fails, as occurs with blockade of a major lymphatic vessel, proteins and fluid accumulate in the interstitium, causing edema. The accumulation of protein in the interstitium is especially important in causing edema because the lymphatics provide the only mechanism for proteins that leak out of the capillaries to re-enter the circulation in significant quantities. When protein accumulates in the interstitial spaces owing to lymphatic failure, there is an increase in colloid osmotic pressure of the interstitial fluid that tends to allow more fluid filtration into the interstitium. As a result, complete blockade of the lymphatic vessels results in severe edema.

Bacteria and Debris from the Tissues Are Removed by the Lymphatic System at Lymph Nodes. Because of the very high permeability of the lymphatic capillaries, bacteria and other small particulate matter in the tissues can pass into the lymph. The lymph passes through a series of nodes on its way out to the blood. It is in these nodes that bacteria and other debris are filtered out, phagocytized by macrophages in the nodes, and finally digested and converted to amino acids, glucose, fatty acids, and other low-molecular-weight substances before being released into the blood.

CHAPTER 17

Local and Humoral Control of Tissue Blood Flow

Local Tissues Autoregulate Blood Flow in Response to Their Individual Needs. In most tissues, blood flow is autoregulated, which means that the tissue regulates its own blood flow. This is beneficial to the tissue because it allows the delivery of oxygen and nutrients and removal of waste products to parallel the rate of tissue activity. Autoregulation permits blood flow from one tissue to be regulated independently of flow to another tissue.

In certain organs, blood flow serves purposes other than supplying nutrients and removing waste products. For instance, blood flow to the skin influences heat loss from the body and in this way helps control body temperature. Delivery of adequate quantities of blood to the kidneys allows them to excrete rapidly the waste products of the body.

The ability of the tissues to regulate their own flow permits them to maintain adequate nutrition and perform necessary functions to maintain homeostasis. In general, the greater the rate of metabolism in an organ, the greater its blood flow. Table 17–1, for example, shows that there is high blood flow in glandular organs such as the thyroid and adrenal glands, which have a high metabolic rate. In contrast, blood flow in resting skeletal muscles is low because metabolic activity of the muscle is also low in the resting state; however, during heavy exercise skeletal muscle metabolic activity can increase by more than 60-fold and the blood flow can increase by as much as 20-fold.

Mechanisms of Local Blood Flow Control (p. 191)

Local tissue blood flow control can be divided into two phases: (1) *acute control* and (2) *long-term control.* Acute control occurs within seconds to minutes via constriction or dilation of arterioles, metarterioles, and precapillary sphincters. Long-term control occurs over a period of days, weeks, or even months and, in general, provides even better control of flow in proportion to the needs of the tissues. Long-term control occurs mainly as a result of increases or decreases in the physical size and number of blood vessels supplying the tissues.

Table 17–1.   Blood Flow to Various Organs and Tissues under Basal Conditions

Organ	Cardiac Output (%)	Flow (mL/min)	mL/min/ 100 g of Tissue
Brain	14	700	50
Heart	4	200	70
Bronchi	2	100	25
Kidneys	22	1100	360
Liver	27	1350	95
Portal	(21)	(1050)	
Arterial	(6)	(300)	
Muscle (inactive state)	15	750	4
Bone	5	250	3
Skin (cool weather)	6	300	3
Thyroid gland	1	50	160
Adrenal glands	0.5	25	300
Other tissues	3.5	175	1.3
Total	100.0	5000	

Acute Control of Local Blood Flow (p. 192)

Increased Tissue Metabolic Rate Usually Increases Local Blood Flow. In many tissues, such as skeletal muscle, increases in metabolism up to eight times normal acutely increase the blood flow about fourfold. Initially, the rise in flow is less than that of the metabolism, but once the metabolism increases sufficiently to remove most of the nutrients from the blood a further rise in metabolism can occur only with a concomitant increase in blood flow to supply the required nutrients.

Decreased Oxygen Availability Increases Tissue Blood Flow. One of the required nutrients for tissue metabolism is oxygen. Whenever the availability of oxygen in the tissues decreases, such as at high altitude, in the presence of pneumonia, or with carbon monoxide poisoning (which inhibits the ability of hemoglobin to transport oxygen), the tissue blood flow increases markedly. Cyanide poisoning, for instance, which reduces the ability of the tissues to utilize oxygen, can increase tissue blood flow by as much as sevenfold.

Increased Demand for Oxygen and Nutrients Increases Tissue Blood Flow. In the absence of an adequate supply of oxygen and nutrients as a result of either increased tissue metabolism, the arterioles, metarterioles, and precapillary sphincters relax, thereby decreasing vascular resistance and allowing more flow to the tissues. The relaxation of precapillary sphincters allows flow to occur more often in capillaries that are closed because of periodic contraction of precapillary sphincters *(vasomotion)*.

Accumulation of Vasodilator Metabolites Increases Tissue Blood Flow. The greater the rate of metabolism in the tissue, the greater is the rate of production of tissue metabolites, such as *adenosine, adenosine phosphate compounds, carbon dioxide, lactic acid, potassium ions,* and *hydrogen ions.* Each of these substances has been suggested to act as a *vasodilator* that contributes to increased blood flow associated with stimulation of tissue metabolism.

Lack of Other Nutrients May Cause Vasodilation. For example, a deficiency of glucose, amino acids, or fatty acids may contribute to local vasodilation, although this has not been proven. Vasodilation occurs with *beriberi,* in which the patient usually has a deficiency of the vitamin B substances thiamine, niacin, and riboflavin. Because these vitamins are all involved in the oxidative phosphorylation mechanism for generating adenosine triphosphate (ATP), a deficiency of these vitamins may lead to diminished ability of the smooth muscle to contract, thereby causing local vasodilation.

Special Examples of Local Blood Flow Control *(p.194)*

"Reactive Hyperemia" Occurs after the Blood Supply to a Tissue Is Blocked for a Short Time. If blood flow is blocked for a few seconds to several hours and then unblocked, flow to the tissue usually increases to four to seven times normal; the increased flow continues for a few seconds or much longer if the flow has been stopped for 1 hour or longer. This phenomenon is called *reactive hyperemia* and appears to be a manifestation of local "metabolic" blood flow regulation mechanisms. After vascular occlusion, there is an accumulation of tissue vasodilator metabolites and the development of oxygen deficiency in the tissues. The extra blood flow during reactive hyperemia lasts long enough to almost exactly repay the tissue oxygen deficiency and to wash out the accumulated vasodilator metabolites.

"Active Hyperemia" Occurs When the Tissue Metabolic Rate Increases. When a tissue becomes highly active, such as muscle during exercise or even the brain during increased mental activity, blood flow to the tissue increases. Again, this appears to be related to increases in local tissue metabolism that cause accumulation of vasodilator substances and possibly a slight oxygen deficit. The dilation of local blood vessels helps the tissue receive the additional nutrients required to sustain its new level of function.

Tissue Blood Flow Is "Autoregulated" during Changes in Arterial Pressure. In any tissue of the body, acute increases in arterial pressure cause an immediate increase in blood flow. Within less than 1 minute, however, the blood flow in many tissues returns toward the normal level even though the arterial pressure remains elevated. This is called "autoregulation of blood flow."

- *The metabolic theory of autoregulation* suggests that when arterial pressure rises and blood flow becomes too great, the excess provides too much oxygen and too many nutrients to the tissues, causing the blood vessels to constrict and the flow to return toward normal despite the increased arterial pressure.

- *The myogenic theory of autoregulation* suggests that sudden stretch of small blood vessels causes the smooth muscles in the vessel walls to contract automatically. This is an intrinsic property of smooth muscles that allows them to resist excessive stretching. Conversely, at low pressures the degree of stretch of the vessel is less, and the smooth muscle relaxes, decreasing vascular resistance and allowing flow to be maintained relatively constant despite the lower blood pressure.

The relative importance of these two mechanisms for autoregulation of blood flow is still debated by physiologists. It seems likely that both mechanisms contribute to maintaining a relatively stable blood flow during variations in arterial pressure.

Additional Mechanisms for Blood Flow Control in Specific Tissues. Although the general mechanisms for local blood flow control discussed thus far are present in most tissues of the body, there are special mechanisms that control blood flow in special areas. These mechanisms are discussed in relation to specific organs, but the following two are notable:

- *In the kidneys, blood flow control is vested, in part, in a mechanism called tubuloglomerular feedback,* in which the composition of fluid in the early distal tubule is detected by the *macula densa,* which is located where the tubule abuts the afferent and efferent arterioles at the *juxtaglomerular apparatus.* When too much fluid filters from the blood through the glomerulus into the tubular system, feedback signals from the macula densa cause constriction of the *afferent arterioles,* thereby reducing renal blood flow and returning the glomerular filtration rate toward normal (see Chapter 26 for further discussion).

- *In the brain, the concentrations of carbon dioxide and hydrogen play prominent roles in local blood flow control.* An increase in either dilates the cerebral blood vessels, which allows rapid washout of the excess carbon dioxide and hydrogen ions.

- *In the skin, blood flow control is closely linked to body temperature* and is controlled largely by the central nervous system through the sympathetic nerves as discussed in Chapter 73. When humans are exposed to body heating, skin blood flow may increase manyfold, to as high as *7 to 8 L/min* for the entire body. When body temperature is reduced, skin blood flow decreases, falling to barely above zero at very low temperatures. Control of Blood Flow by Endothelium-Derived Relaxing or Constricting Factors.

The local mechanisms for controlling tissue blood flow act mainly on the very small microvessels of the tissues because local feedback by vasodilator substances or oxygen deficiency can reach only these vessels, not the larger arteries upstream. When blood flow through the microvascular portion of the circulation increases, however, the endothelial cells lining the larger vessels release a vasodilator substance called *endothelium-derived relaxing factor,* which appears to be mainly *nitric oxide.* This release of nitric oxide is caused, in part, by increased *shear stress* on the endothelial walls, which occurs as blood flows more rapidly through the larger vessels. The release of nitric oxide then relaxes the larger vessels, causing them to dilate. Without the dilation of larger vessels, the effectiveness of local blood flow would be compromised because a significant part of the resistance in blood flow is in the upstream arterioles and small arteries.

Endothelial Cells Also Release Vasoconstrictor Substances. The most important of these is *endothelin,* a peptide that is released by when blood vessels are injured. The usual stimulus for release is damage to the endothelium, such as that caused by crushing the tissues or injecting a traumatizing chemical into the blood vessel. After severe blood vessel damage, release of local endothelin and subsequent vasoconstriction helps to prevent extensive bleeding from arteries.

Long-Term Blood Flow Regulation *(p. 196)*

Most of the mechanisms that have been discussed thus far act within a few seconds to a few minutes after the local tissue conditions have changed. Even with full function of these acute mechanisms, blood flow usually is adjusted only about three fourths of the way back to the exact requirements of the tissues. Over a period of hours, days, and weeks, long-term local blood flow regulation develops that helps adjust the blood flow so it matches precisely the metabolic needs of the tissues.

Changes in Tissue Vascularity Contribute to Long-Term Regulation of Blood Flow. If metabolism of a tissue is increased for prolonged periods of time, the physical size of the vessels in a tissue increases; under some conditions, the number of blood vessels also increases. One of the major factors that stimulate this increased vascularity is *low oxygen concentration* in the tissues. Animals that live at high altitudes, for instance, have increased vascularity. Likewise, fetal chicks hatched at low oxygen levels have up to twice as much vascular conductivity as in normal fetal chicks. This growth of new vessels is called *angiogenesis.*

Angiogenesis occurs mainly in response to the presence of angiogenic factors released from (1) ischemic tissues, (2) tissues that are growing rapidly, and (3) tissues that have excessively high metabolic rates.

Many Angiogenic Factors Are Small Peptides. Three of the best characterized angiogenic factors are *vascular endothelial growth factor (VEGF), fibroblast growth factor (FGF),* and *angiogenin,* each of which has been isolated from tumors or other tissues that are rapidly growing or have inadequate blood supply.

Essentially all angiogenic factors promote new vessel growth by causing the vessels to sprout from small venules or, occasionally, capillaries. The basement membrane of the endothelial cells is dissolved, followed by the rapid production of new endothelial cells that stream out of the vessel in extended cords directed toward the source of the angiogenic factor. The cells continue to divide and eventually fold over into a tube. The tube then connects with another tube budding from another donor vessel and forms a capillary loop through which blood begins to flow. If the flow is sufficient, smooth muscle cells eventually invade the wall so that some of these vessels grow to be small arterioles and/or perhaps even larger vessels.

Collateral Blood Vessels Develop When an Artery or a Vein Is Blocked. New vascular channels usually develop around a blocked artery or vein and allow the affected tissue to be at least partially resupplied with blood. An important example is the development of collateral blood vessels after thrombosis of one of the coronary arteries. In many people over age 60, there is blockage of at least one of the smaller coronary vessels; yet most people do not know that it has happened because collateral blood vessels have gradually developed as the vessels have begun to close, thereby providing blood flow to the tissue sufficient to prevent myocardial damage. It is in instances in which thrombosis occurs too rapidly for the development of collaterals that serious heart attacks occur.

Humoral Control of the Circulation *(p. 199)*

Several hormones are secreted into the circulation and transported in the blood throughout the entire body. Some of these hormones have important effects on circulatory function.

- *Norepinephrine* and *epinephrine,* released by the adrenal medulla, act as vasoconstrictors in many tissues by stimulating α-adrenergic receptors; however, epinephrine is much less potent as a vasoconstrictor and may even cause mild vasodilation through stimulation of β-adrenergic receptors in some tissues, such as skeletal muscle.
- *Angiotensin II* is a powerful vasoconstrictor that is usually formed in response to volume depletion or decreased blood pressure.
- *Vasopressin,* also called *antidiuretic hormone,* is one of the most powerful vasoconstrictors in the body. It is formed in the hypothalamus and transported to

the posterior pituitary, where it is released in response to decreased blood volume, as occurs with hemorrhage, or increased plasma osmolarity, as occurs with dehydration.

- *Prostaglandins* are formed in almost every tissue in the body. These substances have important intracellular effects, but some of them are released in the circulation, especially *prostacyclin* and *prostaglandins of the E series,* which are *vasodilators.* Some prostaglandins, such as *thromboxane A_2* and *prostaglandins of the F series,* are *vasoconstrictors.*

- *Bradykinin,* formed in the blood and in tissue fluids, is a powerful vasodilator that also increases capillary permeability. For this reason, increased levels of bradykinin may cause marked edema as well as increased blood flow in some tissues.

- *Histamine,* a powerful vasodilator, is released into the tissues when they become damaged or inflamed. Most of the histamine is released from *mast cells* in damaged tissues or from *basophils* in the blood. Histamine, like bradykinin, increases capillary permeability and causes tissue edema as well as greater blood flow.

Ions and Other Chemical Factors Can Also Alter Local Blood Flow. Many ions and chemical factors can either dilate or constrict local blood vessels. Their specific effects are as follows:

- *Increased calcium ion concentration* causes vasoconstriction.
- *Increased potassium ion concentration* causes vasodilation.
- *Increased magnesium ion concentration* causes vasodilation.
- *Increased sodium ion concentration* causes vasodilation.
- *Increased osmolarity of the blood,* caused by increased quantities of glucose or other nonvasoactive substances, causes vasodilation.
- *Increased hydrogen ion concentration* (decreased pH) causes vasodilation.
- *Increased carbon dioxide concentration* causes vasodilation in most tissues and marked vasodilation in the brain.

CHAPTER 18

Nervous Regulation of the Circulation, and Rapid Control of Arterial Pressure

Except for certain tissues, such as skin, blood flow regulation is mainly a function of local control mechanisms. Nervous control mainly affects more global functions, such as redistributing blood flow to various parts of the body, increasing the pumping activity of the heart, and providing rapid control of arterial pressure. This control of the circulation by the nervous system is exerted almost entirely through the *autonomic nervous system.*

Autonomic Nervous System (p. 201)

The two components of the autonomic nervous system are the *sympathetic nervous system,* which is most important for controlling the circulation, and the *parasympathetic nervous system,* which contributes to the regulation of heart function.

Sympathetic Stimulation Causes Vasoconstriction, and Increases Heart Rate and Cardiac Contractility. Sympathetic vasomotor fibers exit the spinal cord through all of the thoracic and the first one or two lumbar spinal nerves. They pass into the sympathetic chain and then go via two routes to the circulation: (1) through specific *sympathetic nerves* that innervate mainly the vasculature of the internal viscera and heart and (2) through *spinal nerves* that innervate mainly the vasculature of the peripheral areas. Almost all of the blood vessels, except the capillaries, are innervated by sympathetic nerve fibers. Sympathetic stimulation of the small arteries and arterioles increases the vascular resistance and decreases the rate of blood flow through the tissues. Innervation of large vessels, especially the veins, makes it possible for sympathetic stimulation to decrease the volume of the vessels.

Sympathetic fibers also go to the heart and stimulate its activity, increasing both the rate and strength of pumping.

Parasympathetic Stimulation Decreases Heart Rate and Cardiac Contractility. Although the parasympathetic system plays an important role in controlling many other autonomic functions of the body, its main role in controlling the circulation is to decrease the heart rate markedly and slightly decrease heart muscle contractility.

Control of the Sympathetic Vasoconstrictor System by the Central Nervous System *(p. 201)*

The sympathetic nerves carry large numbers of vaso-constrictor nerve fibers and only a few vasodilator fibers. The vasoconstrictor fibers are distributed to almost all segments of the circulation. Their distribution is greater in some tissues, such as skin, gut, and spleen.

Vasomotor Centers of the Brain Control the Sympathetic Vasoconstrictor System. Located bilaterally in the reticular substance of the medulla and lower third of the pons is an area called the *vasomotor* center, which transmits parasympathetic impulses through the vagus nerves to the heart and sympathetic impulses through the cord and peripheral sympathetic nerves to almost all blood vessels of the body (Figure 18–1).

Although the organization of the vasomotor centers is not completely understood, certain areas appear to be especially important.

- *A vasoconstrictor area* is located bilaterally in the anterolateral portions of the upper medulla. The neurons originating in this area secrete *norepinephrine,* and their fibers are distributed throughout the cord, where they excite vasoconstrictor neurons of the sympathetic nervous system.

- *A vasodilator area* is located bilaterally in the anterolateral portions of the lower half of the medulla. The fibers from these neurons inhibit vasoconstrictor activity of the C-1 area, causing vasodilation.

- *A sensory area* is located bilaterally in the *tractus solitarius* in the posterolateral portions of the medulla and lower pons. The neurons of this area receive sensory nerve signals mainly through the vagus and glossopharyngeal nerves, and the output signals from this sensory area help control the activities of both the vasoconstrictor and vasodilator areas, providing "reflex" control of many circulatory functions. An example is the baroreceptor reflex for controlling arterial pressure (discussed later).

Continuous Sympathetic Vasoconstrictor Tone Causes Partial Constriction of Most Blood Vessels. Normally, the vasoconstrictor area of the vasomotor center transmits signals continuously to the sympathetic vasoconstrictor nerve fibers over the entire body, causing slow firing of these fibers at a rate of about one impulse per second. This *sympathetic vasoconstrictor*

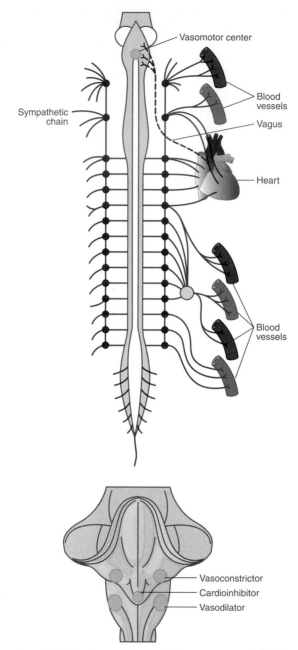

Figure 18–1. Anatomy of *sympathetic nervous* control of the circulation. Also shown by the dashed red line, a vagus nerve that carries *parasympathetic* signals to the heart.

tone maintains a partial state of contraction of the blood vessels. When this tone is blocked (e.g., by spinal anesthesia), the blood vessels throughout the body dilate, and arterial pressure may fall to as low as 50 mm Hg.

The Vasomotor System Is Influenced by Higher Nervous Centers. Large numbers of areas throughout the *reticular substance* of the *pons, mesencephalon,* and *diencephalon* can either excite or inhibit the vasomotor center.

The *hypothalamus* plays a special role in controlling the vasoconstrictor system and can exert powerful excitatory or inhibitory effects on the vasomotor center.

Many parts of the *cerebral cortex* can also excite or inhibit the vasomotor center; for example, stimulation of the *motor cortex* excites the vasomotor center. Many areas of the brain can have profound effects on cardiovascular function.

Norepinephrine Is the Neurotransmitter of the Sympathetic Vasoconstriction System. Norepinephrine, which is secreted at the endings of the vasoconstrictor nerves, acts directly on α-adrenergic receptors of vascular smooth muscle to cause vasoconstriction.

The Adrenal Medulla Releases Norepinephrine and Epinephrine During Sympathetic Stimulation. Sympathetic impulses are usually transmitted to the adrenal medullae at the same time they are transmitted to the blood vessels, stimulating release of epinephrine and norepinephrine into the circulating blood. These two hormones are carried in the bloodstream to all parts of the body, where they act directly on the blood vessels to cause vasoconstriction through stimulation of α-adrenergic receptors. Epinephrine, however, also has potent β-adrenergic effects, which cause vasodilation in certain tissues, such as skeletal muscle.

Role of the Nervous System in Rapid Control of Arterial Pressure *(p. 204)*

One of the most important functions of the sympathetic nervous system is to provide rapid control of arterial pressure by causing vasoconstriction and stimulation of the heart. At the same time that sympathetic activity is increased, there often is reciprocal inhibition of parasympathetic vagal signals to the heart that also contribute to a greater heart rate. As a consequence, there are three major changes that take place to increase arterial pressure through stimulation of the autonomic nervous system.

- *Most arterioles throughout the body are constricted,* causing increased total peripheral resistance and raising the blood pressure.
- *The veins and larger vessels of the circulation are constricted,* displacing blood from the peripheral vessels toward the heart and causing the heart to pump with greater force, which also helps raise the arterial pressure.
- *The heart is directly stimulated by the autonomic nervous system, further enhancing cardiac pumping.* Much of this is caused by an increased heart rate, sometimes to as much as three times normal. In addition, sympathetic stimulation directly increases the contractile force of the heart muscle, thus increasing its ability to pump larger volumes of blood.

An important characteristic of nervous control is that it is rapid, beginning within seconds. Conversely, sudden inhibition of nervous stimulation can decrease the arterial pressure within seconds.

The Autonomic Nervous System Contributes to Increased Arterial Pressure During Muscle Exercise. During heavy exercise, the muscles require greatly increased blood flow. Part of this increase results from local vasodilation, but additional increase in flow results from simultaneous elevation of arterial pressure during exercise. During heavy exercise arterial pressure may rise as much as 30% to 40%.

The rise in arterial pressure during exercise is believed to result mainly from the following effect: At the same time the motor areas of the nervous system become activated to cause exercise, most of the reticular activating system in the brain is also activated, which greatly increases stimulation of the vasoconstrictor and cardioaccelerator areas of the vasomotor center. These effects increase the arterial pressure instantly to keep pace with increased muscle activity. Vasodilation of the muscle, however, is maintained despite increased sympathetic activity because of the overriding effect of local control mechanisms in the muscle.

The Autonomic Nervous System Increases Arterial Pressure During the "Alarm Reaction." For instance, during extreme fright, the arterial pressure often rises to as high as 200 mm Hg within a few seconds. This *alarm reaction* provides the necessary increase in arterial pressure that can immediately supply blood to any of the muscles of the body that might need to respond instantly to flee from the perceived danger.

Reflex Mechanisms Help Maintain Normal Arterial Pressure *(p. 205)*

Aside from special circumstances such as stress and exercise, the autonomic nervous system operates to maintain the arterial pressure at or near its normal level through *negative feedback reflex mechanisms.*

The Arterial Baroreceptor Reflex Control System. This reflex is initiated by stretch receptors, called *baroreceptors,* that are located in the walls of large systemic arteries, particularly in the walls of the *carotid sinus* and the *aortic arch.* Signals from the carotid sinus receptors are transmitted through *Herring's nerve* to the *glossopharyngeal nerve* and then to the *tractus solitarius* in the medullary area of the brain stem. Signals from the aortic arch are transmitted through the *vagus nerves* to the same area of the medulla. The baroreceptors control arterial pressure as follows:

- Increased pressure in blood vessels containing baroreceptors causes increased impulse firing.
- Baroreceptor signals enter the tractus solitarius, inhibit the vasoconstrictor center of the medulla, and excite the vagal center.
- The net effects are inhibition of sympathetic activity and stimulation of parasympathetic activity, which cause (1) *vasodilation of veins and arterioles* and (2) *decreased heart rate* and *strength of heart contraction.*
- This causes the arterial pressure to decrease because of a decline in peripheral vascular resistance and cardiac output.

The Baroreceptors Function as a "Buffer" to Maintain Arterial Pressure Relatively Constant During Changes in Body Posture and Other Daily Activities. When a person stands up after lying down, the arterial pressure in the head and upper parts of the body tends to fall. The reduction in pressure decreases the signals sent from the baroreceptors to the vasomotor centers, eliciting a strong sympathetic discharge that minimizes the reduction in arterial pressure. In the absence of functional baroreceptors, marked reductions in arterial pressure can decrease cerebral blood flow so low that consciousness is lost.

Daily activities that tend to increase blood pressure, such as eating, excitement, defecation, and so forth, can cause extreme increases in blood pressure in the absence of normal baroreceptor reflexes. A primary purpose of the arterial baroreceptor system is to reduce the daily variation in arterial pressure to about one half to one third of the pressure that would occur if the baroreceptor system were not present.

Are the Baroreceptors Important in Long-Term Regulation of Arterial Pressure? The arterial baroreceptors provide powerful moment-to-moment control of arterial pressure, but their importance in long-term blood pressure regulation is still uncertain because they tend to *reset* within 1 to 2 days to the blood pressure to which they are exposed. If, for example, the arterial pressure rises from the normal value of 100 mm Hg to a high 160 mm Hg, very high rates of baroreceptor impulses are at first transmitted. However, the rate of baroreceptor firing returns to nearly normal over a period of 1 to 2 days, even when the mean arterial pressure remains at 160 mm Hg.

This "resetting" of the baroreceptors may attenuate their potency for correcting disturbances that tend to change arterial pressure for longer than a few days. Experimental studies, however, have suggested that the baroreceptors do not completely reset and may therefore contribute to long-term blood pressure regulation, especially by influencing sympathetic nerve activity of the kidneys (see Chapters 19 and 29).

Control of Arterial Pressure by the Carotid and Aortic Chemoreceptors—Effect of Oxygen Lack on Arterial Pressure

Closely associated with the baroreceptor control system is a chemoreceptor reflex that operates in much the same way as the baroreceptor reflex, except that *chemoreceptors*, instead of stretch receptors, initiate the response.

Chemoreceptors Are Sensitive to Oxygen Lack, Carbon Dioxide Excess, or Hydrogen Ion Excess. Chemoreceptors are located in two *carotid bodies*, one of which lies in the bifurcation of each common carotid artery, and in several *aortic bodies* adjacent to the aorta. Whenever the arterial pressure falls below a critical level, the chemoreceptors become stimulated because of diminished blood flow to the bodies and the resulting diminished availability of oxygen and excess buildup of carbon dioxide and hydrogen ions that are not removed by the slow blood flow. Signals transmitted from the chemoreceptors into the vasomotor center *excite* the vasomotor center, which in turn elevates the arterial pressure.

Cardiopulmonary Reflexes Help Regulate Arterial Pressure. Both atria and pulmonary arteries have in their walls stretch receptors called *cardiopulmonary receptors* or *low-pressure receptors* that are similar to the baroreceptor stretch receptors of the systemic arteries. These low-pressure receptors play an important role in minimizing arterial pressure changes in response to blood volume changes. Although the low-pressure receptors do not directly detect systemic arterial pressure, they detect increases in pressure in the heart and pulmonary circulation caused by changes in volume, and they elicit reflexes that parallel the baroreceptor reflexes to make the total reflex system more potent for controlling arterial pressure.

Increased stretch of the atria causes reflex decreases in sympathetic activity to the kidney, which causes vasodilation of the afferent arterioles and increases in the glomerular filtration rate as well as decreases in tubular reabsorption of sodium. These changes cause the kidney to excrete more sodium and water, thereby ridding the body of excess volume.

The Central Nervous System Ischemic Response Raises Arterial Pressure in Response to Diminished Blood Flow in the Brain's Vasomotor Center *(p. 209)*

When blood flow to the vasomotor center in the lower brain stem becomes sufficiently decreased to cause *cerebral ischemia* (i.e., nutritional deficiency), the neurons of the vasomotor center become strongly excited. When this occurs, the systemic arterial pressure often rises to a level as high as the heart can pump. This may be due to the effect of low blood flow, which causes buildup of carbon dioxide in the vasomotor centers. Increased carbon dioxide concentration is a potent agent for stimulating the sympathetic nervous control areas of the medulla of the brain. Other factors, such as build up of lactic acid, may also contribute to marked stimulation of the vasomotor center and increased arterial pressure.

This arterial pressure elevation in response to cerebral ischemia is known as the *central nervous system ischemic response.* This response is an emergency control system that acts rapidly and powerfully to prevent further decline in arterial pressure when blood flow to the brain becomes dangerously decreased; it is sometimes called the "last ditch" mechanism for blood pressure control.

The Cushing Reaction Is a Central Nervous System Ischemic Response That Results from Increased Pressure in the Cranial Vault. When cerebrospinal fluid pressure rises to equal the arterial pressure, a central nervous system ischemic response is initiated that can raise the arterial pressure to as high as 250 mm Hg. This response helps protect the vital centers of the brain from loss of nutrition, which could occur if pressure in the cranial vault exceeds the normal arterial pressure and compresses blood vessels supplying the brain.

If cerebral ischemia becomes so severe that a maximal increase in arterial pressure still cannot relieve the ischemia, the neuronal cells begin to suffer metabolically, and within 3 to 10 minutes they become inactive. This causes the arterial pressure to decrease.

CHAPTER 19

Role of the Kidneys in Long-Term Control of Arterial Pressure and in Hypertension: The Integrated System for Arterial Pressure Regulation

Renal–Body Fluid System for Arterial Pressure Control (p. 213)

The short-term control of arterial pressure by the sympathetic nervous system, discussed in Chapter 18, occurs mainly through changes in vascular resistance and capacitance and cardiac pumping ability. However, the body also has powerful mechanisms for long-term blood pressure regulation that are closely linked to control of body fluid volume by the kidneys, a mechanism known as the *renal–body fluid feedback system*. When arterial pressure rises too high, the kidneys excrete increased quantities of sodium and water because of *pressure natriuresis* and *pressure diuresis*, respectively. As a result of the increased renal excretion, the extracellular fluid volume and blood volume both decrease until blood pressure returns to normal and the kidneys excrete normal amounts of sodium and water.

Conversely, when the arterial pressure falls too low, renal sodium and water excretion are reduced; over a period of hours to days, if the person drinks enough water and eats enough salt to increase the blood volume, the arterial pressure returns to its previous level. This mechanism for blood pressure control is slow to act, sometimes requiring several days, a week, or longer to reach equilibrium; therefore, it is not of major importance in the acute control of arterial pressure. However, it is by far the most potent of all long-term arterial pressure controllers.

Renal Output of Salt and Water Is Balanced with the Intake of Salt and Water under Steady-State Conditions. Figure 19–1 shows the effect of various arterial pressures on urine volume output by an isolated kidney, demonstrating marked increases in the output of volume (pressure diuresis) and sodium (pressure natriuresis) as arterial pressure rises. Note that so long as the arterial pressure is above the normal equilibrium point, renal output exceeds the intake of salt and water, resulting in a progressive decline in extracellular fluid volume. Conversely, if blood pressure falls below the

Figure 19–1. Arterial pressure regulation can be analyzed by
equating the renal output curve with the salt and water intake
curve. The equilibrium point describes the level at which the
arterial pressure is regulated. Curve A *(red line)* shows the
normal renal output curve. Curve B *(pink line)* shows the renal
output curve in hypertension.

equilibrium point, the renal output of water and salt
is lower than the intake, resulting in a progressive
increase in extracellular fluid volume. The only point
on the curve at which a balance between renal output
and intake of salt and water can occur is at the normal
arterial pressure (the equilibrium point).

The Renal–Body Fluid Feedback Mechanism Demonstrates a Near "Infinite Feedback Gain" in Long-Term
Blood Pressure Control. To illustrate why this mechanism demonstrates nearly "infinite gain" in controlling
blood pressure, let us assume that the arterial pressure
rises to 150 mm Hg. At this level, renal output of water
and salt is about three times more than the intake. The
body loses fluid, blood volume decreases, and arterial
pressure decreases. *Furthermore, this loss of fluid
does not cease until the arterial pressure decreases to
the equilibrium point* (see Fig. 19–1A). Conversely,
if blood pressure falls below the equilibrium point,
the kidneys decrease salt and water excretion to a level
below intake, causing accumulation of fluid and blood
volume until the arterial pressure returns to the equilibrium point. Because there is little or no remaining error in arterial pressure after full correction, this
feedback system has nearly *infinite gain.*

There Are Two Primary Determinants of the Long-Term Arterial Pressure. From the curve shown in Figure 19–1, one can see that two factors determine long-term arterial pressure: (1) *the renal output curve for salt and water* and (2) *the level of salt and water intake.* So long as these two factors remain constant, the arterial pressure also remains exactly at the normal level of 100 mm Hg. For arterial pressure to deviate from the normal level for long periods of time, one of these two factors must be altered.

In Figure 19–1, curve B, an abnormality of the kidney has caused the renal output curve to shift 50 mm Hg toward higher blood pressure. This results in a new equilibrium point, and the arterial pressure follows to this new pressure level within a few days. Although greater salt and water intake can theoretically elevate arterial pressure (discussed later), the body has multiple neurohumoral mechanisms that protect against large increases in arterial pressure when salt and water intake is elevated. This is accomplished mainly by decreasing the formation of angiotensin II and aldosterone, which increases the ability of the kidneys to excrete salt and water and results in a steep renal output curve. Therefore, the chronic renal output curve is much steeper than the acute curve shown in Figure 19–1, and in most persons, large increases in salt and water output can be accomplished with minimal increases in arterial pressure.

Increased Total Peripheral Vascular Resistance Cannot Elevate the Long-Term Arterial Pressure if Fluid Intake or Renal Function Does Not Change. When total peripheral vascular resistance is acutely increased, the arterial pressure increases almost immediately. However, if the vascular resistance of the kidneys is not increased and they continue to function normally, the acute rise in arterial pressure is not maintained. The reason is that increasing resistance everywhere in the body except in the kidneys does not change the equilibrium point for blood pressure as dictated by the renal output curve. With increased peripheral resistance and arterial pressure, the kidneys undergo pressure diuresis and pressure natriuresis, causing loss of salt and water from the body. This loss continues until the arterial pressure returns to the normal equilibrium point (see Fig. 19–1, curve *A*).

In many cases, when total peripheral resistance increases, renal vascular resistance also increases; this causes hypertension by shifting the renal function curve to higher blood pressures. When this shift occurs, it is the increase in renal vascular resistance, not the increase in total peripheral resistance, that causes the long-term increase in arterial pressure.

Increased Fluid Volume Can Elevate Arterial Pressure if Vascular Capacity Does Not Increase. The sequential events that link increased extracellular fluid volume and increased arterial pressure are the following (in order of occurrence):

1. Increased extracellular fluid volume and increased blood volume
2. Increased mean circulatory filling pressure
3. Increased venous return of blood to the heart
4. Increased cardiac output
5. Increased arterial pressure

The increased cardiac output, by itself, tends to elevate the arterial pressure; however, the increased cardiac output also causes excess blood flow in many of the tissues of the body that respond by vasoconstriction, which tends to return the blood flow toward normal. This phenomenon is called *autoregulation* and tends to raise the total peripheral vascular resistance. With higher extracellular fluid volume, there is an initial rise in cardiac output and a rise in tissue blood flow; but after several days the total peripheral resistance begins to increase because of autoregulation, and cardiac output usually returns toward normal.

If increases in extracellular fluid volume and blood volume are associated with increased vascular capacity, arterial pressure may not increase. For example, in liver cirrhosis there is often a large increase in extracellular fluid volume resulting from decreased liver synthesis of plasma proteins and subsequent leakage of fluid from the blood into the tissues. Fibrous liver tissue may also impeded blood flow through the liver causing high pressures in the portal circulation, distending the veins, and increasing vascular capacity. Likewise with large varicose veins there is increased vascular capacity. In these instances, the kidneys actually retain salt and water and the increases in extracellulary fluid volume and blood volume serve as a compensatory response that helps to prevent blood pressure from decreasing.

Hypertension (High Blood Pressure) *(p. 218)*

The normal systolic/diastolic arterial pressures are about 120/80 mm Hg, with a mean arterial pressure of 93 mm Hg under resting conditions. Hypertension is said to occur when the diastolic pressure is higher than 90 mm Hg or the systolic pressure is higher than 135 or 140 mm Hg.

Even moderate elevation of the arterial pressure leads to shortened life expectancy by at least three ways:

1. Excessive workload on the heart leads to early heart failure and coronary artery disease, congestive heart disease, or both, often causing death as a result of a *heart attack.*
2. High blood pressure often leads to rupture of a major blood vessel in the brain or hypertrophy and eventual obstruction of a cerebral blood vessel. In either case, this leads to cerebral ischemia and death of a portion of the brain, a condition called *stroke.*
3. High blood pressure often causes damage to the kidneys and can eventually lead to *kidney failure.*

There are multiple ways by which hypertension can occur. With all types of hypertension studied so far, however, there has been a shift of the renal output curve toward higher blood pressures. Lessons learned from one type of hypertension called *volume loading hypertension* have been crucial to understanding the role of the renal–body fluid feedback mechanism for arterial pressure regulation.

Sequential Changes That Occur in Circulatory Function During the Development of Volume-Loading Hypertension. In experimental animals in which the kidney mass has been surgically reduced to about 30% of normal, an increase in the salt and water intake causes marked hypertension. Although reduction of the functional kidney mass, by itself, does not cause significant hypertension, it reduces the ability of the kidney to excrete a large load of salt and water effectively. When salt and water intake are increased, the following sequence of events occur:

- Extracellular fluid volume and blood volume are expanded.
- Increased blood volume increases the mean circulatory filling pressure, venous return, and cardiac output.
- Increased cardiac output raises arterial pressure.
- During the first day after increased salt and water intake, there is a *decrease* in total peripheral resistance, caused mainly by the baroreceptor reflex mechanism, which attempts to prevent the rise in pressure.

- After several days, there is a gradual return of cardiac output toward normal resulting from long-term blood flow autoregulation, which simultaneously causes a secondary increase in total peripheral resistance.
- As arterial pressure increases, the kidneys excrete the excess volume of fluid through pressure diuresis and pressure natriuresis, and a balance between intake and renal output of salt and water is re-established.

This sequence illustrates how an initial abnormality of kidney function and excess salt and water intake can cause hypertension and how the volume-loading aspects of hypertension may not be apparent after the kidneys have had sufficient time to re-establish sodium and water balance and after the autoregulatory mechanisms have caused an increase in total peripheral resistance. The following are two clinical examples of volume-loading hypertension:

- *Volume-loading hypertension can occur in patients who have no kidneys and are being maintained on an artificial kidney.* If the blood volume of a patient maintained on an artificial kidney is not regulated at the normal level and is allowed to increase, hypertension develops in almost exactly the same way as previously discussed.
- *Excessive secretion of aldosterone causes volume-loading hypertension.* Occasionally, a tumor of the adrenal glands causes excessive secretion of aldosterone, which increases reabsorption of salt and water by the tubules of the kidneys (see Chapter 29). This reduces urine output, causing an increase in extracellular fluid volume and initiating the same sequence described previously for volume-loading hypertension.

Renin-Angiotensin System: Its Role in Arterial Pressure Control and Hypertension *(p. 220)*

In addition to its capability of controlling arterial pressure through changes in extracellular fluid volume, the kidneys control pressure through the *renin-angiotensin system*. When the arterial pressure falls too low, the kidneys release a protein enzyme, *renin*, that activates the renin-angiotensin system and helps increase the arterial pressure in several ways, thus helping correct for the initial fall of pressure.

Components of the Renin-Angiotensin System and Role of Angiotensin II in Regulation of Arterial Pressure. The renin-angiotensin system acts in the following manner for acute blood pressure control:

- A decrease in arterial pressure stimulates the secretion of *renin* from the *juxtaglomerular cells* of the kidney into the blood.
- Renin catalyzes the conversion of *renin substrate (angiotensinogen)* to release a 10-amino acid peptide, *angiotensin I.*
- Angiotensin I is converted to *angiotensin II* by the action of a *converting enzyme* present in the endothelium of vessels throughout the body, especially in the lungs and kidneys.
- Angiotensin II, the primary active component of this system, is a potent vasoconstrictor and helps raise the arterial pressure.
- Angiotensin II persists in the blood until it is rapidly inactivated by multiple blood and tissue enzymes collectively called *angiotensinases.*

Angiotensin II has two principal effects that can elevate the arterial pressure:

1. *Angiotensin II constricts arterioles and veins throughout the body,* thereby increasing total peripheral resistance and decreasing vascular capacity, which promotes increased venous return to the heart. These effects are important for preventing excessive reductions in blood pressure during acute circumstances such as hemorrhage.
2. *Angiotensin II decreases salt and water excretion by the kidneys.* This action slowly increases extracellular fluid volume, which increases arterial pressure over a period of hours and days.

The Effects of Angiotensin II That Cause Renal Retention of Salt and Water Are Especially Important for Long-Term Control of Arterial Pressure. Angiotensin II causes salt and water retention by the kidneys in two ways:

- *Angiotensin acts directly on the kidneys to cause salt and water retention.* Angiotensin II constricts the efferent arterioles, which diminishes blood flow through the peritubular capillaries, allowing rapid osmotic reabsorption from the tubules. In addition, angiotensin II directly stimulates the epithelial cells of the renal tubules to increase reabsorption of sodium and water.

• *Angiotensin II stimulates the adrenal glands to secrete aldosterone, and aldosterone increases salt and water reabsorption by the epithelial cells of the renal tubule.*

The Renin-Angiotensin System Helps Maintain Normal Arterial Pressure During Wide Variations in Salt Intake. One of the most important functions of the renin-angiotensin system is to allow a person to ingest either a very small or very large amount of salt without causing great changes in either extracellular fluid volume or arterial pressure. For example, when salt intake is increased, there is a tendency for extracellular fluid volume and arterial pressure to increase. This greater arterial pressure also decreases renin secretion and angiotensin II formation, which in turn decreases renal tubular salt and water reabsorption. The reduced tubular reabsorption allows the person to excrete the extra amounts of salt and water with minimal increases in extracellular fluid volume and arterial pressure.

When salt intake is decreased below normal levels, the opposite effects take place. So long as the renin-angiotensin system is fully operative, salt intake can be as low as 1/10 normal or as high as 10 times normal with only a few millimeters of mercury change in arterial pressure. On the other hand, when the renin-angiotensin system is blocked, the same changes in salt intake cause large variations in blood pressure, often as much as 50 mm Hg.

Excessive Angiotensin II Formation Causes Hypertension. Occasionally, a renin-secreting tumor of the juxtaglomerular cells occurs and causes excessive formation of angiotensin II. This almost invariably leads to severe hypertension.

The effect of angiotensin II to increase total peripheral resistance is the primary cause of the rapid rise in blood pressure that occurs when angiotensin II levels are suddenly elevated. The long-term increase in blood pressure associated with excessive angiotensin II formation is due mainly to the various actions of angiotensin II that cause renal salt and water retention.

Impaired Renal Circulation Causes Hypertension
(p. 223)
Any condition that seriously reduces the ability of the kidneys to excrete salt and water can cause hypertension. One type of renal dysfunction that can cause severe hypertension is renal vascular damage, such as

occurs with (1) stenosis of the renal arteries, (2) constriction of the afferent arterioles, or (3) increased resistance to fluid filtration through the glomerular membrane (i.e., decreased glomerular capillary filtration coefficient). Each of these factors reduces the ability of the kidney to form glomerular filtrate, which in turn causes salt and water retention as well as increased blood volume and increased arterial pressure. The rise in arterial pressure then helps return the glomerular filtration rate toward normal and reduces tubular reabsorption, permitting the kidneys to excrete normal amounts of salt and water despite the vascular disorders.

Constriction of the Renal Arteries Causes Hypertension. When one kidney is removed and a constrictor is placed on the renal artery of the remaining kidney, the immediate effect is greatly reduced pressure in the renal artery beyond the constriction. Within a few minutes, the systemic arterial pressure begins to rise, and it continues to rise for several days until the renal arterial pressure beyond the constriction has returned almost to normal levels. The hypertension produced in this way is called *one-kidney Goldblatt hypertension*, in honor of Harry Goldblatt, who first described the features of hypertension caused by this method in experimental animals.

The rapid rise in arterial pressure in Goldblatt hypertension is caused by activation of the renin-angiotensin vasoconstrictor mechanism. Because of poor blood flow through the kidney after a reduction of renal artery pressure, large quantities of renin are secreted, causing increased angiotensin II formation and a rapid rise in blood pressure. The more delayed rise in blood pressure, occurring over a period of several days, is caused by fluid retention. The fluid retention and expansion of the extracellular fluid volume continue until the arterial pressure has risen sufficiently to return the renal perfusion pressure to almost normal levels.

Hypertension also occurs when the artery of one kidney is constricted and the artery of the other kidney is normal; this is often called *two-kidney Goldblatt hypertension.* The constricted kidney retains salt and water because of decreased arterial pressure in this kidney. The "normal" kidney retains salt and water because of the renin produced in the ischemic kidney and the increase in circulating angiotensin II, which causes the opposite kidney to retain salt and water.

Both kidneys become salt and water retainers, and hypertension develops.

Coarctation of the Aorta above the Renal Arteries Also Causes Hypertension, with Characteristics Similar to Those Described for One-Kidney Goldblatt Hypertension. Aortic coarctation results in decreased perfusion pressure to both kidneys, stimulating the release of renin and angiotensin II formation as well as salt and water retention by the kidneys. These changes increase the arterial pressure in the upper part of the body above the coarctation, thereby helping to return the perfusion pressure of the kidneys toward normal.

Patchy Ischemia of One or Both Kidneys Can Also Cause Hypertension. When this occurs, the characteristics of the hypertension are almost identical to those of two-kidney Goldblatt hypertension; the patchy ischemic kidney tissue secretes renin, which in turn stimulates formation of angiotensin II, causing the remaining kidney mass to retain salt and water. This type of hypertension is much more common than hypertension caused by constriction of the main renal arteries or aortic coarctation, especially in older patients with atherosclerosis.

Toxemia of Pregnancy (Preeclampsia) Is Also Associated with Hypertension. Although the precise cause of hypertension of this condition is not completely understood, many physiologists believe that it is due to ischemia of the placenta and subsequent release by the placenta of toxic factors that cause many of the manifestations of this disorder, including endothelial dysfunction, impaired renal-pressure natriuresis and hypertension in the mother.

Another pathological factor that may cause hypertension in preeclampsia is *thickening of the glomerular membranes* perhaps caused by an autoimmune process, which reduces the glomerular capillary filtration coefficient and rate of fluid filtration from the glomeruli into the renal tubules.

The Causes of Human Primary (Essential) Hypertension Are Unknown

Approximately 25% to 30% of adults in industrialized societies have high blood pressure, although the incidence of hypertension is higher among the elderly. The precise cause of hypertension in about 90% of these people is unknown; this type of hypertension is called *primary or essential hypertension.*

Although the exact causes of primary hypertension are not fully understood, most patients who develop essential hypertension slowly over many years have significant changes in kidney function. Most important, the kidneys cannot excrete adequate quantities of salt and water at normal arterial pressures; instead, they require a high arterial pressure to maintain a normal balance between the intake and output of salt and water unless they are treated with drugs that enhance their ability to excrete salt and water at lower blood pressures.

Abnormal renal excretory capability could be caused by renal vascular disorders that reduce glomerular filtration or tubular disorders that increase reabsorption of salt and water. Because patients with essential hypertension are highly heterogeneous with respect to the characteristics of the hypertension, it seems likely that both disorders contribute to increased blood pressure.

Summary of the Integrated, Multifaceted System for Arterial Pressure Regulation (p. 226)

It is clear that arterial pressure is regulated by several systems, each of which performs a specific function. Some systems are most important for acute regulation of blood pressure and react rapidly, within seconds or minutes. Others respond over a period of minutes or hours. Some provide long-term arterial pressure regulation over days, months, and years.

Nervous System Reflexes Are Rapidly Acting Blood Pressure Control Mechanisms. The three nervous reflexes that act rapidly (within seconds) are (1) the *baroreceptor feedback mechanism,* (2) the *central nervous ischemic mechanism,* and (3) the *chemoreceptor mechanism.* These mechanisms not only act within seconds but also are powerful in preventing acute decreases in blood pressure (e.g., during severe hemorrhage). They also operate to prevent excessive increases in blood pressure, as might occur in response to excessive blood transfusion.

Intermediate Blood Pressure Control Mechanisms That Act after Several Minutes. Three mechanisms that are important in blood pressure control after several minutes of acute pressure change are the (1) *renin-angiotensin vasoconstrictor mechanism,* (2) *stress relaxation of the vasculature,* and (3) *shift of fluid through* *the capillary walls* in and out of the circulation to readjust the blood volume as needed.

The role of the renin-angiotensin vasoconstrictor mechanism has been described. The *stress relaxation mechanism* is demonstrated by the following example: When pressure in the blood vessels becomes too high, the vessels become stretched and continue to stretch for minutes or hours. As a result, the pressure in the vessels tends to fall back toward normal.

The *capillary fluid shift mechanism* means that any time the capillary pressure falls too low fluid is absorbed from the tissue into the capillaries of the circulation, thereby increasing the blood volume and helping to return the blood pressure toward normal. Conversely, when capillary pressure rises too high, fluid is lost out of the circulation, thereby reducing blood volume and arterial pressure.

The Long-Term Mechanism for Arterial Pressure Regulation Involves the Renal–Body Fluid Feedback. The renal–body fluid feedback control mechanism takes several hours to show any significant response, but then it operates powerfully to control arterial pressure over days, weeks, and months. So long as kidney function is unaltered, disturbances that tend to alter arterial pressure, such as increased total peripheral resistance, have minimal effect on blood pressure over long periods of time. Factors that alter the ability of the kidneys to excrete salt and water can cause major long-term changes in arterial pressure. This mechanism, if given sufficient time, controls the arterial pressure at a level that provides normal output of salt and water by the kidneys.

Many factors can affect the renal–body fluid feedback mechanism and therefore long-term blood pressure control. One of the most important factors is the renin-angiotensin system, which allows a person to have very low or very high salt intake with minimal changes in arterial pressure. Thus arterial pressure control begins with lifesaving measures of the nervous reflexes, continues with the sustaining characteristics of the intermediate pressure controls, and finally is stabilized at the long-term pressure level by the renal–body fluid feedback mechanism.

CHAPTER 20

Cardiac Output, Venous Return, and Their Regulation

Cardiac output is the amount of blood pumped into the aorta each minute by the heart. It also represents the quantity of blood that flows to the peripheral circulation; the cardiac output transports substances to and from the tissues. The cardiac output of an average adult is approximately 5 L/min or 3 L/min/m^2 of body surface area.

Venous return is the amount of blood that flows from the veins back to the right atrium each minute.

Control of Cardiac Output by Venous Return—Role of the Frank-Starling Mechanism of the Heart *(p. 229)*

In the absence of changes in cardiac strength, cardiac output is controlled by factors that affect venous return. One of the most important regulators of venous return is metabolism of the tissues. An increase in the tissue metabolic rate results in local vasodilation, which causes a decrease in total peripheral resistance and thus an increase in venous return. This greater venous return causes an increase in diastolic filling pressure in the ventricles, which in turn results in a greater force of contraction by the ventricles. This mechanism for increasing cardiac pumping ability is called the *Frank-Starling law of the heart*. The law states that, within limits, an increase in the volume of blood returning to the heart stretches the cardiac muscle a greater amount, and the heart contracts with greater force and pumps out all the excess venous return.

An important concept that can be learned from the Frank-Starling law is that, except for momentary changes, cardiac output equals venous return. Therefore, factors that control venous return also control cardiac output. If this were not so—for example, if the cardiac output were greater than the venous return—the lungs would quickly be emptied of blood. In contrast, if the cardiac output were less than the venous return, the lung vasculature would rapidly fill with blood.

During increases in venous return, the right atrial stretch elicits two reflexes that help increase the cardiac output. First, the stretch of the sinus node causes a direct effect on the rhythmicity of the node, which causes a 10% to 15% increase in heart rate. This increase in heart rate helps pump the extra blood that is returning to the heart. Second, the extra stretch in the right atrium elicits a *Bainbridge reflex,* with impulses going first to the vasomotor center and then back to the heart by way of sympathetic nerves and the vagi. This reflex causes an increase in heart rate, which also helps pump out the excess venous return. This reflex along with the Frank-Starling law help maintain the volumes of the cardiac chambers within normal limits.

Cardiac Output Regulation Is the Sum of All Tissue Blood Flow Regulation. Because venous return is the sum of all local blood flows, anything that affects local blood flow also affects the venous return and cardiac output.

One of the main ways by which local blood flow can be changed is through local metabolism. For example, if the biceps muscle of the right arm is used repetitively to lift a weight, the metabolic rate of that muscle increases, causing local vasodilation. Blood flow to the biceps muscle thus increases, which in turn causes an increase in venous return and cardiac output. Remarkably, the increased cardiac output goes primarily to the area of increased metabolism, the biceps, because of its vasodilation.

Changes in Cardiac Output Can Be Predicted with the Use of Ohm's Law. Ohm's law, as applied to the circulation, can be stated as the following relationship:

$$\text{Cardiac Output} = \frac{(\text{Arterial Pressure} - \text{Right Atrial Pressure})}{\text{Total Peripheral Resistance}}$$

If the right atrial pressure is equal to its normal value of 0 mm Hg, the relationship can be simplified to the following:

$$\text{Cardiac Output} = \frac{\text{Arterial Pressure}}{\text{Total Peripheral Resistance}}$$

If the arterial pressure is constant, this formula can be accurately used to predict changes in flow that are due to changes in total peripheral resistance. If we return to the example of an increase in the metabolic rate in a peripheral tissue, the increase in oxygen use that also occurs elicits local vasodilation and decreases total peripheral resistance, which causes an increase in oxygen delivery to local tissues, an increase in venous return, and an increase in cardiac output. Thus if the arterial pressure is constant, the long-term cardiac output varies in a reciprocal manner with total peripheral resistance. Therefore a decrease in total peripheral resistance increases the cardiac output, and an increase in total peripheral resistance decreases it.

Maximum Cardiac Output Achieved by the Heart Is Limited by the Plateau of the Cardiac Output Curve (p. 231)

The *cardiac output curve*, in which cardiac output is plotted as a function of right atrial pressure, can be affected by several factors; and their net effect is a change in the plateau level of this curve. Some of these factors are as follows:

- Increased sympathetic stimulation, which increases the plateau
- Decreased parasympathetic stimulation, which increases the plateau
- Cardiac hypertrophy, which increases the plateau
- Myocardial infarction, which decreases the plateau
- Cardiac valvular disease, such as a stenotic or insufficient valve, which decreases the plateau
- Abnormal cardiac rhythm, which may decrease the plateau

Pathologically High and Pathologically Low Cardiac Output (p. 232)

High Cardiac Output Is Almost Always Caused by Reduced Total Peripheral Resistance. A distinguishing feature of many conditions with high cardiac output is that they result from a chronic decrease in total peripheral resistance. Among these conditions are the following:

- *Beriberi.* This disease is caused by a lack of thiamine, and the associated diminished ability to use cellular nutrients results in marked vasodilation, decreased total peripheral resistance, and increased cardiac output.
- *Arteriovenous fistula (shunt).* This condition is caused by a direct opening between an artery and a vein, which decreases total peripheral resistance and thus increases cardiac output.
- *Hyperthyroidism.* This condition causes an increase in oxygen use, which in turn causes release of vasodilatory products as well as a decrease in total peripheral resistance and an increase in cardiac output.

- *Anemia.* The decrease in total peripheral resistance with this condition is caused by (1) the lack of oxygen delivery to tissues, causing vasodilation, and (2) a decrease in the viscosity of blood owing to the lack of red blood cells. The cardiac output thus rises.

Low Cardiac Output Can Be Caused by Cardiac or Peripheral Factors. Severe myocardial infarction, severe valvular disease, myocarditis, cardiac tamponade, and certain metabolic derangements can decrease cardiac output by lowering the plateau of the cardiac output curve (see Chapter 22).

The peripheral factors that acutely reduce cardiac output also reduce venous return; they include the following:

- Decreased blood volume
- Acute venous dilation
- Obstruction of the large veins

A More Quantitative Analysis of Cardiac Output Regulation *(p. 238)*

The cardiac output curve is used to describe the ability of the heart to increase its output when right atrial pressure rises. Figure 20–1 shows the intersection of the cardiac output cube with two venous return curves; the cardiac output curve plateaus at 13 L/min. This is a normal cardiac output curve; sympathetic stimulation elevates the plateau of this curve, whereas sympathetic inhibition or depressed cardiac function lowers the plateau of the curve.

The normal cardiac output curve (see Fig. 20–1) is plotted for an intrapleural pressure of –4 mm Hg (the normal external pressure on the outside of the heart). As the intrapleural pressure increases, the heart tends to collapse, particularly the atria. For example, if the intrapleural pressure increases from –4 mm Hg to –1 mm Hg, the volume of the right atrium decreases. To return the right atrial size to normal, an additional 3 mm Hg of right atrial pressure is required to overcome the extra 3 mm Hg of intrapleural pressure. Therefore, the cardiac output curve shifts to the right by exactly 3 mm Hg. The cardiac output curve can be shifted to the right or left by several factors:

- *Normal inspiration,* which shifts the curve leftward
- *Normal expiration,* which shifts the curve rightward
- *Negative pressure breathing,* which shifts the curve to the left

Figure 20–1. Two solid curves demonstrate an analysis of cardiac output and right atrial pressure when the cardiac output and venous return curves are normal. Transfusion of an amount of blood equal to 20% of the blood volume causes the venous return curve to become the *dashed curve*. As a result, the cardiac output and right atrial pressure shift from point A to point B. Psf, mean systemic filling pressure.

- *Positive pressure breathing*, which shifts the curve to the right
- *Surgical opening of the thoracic cage*, which shifts the curve to the right and causes the intrapleural pressure to increase to 0 mm Hg (atmospheric pressure)
- *Cardiac tamponade*, which shifts the curve to the right and rotates it downward to a degree depending on the amount of fluid in the pericardial sac

The Venous Return Curve Describes the Relationship between Venous Return and Right Atrial Pressure. The normal *venous return curve* (see Fig. 20–1, solid line) intersects the normal cardiac output curve at point A, a right atrial pressure of 0 mm Hg; this is the normal right atrial pressure. The mean systemic filling pressure (P_{sf}) is located where the venous return curve intersects the abscissa; this pressure has a value of 7 mm Hg.

The Mean Systemic Filling Pressure Is a Measure of the Tightness with Which the Circulatory System Is Filled with Blood. This pressure is proportional to the amount of blood volume that exceeds the unstressed vascular volume and is inversely proportional to the total vascular compliance. The slope of the linear portion of the venous return curve is equal to 1 divided by the resistance to venous return. If the mean systemic filling pressure is known, venous return can be determined with the following relationship:

$$\text{Venous Return} = \frac{\left(\begin{array}{cc}\text{Mean Systemic} & \text{Right Atrial} \\ \text{Filling Pressure} & - \text{Pressure}\end{array}\right)}{\text{Resistance to Venous Return}}$$

The numerator of this formula equals the pressure gradient for venous return, which is the average pressure from the peripheral vessels to the heart. Therefore, if the pressure gradient for venous return increases, venous return increases.

In Figure 20–1, the dashed venous return curve represents a condition of excess blood volume. This hypervolemia increased the mean systemic filling pressure to 16 mm Hg and decreased the resistance to venous return because the excess blood volume distended the blood vessels and decreased their resistance.

The Resistance to Venous Return Is the Average Resistance between the Peripheral Vessels and the Heart. Most of the resistance to venous return occurs in the veins, although some occurs in the arterioles and arteries. Venous resistance is an important determinant of the resistance to venous return: If venous resistance increases, blood is dammed up in the highly distensible veins, and venous pressure increases by a small amount. The venous return would therefore decrease dramatically.

The venous return curve is shifted upward and to the right during sympathetic stimulation and is shifted downward and to the left during sympathetic inhibition or decreased blood volume. The cardiac output curve is elevated dramatically during sympathetic stimulation; when combined with this upward- and rightward-shifted venous return curve, the cardiac output increases markedly. Sympathetic stimulation also increases the venous resistance, which by itself increases the resistance to venous return; however, the mean systemic filling pressure increases even more, and therefore the venous return increases.

Methods for Measuring Cardiac Output

Cardiac output can be measured using several methods, including the following:

- Electromagnetic flowmetry
- Ultrasonic flowmetry

- Indicator dilution method
- Oxygen Fick method

The Fick procedure can be used to calculate cardiac output with the following relationship:

$$\text{Cardiac Output (L/min)} = \frac{\left(\begin{array}{c}\text{Oxygen Absorbed in} \\ \text{the Lungs [mL/min]}\end{array}\right)}{\left(\begin{array}{c}\text{Arteriovenous Oxygen} \\ \text{Difference [mL/L of blood]}\end{array}\right)}$$

With this technique, the venous blood sample is removed from the pulmonary artery, and the arterial blood sample is taken from any artery in the body.

CHAPTER 21

Muscle Blood Flow and Cardiac Output During Exercise; the Coronary Circulation and Ischemic Heart Disease

Blood Flow in Skeletal Muscle Increases Markedly During Exercise (p. 243)

Resting blood flows through skeletal muscle at an average rate of 3 to 4 mL/min/100 g of muscle. During exercise, this rate can increase by 15- to 25-fold, and cardiac output may increase up to six or seven times normal. This rise in blood flow is necessary to deliver extra nutrients to the exercising muscle and carry away the byproducts of muscular contraction. During skeletal muscle contraction, the muscle blood flow drops markedly (because of mechanical compression of the vessels), but it rises rapidly between contractions.

Vasodilator Factors Increase Skeletal Muscle Blood Flow During Exercise. Muscle contraction increases the metabolic rate of the tissue, which in turn reduces *oxygen* concentration in the tissues; the decreased oxygen concentration causes blood vessels to vasodilate. More importantly, the exercising skeletal muscle releases vasodilator factors, including the following:

- Adenosine
- Potassium ions
- Hydrogen ions
- Lactic acid
- Carbon dioxide

Sympathetic Activation Reduces Skeletal Muscle Blood Flow. During massive sympathetic stimulation, such as occurs during circulatory shock, blood flow to skeletal muscle can decrease to as little as one fourth of normal. This effect is due to the direct effects of sympathetic nerve stimulation and adrenal release of norepinephrine and epinephrine. The sympathetic nerve stimulation and the norepinephrine release from the adrenals predominantly stimulate α-adrenergic receptors, and the epinephrine release from the adrenal predominantly stimulates β-adrenergic receptors. Stimulation of α receptors causes vasoconstriction, whereas stimulation of peripheral β receptors causes vasodilation.

Cardiovascular Changes During Exercise Deliver More Nutrients and Remove Greater Amounts of Metabolic Byproducts from Exercising Muscle. The cardiovascular changes that occur during exercise include the following:

- *Massive sympathetic discharge,* which increases heart rate and heart strength and causes arteriolar constriction and venoconstriction in all of the vasculature except exercising muscle, brain, and the coronary bed
- *Decreased parasympathetic impulses,* which also increases heart rate
- *Local vasodilation in exercising muscle,* which decreases resistance to venous return
- *Increased mean systemic filling pressure,* due mainly to venoconstriction but also to arteriolar constriction
- *Increased venous return and cardiac output,* resulting from increased mean systemic filling pressure, decreased resistance to venous return, and increased heart strength
- *Increased mean arterial pressure,* an important result of the increased sympathetic activity during exercise. The cause of this elevated pressure is (1) arteriolar and small artery constriction, (2) increased cardiac contractility, and (3) increased mean systemic filling pressure

The increase in arterial pressure can range from 20 to 80 mm Hg depending on the type of exercise being performed. When exercise is performed under tense conditions, such as isometrics, during which many of the muscles are contracted for significant periods of time, there is a large increase in arterial pressure. When a more isotonic exercise is performed, such as swimming or running, the arterial pressure increase is much less.

If arterial pressure is prevented from increasing during exercise, such as in a patient with a congenitally impaired sympathetic nervous system, cardiac output increases only about one third of what it does normally. When arterial pressure is allowed to increase normally, blood flow through skeletal muscle increases normally from about 1 L/min during rest to 20 L/min during exercise. If arterial pressure is prevented from increasing during exercise, skeletal muscle blood flow seldom increases more than about eightfold.

The rise in arterial pressure helps increase blood flow by (1) pushing the blood through the arterial system and back toward the heart and (2) dilating the arterioles, which reduces total peripheral resistance and allows more blood to flow through the skeletal muscle and back to the heart.

Coronary Circulation (p. 246)

The resting coronary blood flow is about 225 mL/min and can increase by three- to fourfold during exercise. The coronary flow is delivered to the cardiac muscle primarily through the *left coronary artery*, which supplies most of the left ventricle, and the *right coronary artery*, which supplies the right ventricle and part of the posterior part of the left ventricle. Like skeletal muscle, the flow into the cardiac muscle decreases during muscle contraction, which in the heart coincides with systole. Flow particularly decreases a large amount in the subendocardial vessels because they lie in the midportion of the heart muscle. The surface vessels, the *epicardial vessels,* experience a much smaller decrease in flow during systole.

Local Metabolism Is a More Important Controller of Coronary Flow Than Is Nervous Control

Several vasodilator factors are released during decreases in the cardiac muscle oxygen concentration, including the following:

- Adenosine
- Adenosine phosphate compounds
- Potassium ions
- Hydrogen ions
- Carbon dioxide
- Bradykinin
- Prostaglandins

The release of these vasodilator factors occurs in response to changes in local metabolism and is an important regulator of coronary flow; most of these factors contribute to vasodilation in exercising skeletal muscle. One of the most important regulators of coronary flow is adenosine. There also are some sympathetic effects on coronary flow. Compared with the vasodilator factors, the sympathetic effects on coronary flow are usually modest. The epicardial vessels have a preponderance of α receptors and therefore are constricted during sympathetic stimulation. In contrast, the subendocardial arteries have more β receptors and are vasodilated during sympathetic stimulation. The overall effect of sympathetic stimulation is usually a small decrease in coronary flow.

The control of coronary flow is important because constant of delivery of oxygen is necessary for normal cardiac metabolism. Fat metabolism, which requires oxygen, normally supplies 70% of the energy for the heart. Under moderate ischemic conditions, anaerobic glycolysis can supply energy for cardiac metabolism.

Ischemic Heart Disease Is Responsible for About 35% of Deaths in the United States Each Year

Atherosclerosis Is the Primary Cause of Ischemic Heart Disease. People who eat excessive quantities of fat or cholesterol and are overweight have a high risk of developing atherosclerosis. The stages of development of atherosclerosis and its effects on the heart are as follows:

1. First, large quantities of cholesterol are deposited underneath the endothelium in arteries throughout the body, including the coronary arteries.
2. Later, these areas are invaded by fibrous tissue.
3. This change is followed by a necrotic stage.
4. Finally, a stage of calcification occurs.
5. The final result is the development of atherosclerotic plaque, which can protrude into the lumen of the vessel. The plaque's rough surface initiates formation of blood clots.
6. The blood clot is called a *thrombus* and can partially or fully occlude the coronary vessels.
7. Sometimes the clot breaks away and flows downstream; this is an *embolism.*
8. A thrombus or embolism can totally block blood flow to an area of the heart, which causes death (infarction) of myocardial tissue.
9. The final result is a myocardial infarction.

When atherosclerosis slowly constricts coronary vessels over many years, collateral vessels can develop and maintain coronary flow at a nearly normal level. Such development of vessels can prevent or even postpone a myocardial infarction for many years.

Coronary Spasm Can Also Cause a Myocardial Infarction. Coronary spasm can cause a temporary occlusion in the coronary vessels and thus cause a myocardial infarction. The etiology of the spasm can be irritation of a vessel by roughened atherosclerotic plaque or the result of nervous reflexes or circulating factors. Coronary spasm can also occur in vessels that have no atherosclerotic damage.

Death May Occur after a Myocardial Infarction. There are several causes of death after myocardial infarction:

- Decreased cardiac output
- Pulmonary edema

- Ventricular fibrillation
- Rupture of the heart

Decreased cardiac output occurs after myocardial infarction because the mass of cardiac tissue that contracts normally is decreased. Further weakening of the heart may occur as some of the ischemic muscle bulges outward during the high intraventricular pressure of systole; this is called *systolic stretch.* If a large portion of the heart is damaged, cardiac output may decline to very low levels, which can reduce arterial pressure. The decreased pressure, in turn, reduces coronary flow and further weakens the heart. This vicious cycle of events is called *cardiogenic shock.*

If the left side of the heart is damaged severely, blood backs up into the pulmonary system and causes *pulmonary edema.* Pulmonary capillary pressure increases in this condition, which can cause leakage of fluid into the pulmonary interstitium. This edema prevents proper oxygenation of blood and can lead to death.

Ventricular fibrillation, or uncoordinated contraction of the ventricle, usually occurs within 10 minutes of a myocardial infarction. The factors that increase the tendency of the heart to fibrillate are the following:

- *Increased extracellular potassium concentration* resulting from loss of potassium from ischemic cardiac muscle
- *Current of injury* from the infarcted area
- *Increased irritability of cardiac muscle* resulting from sympathetic reflexes after a myocardial infarction
- *Circus movements,* which occur because dilation of the heart after a myocardial infarction causes an increased pathway length for impulse conduction in the heart

Cardiac rupture is another cause of death after a myocardial infarction. If systolic stretch is severe after an infarction, the area sometimes ruptures and causes rapid blood loss into the pericardial area. Cardiac tamponade results, which causes marked decreases in cardiac output because of the inability of the heart to fill properly during diastole.

Proper Treatment of a Patient with Myocardial Infarction Often Leads to Recovery of Much of the Myocardial Function. If a patient lives past the critical early period after a myocardial infarction, proper medical treatment can enhance the probability of recovery. After an infarct occurs, the necrotic tissue in the center of the damaged area of the myocardium is gradually replaced by fibrous tissue. During the early phases of recovery from a myocardial infarction, tissues on the margin of the infarct usually have just the minimal amount of blood flow necessary to prevent tissue death. Any increase in the activity of the heart may cause normal cardiac tissue to rob the marginal tissue of its blood flow and cause *coronary steal syndrome*. This condition can cause ischemia of the tissue on the margins of the infarct and may cause death. Therefore it is critical that patients maintain complete bed rest after experiencing a myocardial infarction. In addition, patients are usually administered oxygen to breathe during recovery, which may help deliver a little more oxygen to the heart and can help improve cardiac function. Over weeks and months, some of the normal cardiac tissue hypertrophies and thereby helps return cardiac function to normal.

Occasionally, after recovery from an extensive myocardial infarction, cardiac function returns nearly to normal. In most cases, however, cardiac function remains below that of a normal heart. Cardiac reserve is significantly decreased below the normal level of 300% in these patients, which means that the heart can normally pump 300% more blood per minute than is needed during rest. Although the resting cardiac output may be normal after partial recovery from a myocardial infarction, the amount of strenuous activity that can be performed is limited.

Angina Pectoris Is Pain That Originates in the Heart. In many cases, patients with partially recovered hearts and patients without myocardial infarction but ischemic heart disease experience heart pain, called *angina pectoris*. This occurs when the heart is overloaded in relation to the amount of coronary blood flow supplied. Cardiac ischemia occurs. The pain associated with this ischemia is felt underneath the sternum but may be referred to the surface areas of the body, such as the left arm, left shoulder, neck, face, and sometimes the right arm and shoulder.

This anginal pain is caused by a lack of oxygen supply to the heart. Anaerobic glycolysis occurs, which produces lactic acid or other pain-producing compounds. Several treatments for angina pain and cardiac ischemia may be helpful, including the following:

- *Nitrovasodilators*, such as nitroglycerin
- *β-Blockers*, which decrease the need of the heart for oxygen during stressful conditions

- *Coronary angioplasty,* in which a balloon is inflated in a coronary artery that has atherosclerotic narrowing in an attempt to increase the lumen diameter
- *Coronary artery stent,* which is an cylindrical stainless steel tube with slots, is placed in an atherosclerotic coronary artery following angioplasty to help maintain a patent artery
- *Coronary bypass surgery,* during which vascular grafts are attached from the aorta to a point on the coronary artery distal to the constricted area

CHAPTER 22

Cardiac Failure

The term cardiac failure means that the heart is unable to pump sufficient blood to satisfy the needs of the body. The cause usually is decreased myocardial contractility resulting from diminished coronary blood flow. However, failure can also result from heart valve damage, external pressure around the heart, vitamin B deficiency, or primary cardiac muscle disease.

Dynamics of the Circulation in Cardiac Failure (p. 255)

Rapid Compensation for Heart Failure Occurs Primarily via the Sympathetic Nervous System. Immediately after the heart becomes damaged in patients with heart failure, myocardial contractility decreases dramatically. This results in a lower plateau of the cardiac output curve. Within a few seconds, the sympathetic reflexes are activated, and the parasympathetic reflexes are reciprocally inhibited at the same time. Sympathetic stimulation has two major effects on the circulation:

- The heart is strongly stimulated.
- The peripheral vasculature is constricted.

Under the influence of increased sympathetic impulses, the heart becomes a much stronger pump, increasing the plateau of the cardiac output curve. This increased contractility helps restore the cardiac output.

Sympathetic stimulation during heart failure also increases the vascular tone of the peripheral blood vessels, especially the veins, which aids in the restoration of cardiac output. The mean systemic filling pressure increases to 12 to 14 mm Hg, which increases the tendency of the blood to flow back to the heart in spite of increased arterial and venous resistance.

Chronic Responses to Heart Failure Involve Renal Sodium and Water Retention. The depressed cardiac output that occurs during heart failure reduces arterial pressure and urinary output. This results in sodium and water retention and an increase in blood volume. The resulting hypervolemia increases the mean systemic filling pressure and the pressure gradient for venous return, which in turn increases venous return. The hypervolemia distends the veins and thus decreases venous resistance, further adding to the increase in venous return.

Recovery of the Heart Also Helps Restore Cardiac Output During Heart Failure. The cardiac recovery process depends on the factors that initiated cardiac failure. If the initiating factor was, for example, a myocardial infarction, a collateral blood supply rapidly begins to develop after the initial cardiac damage. The undamaged myocardium hypertrophies, which offsets much of the cardiac damage and helps increase the cardiac output. Recovery of the cardiac output to normal levels for sustained periods of time is referred to as *compensated failure.* The features of compensated failure are the following:

- Relatively normal cardiac output so long as the person remains at rest and places no additional demands on the heart
- Increased right atrial pressure, which causes engorgement of the jugular veins
- Decreased cardiac reserve
- Increased heart rate
- Pale or clammy skin (which normalizes after recovery)
- Sweating and nausea (which also normalize after recovery)
- Air hunger (dyspnea)
- Weight gain as a result of fluid retention

One of the key diagnostic features of a patient in compensated heart failure is increased right atrial pressure and the resultant distended neck veins. The increase in right atrial pressure during compensated failure occurs because (1) blood from the damaged heart backs up into the right atrium, (2) venous return increases because of sympathetic stimulation, and (3) the kidney retains sodium and water and thus increases the blood volume and venous return.

Sodium and Water Retention Occur During Heart Failure Because of Sympathetic Reflexes, Decreased Arterial Pressure, and Stimulation of the Renin-Angiotensin-Aldosterone System. Retention of sodium and water by the kidneys during heart failure is a critical factor in the compensatory increases in blood volume and mean systemic filling pressure. The causes of sodium and water retention are as follows:

- *Decreased arterial pressure,* which decreases the glomerular filtration rate
- *Sympathetic constriction of the afferent arterioles,* which also decreases the glomerular filtration rate
- *Increased angiotensin II formation,* which occurs in the kidney because of an increase in renin release.

Decreases in arterial pressure and renal blood flow, as well as an increase in sympathetic output, contribute to the increase in renin release. The increased angiotensin II blood concentration constricts the efferent arterioles in the kidney, which decreases peritubular capillary pressure and thus promotes sodium and water retention

- *Increased aldosterone release,* which occurs because of stimulation of the adrenal gland by the increased angiotensin II in blood and the elevated plasma potassium concentrations that occur during heart failure. This increased aldosterone concentration causes renal sodium retention in the distal parts of the nephron
- *Increased antidiuretic hormone release,* which occurs because of renal sodium retention during heart failure; this hormone promotes water retention in the kidney

With Decompensated Heart Failure, Compensatory Responses Cannot Maintain Adequate Cardiac Output. In some patients, the heart is too weak to restore cardiac output to a level adequate to maintain the nutritional needs of the body and to make the kidneys excrete the necessary daily amounts of fluid. Therefore, the kidneys continue to retain fluid, and the heart muscle continues to be stretched until the interdigitation of the actin and myosin filaments is past optimal levels. Cardiac contractility then decreases further, and a vicious cycle ensues. The causes of decompensated heart failure are believed to be the following:

- Longitudinal tubules of the sarcoplasmic reticulum fail to accumulate sufficient calcium, which is one of the basic causes of myocardial weakness.
- Myocardial weakness causes excess fluid retention, which in turn causes overstretched sarcomeres and further decreases cardiac contractility.
- Excess fluid retention also causes edema of the heart muscle, which results in a stiffened ventricular wall of the heart and in turn inhibits diastolic filling.
- Norepinephrine content of the sympathetic nerve endings of the heart decreases to very low levels, which further decreases cardiac contractility.

There are several treatments for decompensated heart failure, including the following:

- Use of a *cardiotonic drug* such as digitalis. This drug is believed to decrease calcium transport out of the myocardial cells by the Na-Ca exchanger. More calcium then accumulates in the cell, which increases cardiac contractility.

- *Use of diuretics* such as furosemide. This agent also causes venodilation, which decreases the preload on the heart.
- *Decreased sodium and water intake.* When combined with the use of diuretics, decreased sodium and water intake reduces the excess fluid in the body, which improves cardiac function and allows a balance between fluid intake and output despite a low cardiac output.

Unilateral Left Heart Failure *(p. 259)*

With unilateral left heart failure, the blood backs up into the lungs, which increases pulmonary capillary pressure and the tendency for pulmonary edema to develop. The features of left-sided heart failure are as follows:

- Increased left atrial pressure
- Pulmonary congestion
- Pulmonary edema if pulmonary capillary pressure exceeds approximately 28 mm Hg
- Arterial pressure and cardiac output remain near normal so long as the patient remains at rest
- Intolerance to exercise, which if attempted may worsen the pulmonary edema

In contrast, unilateral right-sided heart failure is accompanied by increased right atrial pressure and peripheral edema. Elevated left atrial pressure and pulmonary edema are not present.

"High-Output Cardiac Failure"—This Can Occur Even in a Normal Heart That Is Overloaded *(p. 263)*

With many types of high-output failure, the pumping ability of the heart is not diminished but is overloaded by excess venous return. Most often, this is caused by a circulatory abnormality that drastically decreases total peripheral resistance, such as the following:

- *Arteriovenous fistulas*
- *Beriberi*—The lack of B vitamins in this condition, especially thiamine, markedly decreases peripheral resistance, which increases the venous return. Also, the cardiac output curve is depressed, reflecting a decrease in cardiac contractility. However, cardiac

output remains elevated because of the increased venous return

- *Thyrotoxicosis*—The increased metabolic rate resulting from the increase in thyroid hormone causes an autoregulatory decrease in total peripheral resistance and an increase in venous return. The cardiac output curve is often depressed because of a weakened heart muscle, but the cardiac output still increases because of increased venous return of blood to the heart

Low-Output Cardiac Failure—Cardiogenic Shock *(p. 259)*

Cardiogenic shock can occur in a number of conditions associated with depressed myocardial function, but the most common occurrence is after a myocardial infarction, when cardiac output and arterial pressure often decrease rapidly. The decreased pressure results in a decrease in coronary flow, which can weaken the heart and further decrease cardiac output and arterial pressure. To break this vicious cycle, the following treatments are used:

- *Digitalis* is used to increase cardiac strength.
- *A vasopressor* drug is given to increase arterial pressure.
- *Blood or plasma* is given to increase arterial pressure. This increase in pressure helps increase coronary flow.
- *Tissue plasminogen activator* can be infused to dissolve the coronary thrombosis if treatment is started during or soon after the clot forms.

Acute Progressive Pulmonary Edema Sometimes Occurs in Patients with Long-Standing Heart Failure. If a patient already has some degree of pulmonary edema and an acute event further depresses left ventricular function, more pulmonary edema fluid can quickly form. This increase in edema fluid reduces the oxygenation of blood, which in peripheral tissues causes vasodilation. An increase in venous return thus results from the vasodilation, and the resulting increase in pulmonary capillary pressure can cause more pulmonary edema fluid to form and further reduce blood oxygenation. The treatment of this cycle of pulmonary edema in many ways requires heroic measures and in some ways is opposite of that for cardiogenic shock.

- Applying tourniquets to both arms and legs, which sequesters blood in these limbs and thus reduces

the pulmonary blood volume; the amount of pulmonary edema is thus decreased
- Bleeding the patient
- Administering a rapidly acting diuretic such as furosemide
- Administering oxygen for the patient to breathe
- Administering digitalis to increase heart strength

Although volume-expanding agents are sometimes given for cardiogenic shock to increase arterial pressure, volume-reducing measures are used to decrease edema fluid in the lungs when there is acute, progressive pulmonary edema.

Cardiac Reserve Decreases with All Types of Heart Failure. Cardiac reserve is the percentage increase in cardiac output that can be achieved during maximum exertion; it can be calculated with the following relationship:

Cardiac Reserve

$$= \frac{\left[\left(\frac{\text{Maximum}}{\text{Cardiac Output}} - \frac{\text{Normal}}{\text{Cardiac Output}}\right) \times 100\right]}{\text{Normal Cardiac Output}}$$

If a patient with decreased cardiac reserve undergoes an exercise test, the following often occur:

- Dyspnea (shortness of breath and air hunger)
- Extreme muscle fatigue
- Excessively increased heart rate

CHAPTER 23

Heart Valves and Heart Sounds; Valvular and Congenital Heart Defects

Heart Sounds (p. 265)

Listening to the sounds of the heart is one of the oldest methods used to examine a patient. Heart sounds are associated with *closure of the heart valves;* no sounds occur when the valves are open except that a mitral snap can sometimes be heard on opening of the mitral value.

When one listens to the heart with a stethoscope, the sounds are described as *lub, dub, lub, dub.* The lub is associated with closure of the atrioventricular (A-V) valves at the beginning of systole; the dub occurs at the end of systole, caused by closure of the aortic and pulmonary valves.

The *First Heart Sound* Is Associated with Closure of the A-V Valves. Vibration of the valves and surrounding blood, ventricular wall, and major vessels around the heart causes the first heart sound. The closure of these valves at the beginning of systole is caused by the effects of ventricular contraction, which increases intraventricular pressure and results in a backflow of blood against the A-V valves. After these valves close, the back-and-forth vibration of the elastic valve leaflets and chordae tendineae causes reverberation of the surrounding blood and ventricular walls. The mitral valve closes first followed by the tricuspid valve.

The *Second Heart Sound* Is Associated with Closure of the Aortic and Pulmonary Valves. The second heart sound occurs at the end of systole, when the total energy of the blood in the ventricles is less than that in the aorta and pulmonary artery. This causes the semilunar valves (aortic and pulmonary) to close and again starts a vibration in the valve leaflets and the surrounding blood, ventricular wall, and blood vessels. When the vibration of these structures contacts the chest wall, the sound, with proper amplification, can be heard from outside the body. The aortic valve closes first followed by the pulmonary valve.

Comparison of the first and second heart sounds shows that the first sound, the *lub,* is louder because of the high rate of change of pressure across the A-V valves. In addition, the first heart sound has a lower pitch than that of the second heart sound because of the low elastic modulus of the valves and greater amount of blood vibrating in the ventricles than in the aorta and pulmonary artery. This effect is analogous to the lower pitch made by the thick strings of a piano or guitar after being struck.

The *Third Heart Sound* Occurs at the Beginning of the Middle Third of Diastole. The cause of the sound is thought to be an in-rushing of blood into the ventricles. Little sound occurs at the beginning of diastole because insufficient blood has entered the ventricles to create much elastic tension in the walls, which is necessary for reverberation. This sound can be heard with the bell of the stethoscope in normal children and young adults or in individuals older than 40 years with heart disease, and it can be recorded with a phonocardiogram.

The *Fourth Heart Sound* Is Associated with Atrial Contraction. An atrial heart sound is difficult to hear with a stethoscope, and it can be recorded with a phonocardiogram. The sound is associated with atrial contraction and the associated inflow of blood into the ventricles. It occurs during the last third of diastole.

Most Cardiac Valvular Lesions Result from Rheumatic Fever *(p. 266)*

Rheumatic fever is an autoimmune disease in which a patient's immune system damages or destroys the heart valves. Patients with this disease contract a group A hemolytic streptococcal infection, and *M antigen* is released by the streptococci. Antibodies form against the M antigen, and the antigen-antibody complex has a propensity for attaching to the heart valves. The immune system then attacks the M antigen-antibody-heart valve complex and causes damage, including hemorrhagic, fibrinous, bulbous lesions.

Two heart valve lesions occur with rheumatic fever:

- *Stenotic valves* occur if damage to the valves causes the leaflets to adhere to one another.
- *Insufficient or regurgitant valves* result if the valves are partially destroyed or cannot properly close; back-leak of blood results.

Heart Murmurs Are Abnormal Heart Sounds Caused by Valvular Lesions *(p. 267)*

Aortic Stenosis Causes a Harsh-Sounding Systolic Murmur. Because of the small opening in the aortic valve in this condition, intraventricular pressure must increase to as much as 300 to 400 mm Hg to eject the ventricular blood through the small opening. The jetlike ejection of blood intensely vibrates the aortic wall. The resultant sound is harsh and sometimes can be heard from several feet away. The vibration can be felt on the upper chest. The following are common features of aortic stenosis:

- *Intense left ventricular hypertrophy* occurs because of the increased ventricular workload.
- *Chronic increase in blood volume* occurs as renal compensation to an initial decrease in arterial pressure; the red blood cell mass also increases because of mild hypoxia.
- *Chronic increase in left atrial pressure* is present secondary to hypervolemia, which increases venous return to the heart. The larger venous return also increases the ventricular end-diastolic volume and end-diastolic pressure, which are necessary for the heart to contract forcefully enough to overcome the outflow resistance.
- *Angina pectoris pain* occurs with severe stenosis.

Aortic Regurgitation Causes a "Blowing" Type of Diastolic Murmur. Because of the lack of ability to close the aortic valve completely, blood leaks backward through this valve and into the left ventricle during diastole. The murmur has a relatively high pitch that is caused by the jetting of blood back into the ventricle. The associated vibration is best heard over the left ventricle. The following are features of aortic regurgitation:

- *Stroke volume increases* to as high as 300 mL with 70 mL to the periphery and 230 mL leaking back into the heart.
- *Left ventricular hypertrophy* is caused by the increased stroke volume required by the heart.
- *Aortic diastolic pressure decreases rapidly* because of back-leaking of blood into the left ventricle.
- *Blood volume chronically increases.*

Coronary Ischemia Is Often Associated with Aortic Valvular Lesions. The amount of left ventricular hypertrophy is particularly large during both aortic stenosis and regurgitation and often is associated with coronary ischemia. During aortic stenosis, the ventricular muscle must develop a very high tension to create the high intraventricular pressure needed to force blood through the stenosed aortic valve. The oxygen consumption of the ventricle increases, necessitating a rise in coronary flow to deliver this oxygen. The high wall tension of the ventricle causes marked decreases in coronary flow during systole, particularly in the subendocardial vessels.

Intraventricular diastolic pressure is increased in this condition, which may cause compression of the inner layers of the heart muscle and result in reduced coronary flow. Coronary ischemia is likely to occur with severe aortic stenosis. With aortic regurgitation, the intraventricular diastolic pressure also increases, which compresses the inner layer of the heart muscle and decreases coronary flow. Aortic diastolic pressure falls during aortic regurgitation, which can cause a direct decrease in coronary flow. Both of these mechanisms can lead to a decrease in coronary flow and result in coronary ischemia.

***Mitral Stenosis* Is a Weak-Sounding Diastolic Murmur That Is Heard Best During Mid to Late Diastole.** With mitral stenosis, blood passes with difficulty from the left atrium to the left ventricle. The left atrium is unable to develop a pressure of much more than 30 mm Hg; therefore the velocity of blood flow through the mitral valve never increases dramatically. Sufficient velocity develops to create a low frequency, weak, rumbling murmur that is best detected using phonocardiography. The following are features of mitral stenosis:

• *Cardiac output and mean arterial pressure decrease* but not as much as with aortic stenosis.
• *Atrial volume increases* and may lead to atrial fibrillation.
• *Left atrial pressure increases* and may cause pulmonary edema.
• *Right ventricular failure* occurs with severe stenosis because the right ventricle must pump much harder owing to an increase in pulmonary artery pressure.

Abnormal Circulatory Dynamics Associated with Congenital Cardiac Defects *(p. 269)*

Occasionally, the heart and associated blood vessels are malformed during fetal life. The three major congenital abnormalities are the following:

• *Stenosis* of a channel of blood flow in the heart or one of the surrounding blood vessels
• A *left-to-right shunt,* an abnormality in which blood flows from the left side of the heart or aorta to the right side of the heart or pulmonary artery

- A *right-to-left shunt (tetralogy of Fallot),* an abnormality in which blood bypasses the lungs and goes directly to the left side of the heart

One of the most common causes of congenital heart defects is viral infection, such as German measles, during the first trimester of pregnancy. The fetal heart is being formed at this time and is susceptible to damage.

Patent Ductus Arteriosus Is a Left-to-Right Shunt. Because the lungs are collapsed during fetal life, most blood flow bypasses the lungs and enters the aorta through the ductus arteriosus, which connects the pulmonary artery and aorta. After birth, the high oxygen concentration in the aortic blood that passes through the ductus causes closure of the ductus in most newborns. Occasionally the ductus does not close, and the condition is called *patent ductus arteriosus.*

With patent ductus arteriosus, the high pressure in the aorta forces blood through the open ductus and into the pulmonary artery, and blood recirculates several times through the lungs. Arterial blood oxygen saturation is therefore greater than normal unless heart failure has occurred. The following are features of patent ductus arteriosus:

- *Blood volume increases* to compensate for the decrease in cardiac output.
- *This murmur is heard throughout systole and diastole.*
- *Cardiac reserve decreases.*
- *Left ventricular hypertrophy* occurs because of the extra blood the left ventricle must pump.
- *Right ventricular hypertrophy* occurs because of high pulmonary artery pressure.
- *Pulmonary edema* can occur if the left heart is too overloaded.

Other left-to-right shunts that can occur include the *interventricular septal defect* and *interatrial septal defect.*

Tetralogy of Fallot Is a Right-to-Left Shunt. With *tetralogy of Fallot,* four abnormalities of the heart occur simultaneously:

1. The aorta is displaced over the ventricular septum and originates from the right ventricle.
2. A ventricular septal defect is also present, causing the right ventricle to pump both left and right ventricular blood through the aorta.

3. Pulmonary artery or pulmonary valve stenosis is also present, and because of the high pulmonary arterial resistance, much of the right ventricular blood shunts around the lungs and enters the aorta.
4. Right ventricular hypertrophy occurs because the right side of the heart must pump large quantities of blood against the high pressure in the aorta.

Surgical treatment of this condition is very helpful.

CHAPTER 24

Circulatory Shock and Its Treatment

Circulatory shock occurs when blood flow is inadequate to meet tissue demands leading to widespread tissue damage occurs throughout the body. Damage to the tissues of the cardiovascular system, including the heart, blood vessels, and sympathetic nervous system, causes the shock to become progressively worse.

Because shock results from inadequate cardiac output, factors that decrease cardiac output can lead to shock, including the following:

- *Cardiac abnormalities* that decrease the pumping ability of the heart, including myocardial infarction, toxic states of the heart, dysfunction of the heart and heart valves, and cardiac arrhythmias
- *Factors that reduce venous return,* including decreased blood volume, decreased vascular tone (especially that of the veins), and obstruction to blood flow

Cardiac output does not always decrease during shock. Inadequate cardiac output can result from excessive increases in metabolic rate or from abnormal perfusion patterns that route blood through vessels other than those that supply the local tissues with nutrition. In these cases, normal cardiac output is not sufficient to meet the needs of the tissues.

Shock Caused by Hypovolemia— Hemorrhagic Shock *(p. 274)*

Nonprogressive (Compensated) Shock

One of the most common causes of shock is rapid loss of blood. If the sympathetic reflexes and other factors compensate sufficiently to prevent further deterioration of the circulation, this type of reversible shock is called *compensated shock.* The mechanisms that compensate for the blood loss and its cardiovascular effects are the following:

- *The sympathetic nervous system,* which is the first reflex mechanism that increases arterial pressure, helps the pressure increase toward normal; the baroreceptors are the main activators of the sympathetic nervous system during moderate hypotension. The decreased blood volume in compensated shock causes a decrease in mean systemic filling pressure, cardiac output, and arterial pressure. The arterial pressure reduction stimulates the sympathetic nervous system through the baroreceptors, which in turn causes several cardiovascular effects, including constriction of the arterioles (increasing the total peripheral vascular resistance), constriction of the veins (increasing the mean systemic filling pressure and venous return), and a faster heart rate. Without these reflexes, a person would die after a loss of only 15% to 20% of the blood volume over a period of 30 minutes; this is in contrast to the 30% to 40% loss in blood volume that a person with normal sympathetic reflexes can sustain

- *Central nervous system ischemic response,* which occurs during severe hypotension, when arterial pressure falls below 50 mm Hg
- *Reverse stress-relaxation,* which causes the blood vessels, especially the veins, to contract down around the diminished volume and so helps prevent the decrease in arterial pressure and cardiac output
- *Increased angiotensin II formation,* which constricts peripheral arterioles and causes sodium and water retention by the kidneys
- *Increased vasopressin release,* which constricts the peripheral blood vessels and causes water retention by the kidneys
- *Other mechanisms that increase blood volume back toward normal,* including absorption of fluid from the intestines and interstitial spaces, decreased urinary volume output, increased thirst, and increased appetite for sodium

Progressive Shock Is Caused by a Vicious Circle of Cardiovascular Deterioration *(p. 276)*

When shock becomes sufficiently severe, various circulatory system structures begin to deteriorate, causing a progressive vicious circle of decreasing cardiac output.

Cardiac Deterioration in Progressive Shock Is Due to Poor Coronary Flow. With severe decreases in arterial pressure, particularly diastolic pressure, the coronary blood flow also decreases, and coronary ischemia occurs. This weakens the myocardium and further decreases cardiac output. A positive feedback cycle can develop and cause progressive cardiac deterioration.

Peripheral Circulatory Failure Can Also Occur During Progressive Hemorrhagic Shock. During moderate decreases in cardiac output, the flow to the brain and heart are usually preserved. When the arterial pressure falls sufficiently low, the cerebral blood flow begins to decrease, and flow to the vasomotor center also decreases. If flow decreases sufficiently, the sympathetic discharge of the vasomotor center falls dramatically, which can result in further reductions in arterial pressure and progressive peripheral circulatory failure.

Blood Clotting in Minute Vessels Also Occurs During Progressive Hemorrhagic Shock. Because of the low blood flow during shock, tissue metabolites, including large amounts of carbonic and lactic acid, are not carried away from the tissues properly, allowing local acid concentrations to build up. The resulting increased concentration of hydrogen ions and other ischemic products cause local agglutination of blood and formation of blood clots. The thickened blood in these minute blood vessels is called *sludged blood.*

Increased Capillary Permeability Causes a Further Decrease in Blood Volume During Progressive Hemorrhagic Shock. Because of capillary hypoxia and lack of other nutrients during shock, the capillary permeability increases, allowing fluid and protein to transude into the tissues. This loss of fluid into the interstitium decreases blood volume thus progressively worsening the shock.

Release of Toxins May Cause Cardiac Depression in Progressive Hemorrhagic Shock. Dead gram-negative bacteria in the intestines release a toxin called *endotoxin.* This toxin, in turn, causes an increase in cellular metabolism that can be harmful in shock because the cells that are alive have barely adequate nutrition. Endotoxin specifically depresses the heart. Both of these factors can lead to progressive cellular damage and shock.

Widespread Cellular Deterioration Occurs During Progressive Hemorrhagic Shock. During shock, generalized cellular damage usually occurs first in highly metabolic tissues, such as the liver. Among the damaging cellular effects are the following:

- Decreases occur in active transport of sodium and potassium through cell membranes; sodium accumulates in the cells and potassium is lost, and the cells begin to swell.
- Mitochondrial activity decreases.
- Lysosomes begin to split in tissues throughout the body, releasing hydrolases, which then cause widespread intracellular damage.
- The cellular metabolism of glucose decreases.

Irreversible Shock *(p. 278)*

During *irreversible shock,* even though a transfusion of blood may temporarily increase cardiac output and arterial pressure to normal levels, the cardiac output begins to fall, and death soon ensues. The temporary increase in cardiac output does not prevent the widespread tissue damage caused by acidosis, release of hydrolases, blood clots, and other destructive factors. Therefore a stage is reached after which even rigorous therapy is of no avail.

One of the main causes of irreversible shock is the *depletion of high-energy phosphate compounds.* Once adenosine triphosphate (ATP) has been degraded in the cell to adenosine diphosphate, adenosine monophosphate, and finally adenosine, the adenosine diffuses out of the cell and is converted to uric acid, which cannot re-enter the cell. New adenosine can be synthesized at a rate of only 2% of the total cellular amount per hour. The high-energy phosphate compounds are therefore difficult to regenerate during shock, and this contributes to the final stage of irreversible shock.

Physiology of Treatment in Shock *(p. 280)*

Replacement Therapy

Because Blood Loss Is the Cause of Hemorrhagic Shock, the Appropriate Therapy Is to Replace the Blood. Intravenous infusion of whole blood has proved extremely helpful for treating hemorrhagic shock. Most blood banks store blood as packed red blood cells, although fresh frozen plasma is also available. The combination of packed red cells and plasma is currently used to treat hypovolemic shock instead of whole blood. Other therapies, such as norepinephrine infusion, have been of little benefit. Under battlefield conditions, packed red blood cells are often not available, and plasma has been substituted. Plasma maintains the colloid osmotic pressure of the blood, but the hematocrit decreases with this therapy, placing an extra load on the heart because cardiac output must increase to maintain oxygen delivery to the tissues. Blood administration is therefore the better therapy for hemorrhagic shock.

If neither packed red cells nor plasma is available for a patient in hemorrhagic shock, a plasma substitute may be used. The substitute must have a high colloid osmotic pressure so the fluid does not rapidly transude through the capillary pores into the interstitium. *Dextran* and other high-molecular-weight polysaccharide polymers have been developed and have proved to remain in the blood compartment after intravenous infusion.

Because Plasma Loss Is the Cause of Hypovolemic Shock in Patients with Intestinal Destruction or Burns, Plasma Infusion Is the Appropriate Therapy. During intestinal obstruction, blockage and distention of the intestines partly impede the venous blood flow and thus increase capillary pressure and leakage of highly proteinaceous fluid into the intestinal lumen. With severe intestinal blockage, shock can ensue; however, if an intravenous plasma infusion is started soon, hemodynamic conditions are rapidly restored to normal. In patients with severe burns, plasma transudes through the damaged areas of the skin, causing a marked decrease in plasma volume. The appropriate therapy for the shock that might occur in a burn patient therefore is intravenous infusion of plasma.

Because Water and Electrolyte Loss Is the Cause of Hypovolemic Shock in Patients with Dehydration, Intravenous Infusion of a Balanced Electrolyte Solution Is the Appropriate Therapy. A number of conditions can result in dehydration, including vomiting, diarrhea, excess perspiration, diabetes mellitus, diabetes insipidus, excessive use of diuretics, destruction of the adrenal cortices with loss of aldosterone, and loss of fluid by nephrotic kidneys. If the dehydration is severe, shock can occur. If a balanced electrolyte solution such as lactated Ringer's solution is rapidly infused intravenously, the problem can be corrected.

Traumatic Shock Can Be Caused by Hypovolemia and Pain. Often, a patient with trauma resulting from severe contusion of the body also experiences hypovolemia. Blood administration can correct this hypovolemia, but the pain associated with trauma is an additional aggravating factor. This pain sometimes inhibits the vasomotor center, resulting in a decrease in sympathetic output, which can reduce arterial pressure and venous return of blood to the heart. Administration of a proper analgesic can help alleviate the pain and its effects on the sympathetic nervous system.

Neurogenic Shock Is Caused by Increased Vascular Capacity; Therefore, Therapy Should Decrease This Capacity Toward Normal. *Neurogenic shock* results from a sudden loss of vasomotor tone throughout the body, thereby increasing total vascular capacity. The normal blood volume is inadequate to fill the circulatory system properly, and a decrease in the mean systemic filling pressure results. Some causes of neurogenic shock include the following:

- *Deep general anesthesia*, which depresses the vasomotor center
- *Spinal anesthesia*, especially when the anesthetic migrates all the way up the spinal cord, blocking sympathetic outflow
- *Brain damage*, such as a brain concussion or contusion in the basal areas of the brain near the vasomotor center, that dramatically decreases sympathetic outflow from the vasomotor center

The therapy of choice for neurogenic shock is intravenous infusion of a sympathomimetic drug, such as norepinephrine or epinephrine, that replaces the lost neurogenic vascular tone.

Anaphylactic Shock Is Caused by an Allergic Reaction. When an antigen enters the bloodstream in a person who is highly allergic, an antigen-antibody reaction takes place. One of the main effects is the release of histamine or histamine-like substances from basophils and mast cells. The histamine has several effects, including the following:

- Increased vascular capacity because of venodilation
- Arteriolar dilation, which decreases arterial pressure
- Increased capillary permeability, causing loss of fluid from the vascular compartment

These effects of histamine can decrease arterial pressure and venous return, leading to anaphylactic shock. A person may die minutes after anaphylactic shock symptoms appear. Rapid administration of a sympathomimetic drug, which decreases vascular capacity and constricts the arterioles, is often lifesaving.

Septic Shock Is Caused by Widespread Dissemination of Bacteria in the Body. There are many causes of *septic shock*, all of which start with a bacterial infection. When sufficient bacteria spread throughout the body, there are many effects, including the following:

- High fever
- High metabolic rate
- Marked vasodilation throughout the body
- High cardiac output, caused by peripheral vasodilation, in perhaps one half of patients

- Sludging of blood resulting from red blood cell agglutination
- Disseminated intravascular coagulation

A special case of septic shock occurs when the colon bacteria, containing a toxin called *endotoxin*, are released during strangulation of the gut.

Therapy for shock other than that previously mentioned includes the following:

- Placing the patient in a head-down position, which promotes venous return
- Oxygen
- Glucocorticoids, which stabilize the lysosomes (also shown to be helpful during anaphylactic shock)

Other Effects of Shock on the Body

During shock, especially hypovolemic shock, the decrease in cardiac output reduces the delivery of oxygen and other nutrients to the tissues and also removal of carbon dioxide and other waste products from tissues. Widespread cellular damage may occur, including impaired ability of the mitochondria to synthesize ATP and a depressed sodium-potassium cellular membrane pump. Other effects include the following:

- Muscle weakness
- Decreased body temperature because of decreased metabolism
- Depressed mental function
- Decreased renal function and renal deterioration

V

The Body Fluids and Kidneys

CHAPTER 25

The Body Fluid Compartments: Extracellular and Intracellular Fluids; Edema

The total amount and composition of the body fluids are maintained relatively constant under most physiological conditions, as required for homeostasis. Some of the most important problems in clinical medicine, however, arise because of abnormalities in the control systems that maintain this constancy. In this section, we discuss the overall regulation of body fluid volume, control of the constituents of the extracellular fluid, regulation of the fluid exchange between the extracellular and intracellular compartments, and regulation of the acid-base balance.

Fluid Intake and Output Are Balanced During Steady-State Conditions (p. 285)

The total intakes of water and electrolytes must be carefully matched by equal outputs from the body to prevent fluid volumes and electrolyte concentrations from increasing or decreasing. Table 25–1 shows the routes of daily water intake and output from the body. Under most conditions, the primary means of regulating output is by altering renal excretion. Urine volume can be as low as 0.5 L/day in a dehydrated person or as high as 20 L/day in a person who has been drinking large amounts of fluids. This ability of the kidneys to adjust the output to such an extreme to match intake also occurs for the electrolytes of the body such as sodium, chloride, and potassium.

Total Body Fluid Is Distributed between the Extracellular Fluid and the Intracellular Fluid (p. 286)

The total amount of body water averages about 60% of the body weight, or about 42 L in a 70-kg adult man. Because women normally have more body fat than men, their total body water averages about 50% of the body weight. In premature and newborn babies, the total body water ranges from 70% to 75% of body weight. Therefore, when discussing the "average" body fluid compartments, we should realize that variations exist, depending on age, gender, and percentage of body fat.

Table 25–1.   Daily Intake and Output of Water

Parameter	Normal (mL/day)	With Prolonged Heavy Exercise (mL/day)
Intake		
Fluids ingested	2100	?
From metabolism	200	200
Total intake	2300	?
Output		
Insensible skin	350	350
Insensible lungs	350	650
Sweat	100	5000
Feces	100	100
Urine	1400	500
Total output	2300	6600

Total body fluid is distributed into two main compartments: (1) the *intracellular fluid,* which is about 40% of body weight or 28 L, and (2) the *extracellular fluid,* which is about 20% of body weight, or 14 L in a 70-kg person.

The two main compartments of the extracellular fluid are the *interstitial fluid,* which makes up about three fourths of the extracellular fluid, and the *plasma,* which makes up about one fourth of the extracellular fluid, or about 3 L. The plasma is the noncellular portion of the blood that mixes continuously with interstitial fluid through the pores of the capillary membranes.

Blood Contains Extracellular and Intracellular Fluids. The average blood volume in a normal adult human is 8% of the body weight, or about 5 L. About 60% of the blood is plasma, and about 40% is red blood cells. The *hematocrit,* the fraction of blood that is composed of red blood cells, is normally about 0.42 in men and about 0.38 in women. With severe *anemia,* the hematocrit may fall to as low as 0.10, which is barely sufficient to sustain life. When there is excessive production of red blood cells, resulting in *polycythemia,* the hematocrit can rise to as high as 0.65.

The Constituents of Extracellular and Intracellular Fluids Differ. Table 25–2 compares the compositions of the intracellular and extracellular fluids.

The plasma and interstitial fluid of the extracellular compartment are separated by highly permeable capillary membranes, so their ionic compositions are similar. The most important difference between these two compartments is that the plasma has a higher protein concentration. The capillaries have low permeability to proteins and therefore leak only small amounts of protein into the interstitial spaces in most tissues.

The intracellular fluid is separated from the extracellular fluid by a highly selective cell membrane that is permeable to water but not to most electrolytes found in the body. For this reason, the concentration of water and the osmolarity of intracellular and extracellular fluids are approximately equal under steady-state conditions, although the concentrations of various solutes are markedly different in these fluid compartments.

The Indicator-Dilution Principle Can Be Used to Measure Volumes of Body Fluid Compartments (p. 287)

The volume of a fluid in a compartment in the body can be estimated by injecting a substance into the compartment, allowing it to disperse evenly, and then

Table 25–2. Chemical Compositions of Extracellular and Intracellular Fluids

Chemical	Intracellular Fluid	Extracellular Fluid
Na^+ (mmol/L)	10	142
K^+ (mmol/L)	140	4
Cl^- (mmol/L)	4	108
HCO_3^- (mmol/L)	10	24
Ca^{2+} (mmol/L)	0.0001	2.4
Mg^{2+} (mmol/L)	58	1.2
SO_4^{2-} (mmol/L)	2	1
Phosphates (mmol/L)	75	4
Glucose (mg/dL)	0–20	90
Amino acids (mg/dL)	200?	30
Protein (g/dL)	16	2

analyzing the extent to which the substance has become diluted. This method is based on the assumption that the total amount of substance remaining in the fluid compartment after dispersion is the same as the total amount that was injected into the compartment. Thus when a small amount of substance contained in syringe A is injected into compartment B and the substance is allowed to disperse throughout the compartment until it becomes mixed in equal concentrations in all areas, the following relation can be expressed:

$$\text{Volume B} = \frac{\text{Volume A} \times \text{Concentration A}}{\text{Concentration B}}$$

This method can be used to measure the volume of virtually any compartment in the body if (1) the amount of indicator injected into the compartment (the numerator of the equation) is known, (2) the concentration of the indicator in the compartment is known, (3) the indicator disperses evenly throughout the compartment, and (4) the indicator disperses only in the compartment that is being measured.

Table 25–3 shows some of the indicators that can be used to measure the fluid volumes of the body compartments. The volumes of two of the compartments, the intracellular and extracellular interstitial fluids, cannot be measured directly but, instead, are calculated from the values for other body fluid volumes.

Table 25–3. Measurement of Body Fluid Volume

Volume	Indicators
Total body water	^3H_2O, ^2H_2O, antipyrine
Extracellular fluid	^{22}Na, ^{125}I-iothalamate, inulin
Intracellular fluid	Calculated as: Total Body Water − Extracellular Fluid Volume
Plasma volume	^{125}I-albumin, Evans blue dye (T-1824)
Blood volume	^{51}Cr-labeled red blood cells; calculated as: Blood Volume = Plasma Volume/(1 − Hematocrit)
Interstitial fluid	Calculated as: Extracellular Fluid Volume − Plasma Volume

Intracellular and Extracellular Fluid Distribution Is Determined Mainly by the Osmotic Effect of Electrolytes Acting across the Cell Membrane *(p. 290)*

Because the cell membrane is highly permeable to water but relatively impermeable to even small ions, such as sodium and chloride, the distribution of fluid between the intracellular and extracellular compartments is determined mainly by the osmotic effects of these ions. The basic principles of osmosis and osmotic pressure are presented in Chapter 4. Therefore, only the most important principles as they apply to volume regulation are discussed in this section.

Osmosis Is the Net Diffusion of Water across a Selectively Permeable Membrane from a Region of High Water Concentration to One of Lower Water Concentration. The addition of a solute to pure water reduces the water concentration and causes water to move toward the region of high solute concentration. The concentration term used to measure the total number of solute particles in solution is the *osmole:* 1 osmole is equal to 1 mole (6.02×10^{23}) of solute particles. For biological solutions, the term *milliosmole* (mOsm), which equals 1/1000 osmole, is commonly used.

The osmolar concentration of a solution is called its *osmolality* when the concentration is expressed as osmoles per kilogram of water and *osmolarity* when it is expressed as osmoles per liter of solution. The amount of pressure required to prevent osmosis of water through a semipermeable membrane is called the *osmotic pressure.* Expressed mathematically, the osmotic pressure (π) is directly proportional to the concentration of osmotically active particles in that solution.

$$\pi = CRT$$

where C is the concentration of solutes in osmoles per liter, R is the ideal gas constant, and T is the absolute temperature in degrees Kelvin. If π is expressed in millimeters of mercury (the unit of pressure commonly used for biologic fluids), π calculates to be about 19.3 mm Hg for a solution with an osmolarity of 1 mOsm/L. Thus, for each milliosmole concentration gradient across the cell membrane, 19.3 mm Hg of force is required to prevent water diffusion across the membrane. Very small differences in solute concentration across the cell membrane can therefore cause rapid osmosis of water.

Isotonic, Hypotonic, and Hypertonic Fluids. A solution is said to be *isotonic* if no osmotic force develops across the cell membrane when a normal cell is placed in the solution. An isotonic solution has the same osmolarity as the cell, and the cells do not shrink or swell if placed in the solution. Examples of isotonic solutions include a 0.9% sodium chloride solution and a 5% glucose solution.

A solution is said to be *hypertonic* when it contains a higher concentration of osmotic substances than does the cell. In this case, an osmotic force develops that causes water to flow out of the cell into the solution, thereby reducing the intracellular fluid volume and increasing the intracellular fluid concentration.

A solution is said to be *hypotonic* if the osmotic concentration of substances in the solution is less than the concentration of the cell. The osmotic force develops immediately when the cell is exposed to the solution, causing water to flow by osmosis into the cell until the intracellular fluid has about the same concentration as the extracellular fluid or until the cell bursts as a result of excessive swelling.

Volumes and Osmolarities of Extracellular and Intracellular Fluids in Abnormal States *(p. 292)*

Some of the factors that can cause extracellular and intracellular volumes to change markedly are ingestion of large amounts of water, dehydration, intravenous infusion of various solutions, loss of large amounts of fluid from the gastrointestinal tract, and loss of abnormal amounts of fluid via sweating or from the kidneys.

One can approximate the changes in intracellular and extracellular fluid volumes and the therapy that must be instituted if the following basic principles are kept in mind:

- *Water moves rapidly across cell membranes;* therefore, the osmolarities of intracellular and extracellular fluids remain almost exactly equal to each other except for a few minutes after a change in one of the compartments.

- *Cell membranes are almost completely impermeable to most solutes;* therefore, the number of osmoles in the extracellular and intracellular fluids remains relatively constant unless solutes are added to or lost from the extracellular compartment.

Effect of Adding *Isotonic,* Hypertonic, and Hypotonic Saline Solutions to Extracellular Fluid

If an *isotonic* solution is added to the extracellular fluid compartment, the osmolarity of the extracellular fluid does not change, and there is no osmosis through the cell membranes. The only effect is an increase in the extracellular fluid volume (Fig. 25–1). Sodium and chloride mainly remain in the extracellular fluid because the cell membrane behaves as though it were virtually impermeable to sodium chloride.

If a *hypertonic* solution is added to the extracellular fluid, the extracellular fluid osmolarity increases and causes osmosis of water out of the cells into the extracellular compartment. The net effect is an increase in extracellular volume (greater than the volume of fluid that was added), a decrease in intracellular fluid volume, and an increase in the osmolarity of both compartments.

If a *hypotonic* solution is added to the extracellular fluid, the osmolarity of the extracellular fluid decreases, and some of the extracellular water diffuses into the cells until the intracellular and extracellular compartments have the same osmolarity. Both the intracellular and extracellular volumes are increased by addition of hypotonic fluid, although the intracellular volume is increased to a greater extent.

Edema: Excess Fluid in the Tissues *(p. 296)*

Intracellular Edema: Increased Intracellular Fluid

Three conditions especially likely to cause intracellular swelling are (1) hyponatremia, (2) depression of the metabolic systems of the tissues, and (3) lack of adequate nutrition to the cells. When the cell's metabolic systems are depressed or they receive inadequate nutrition, sodium ions that normally leak into the interior of the cells can no longer be effectively pumped out of the cells, and the excess sodium ions cause osmosis of water into the cells.

Intracellular edema can also occur in inflamed tissues. Inflammation usually has a direct effect on the cell membranes to increase their permeability, allowing sodium and other ions to diffuse into the interior of the cells with subsequent osmosis of water into the cells.

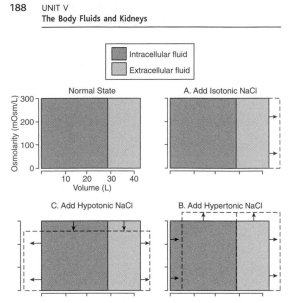

Figure 25–1. Effect of adding isotonic, hypertonic, and hypotonic solutions to extracellular fluid after osmotic equilibrium. The normal state is indicated by the *solid lines*, and the shifts from normal are shown by the *dashed lines*. The volumes of intracellular and extracellular fluid compartments are shown on the abscissa of each diagram, and the osmolarities of these compartments are shown on the ordinates.

Extracellular Edema: Increased Fluid in Interstitial Spaces

The two general causes of extracellular edema are (1) abnormal leakage of fluid from the plasma to the interstitial spaces across the capillaries and (2) failure of the lymphatics to return fluid from the interstitium to the blood, often called *lymphedema.*

Factors Can Increase Capillary Filtration and Cause Interstitial Fluid Edema. To understand the causes of excessive capillary filtration, it is useful to review the determinants of capillary filtration discussed in Chapter 16 as shown in the following equation:

$$\text{Filtration} = K_f \times (P_c - P_{if} - \pi_c + \pi_{if})$$

where K_f is the capillary filtration coefficient (the product of the permeability and surface area of the capillaries), P_{if} is the interstitial fluid hydrostatic pressure, π_c is the capillary plasma colloid osmotic pressure, and π_{if}

is the interstitial fluid colloid osmotic pressure. Thus, any of the following changes can increase the capillary filtration rate:

1. *Increased capillary filtration coefficient,* which allows increased leakage of fluids and plasma proteins through the capillary membranes. This can occur as a result of allergic reactions, bacterial infections, and toxic substances that injure the capillary membranes and increase their permeability to plasma proteins.
2. *Increased capillary hydrostatic pressure,* which can result from obstruction of veins, excessive flow of blood from the arteries into the capillaries, or failure of the heart to pump blood rapidly out of the veins (heart failure).
3. *Decreased plasma colloid osmotic pressure,* which may result from failure of the liver to produce sufficient quantities of plasma proteins (cirrhosis), loss of large amounts of protein in the urine with certain kidney diseases (nephrotic syndrome), or loss of large quantities of protein through burned areas of the skin or other denuding lesions.
4. *Increased interstitial fluid colloid osmotic pressure,* which draws fluid out of the plasma into the tissues spaces. This situation occurs most often as a result of lymphatic blockage, which prevents the return of protein from interstitial spaces to the blood (discussed in the following sections).

Lymphatic Blockage Causes Edema. When lymphatic blockage occurs, edema can become especially severe because plasma proteins that leak into the interstitium have no other way to be returned to the plasma. The rise in protein concentration increases the colloid osmotic pressure of the interstitial fluid, which draws even more fluid out of the capillaries.

Blockage of lymph flow can be especially severe with infections of the lymph nodes, such as occurs with infection by *filarial nematodes.* Lymph vessels may also be blocked with certain types of cancer or after surgery in which the lymph vessels are removed or obstructed.

Safety Factors That Normally Prevent Edema

Although many abnormalities can cause fluid accumulation in interstitial spaces, the disturbances must be substantial before clinically significant edema develops. *Three major safety factors normally prevent fluid accumulation in the interstitial spaces:*

1. *The compliance of the tissues is low so long as interstitial fluid hydrostatic pressure is in the negative range.* Low compliance (defined as the change in volume per millimeter of mercury pressure change) means that small increases in interstitial fluid volume are associated with relatively large increases in interstitial fluid hydrostatic pressure. When the interstitial fluid volume increases, the interstitial fluid hydrostatic pressure increases markedly, which opposes further excessive capillary filtration. The safety factor that protects against edema for this effect is about 3 mm Hg in many tissues such as skin.

2. *Lymph flow can increase as much as 10- to 50-fold.* Lymph vessels carry away large amounts of fluid and proteins in response to increased capillary filtration. The safety factor for this effect has been calculated to be about 7 mm Hg.

3. *There is a "wash-down" of interstitial fluid protein as lymph flow increases.* As increased amounts of fluid are filtered into the interstitium the interstitial fluid pressure increases, causing greater lymph flow. This decreases the protein concentration of the interstitium because more protein is carried away than can be filtered by the capillaries. A decrease in tissue fluid protein concentration lowers the net filtration force across the capillaries and tends to prevent further fluid accumulation. The safety factor for this effect has been calculated to be about 7 mm Hg in most tissues.

Combining all of the safety factors, the total safety factor that protects against edema is about 17 mm Hg. Capillary pressure in peripheral tissues could therefore theoretically rise 17 mm Hg before significant interstitial edema would occur.

CHAPTER 26

Urine Formation by the Kidneys: I. Glomerular Filtration, Renal Blood Flow, and Their Control

The multiple functions of the kidney in the maintenance of homeostasis include the following:

- Excretion of metabolic waste products and foreign chemicals
- Regulation of water and electrolyte balances
- Regulation of body fluid osmolarity and electrolyte concentrations
- Regulation of arterial pressure through excretion of varying amounts of sodium and water and secretion of substances such as renin that lead to formation of vasoactive products such as angiotensin II
- Regulation of acid-base balance through excretion of acids and regulation of body fluid buffer stores
- Regulation of erythrocyte production through secretion of erythropoietin, which stimulates red blood cell production
- Regulation of 1,25-dihydroxy vitamin D_3 production
- Synthesis of glucose from amino acids (gluconeogenesis) during prolonged fasting
- Secretion, metabolism, and excretion of hormones

Urine Formation Results from Glomerular Filtration, Tubular Reabsorption, and Tubular Secretion (p. 310)

A primary function of the kidney is to "clear" unneeded substances from the blood and excrete them in the urine and to return needed substances to the blood. The first step in the performance of this function is filtration of fluid from the glomerular capillaries into the renal tubules, a process called *glomerular filtration*. As the glomerular filtrate flows through the tubules, the volume of filtrate is reduced, and its composition is altered by *tubular reabsorption* (the return of water and solutes from the tubules back into the blood) and by *tubular secretion* (the net movement of water and solutes into the tubules), each of which is highly variable depending on the body's needs. Thus excretion of each substance in the urine involves a specific combination of filtration, reabsorption, and secretion (Fig. 26–1), as expressed by the following relation.

Excretion = Filtration − Reabsorption + Secretion

Figure 26–1. Basic kidney processes that determine the composition of the urine. The urinary excretion rate of a substance is equal to the rate at which the substance is filtered minus its reabsorption rate plus the rate at which it is secreted from the peritubular capillary blood into the tubules.

Urinary Excretion Rate

= Filtration Rate − Reabsorption Rate

+ Secretion Rate

Each of these processes is physiologically controlled, and changes in the excretion rate can obviously occur via changes in glomerular filtration, tubular reabsorption, or tubular secretion.

Renal Blood Flow Constitutes about 22% of the Cardiac Output. Blood flows to each kidney through a renal artery, which branches progressively to form the *interlobar arteries, arcuate arteries, interlobular arteries,* and *afferent arterioles,* which lead to the glomerular capillaries, where filtration of fluid and solutes begins. The capillaries of each glomerulus coalesce to form an *efferent arteriole,* which leads to a second capillary network, the *peritubular capillaries,* which surround the tubules. The peritubular capillaries empty into the vessels of the venous system, which run parallel to the arteriolar vessels, and progressively form the *interlobular vein, arcuate vein, interlobar vein,* and *renal vein,* which leaves the kidney along the renal artery and ureter. The *vasa recta* are specialized peritubular capillaries that dip into the renal medulla and run parallel to the loops of Henle. The outer portion of the kidney, the renal cortex, receives most of the blood flow of the kidney; only 1% to 2% of the total renal blood flow passes through the vasa recta, which supply the renal medulla.

Two distinguishing features of the renal circulation are (1) the high rate of blood flow (about 1100 mL/min for a 70-kg man) relative to the tissue weight (about 300 g for the two kidneys) and (2) the presence of two capillary beds, the glomerular and peritubular capillaries, which are arranged in series and separated by efferent arterioles. The glomerular capillaries filter large amounts of fluid and solutes, most of which are reabsorbed from the renal tubules into the peritubular capillaries.

Renal blood flow is determined according to the pressure gradient across the renal vasculature and the total renal vascular resistance, as expressed by the following relation:

$$\text{Renal Blood Flow} = \frac{(\text{Renal Artery Pressure} - \text{Renal Vein Pressure})}{\text{Total Renal Vascular Resistance}}$$

The total renal vascular resistance is the sum of the resistances of the individual vascular segments, including the arteries, arterioles, capillaries, and veins. Most of the renal vascular resistance resides in three major segments: interlobular arteries, afferent arterioles, and efferent arterioles.

The Nephron Is the Structural and Functional Unit of the Kidney. Each kidney has about 800,000 to 1,000,000 nephrons, each of which is capable of forming urine. A nephron is comprised of a tuft of *glomerular capillaries* called the *glomerulus* in which large amounts of fluid are filtered from the blood, a capsule around the glomerulus called *Bowman's capsule,* and a long *tubule* in which the filtered fluid is converted to urine on its way to the *renal pelvis,* which receives urine from all of the nephrons.

The renal tubule is subdivided into the following major sections, each of which has different structural and functional characteristics: (1) the *proximal tubule,* which lies in the outer portion of the kidney (cortex); (2) the *loop of Henle,* which includes descending and ascending limbs that dip into the inner part of the kidney (medulla); (3) the *distal tubule,* which lies in the renal cortex; and (4) the *connecting tubule,* the *cortical collecting tubule,* and the *cortical collecting duct,* which begin in the cortex and run downward into the medulla to become (5) the *medullary collecting duct.* Urine passes from the renal pelvis to the bladder, where it is stored until it is eventually expelled from the body through the process of *micturition,* or urination.

Micturition *(p. 307)*

Micturition is the process by which the urinary bladder empties when it becomes filled and involves two main steps: (1) the bladder fills progressively until the tension in its walls rises above a threshold level, which elicits the second step, and (2) a nervous reflex, called the *micturition reflex,* is activated and empties the bladder or, if this fails, at least causes a conscious desire to urinate.

Physiologic Anatomy and Nervous Connections of the Bladder

The *ureters* carry the urine from the renal pelvis to the bladder, where they pass obliquely through the bladder wall before emptying into the bladder chamber. There are no major changes in the composition of the urine as it flows through the ureters into the bladder. Peristaltic contractions of the ureter, which are enhanced by parasympathetic stimulation, force the urine from the renal pelvis toward the bladder.

The urinary bladder is a smooth muscle chamber composed of two main parts: (1) *the body,* which is the major portion of the bladder in which urine collects, and (2) *the neck,* which is a funnel-shaped extension of the body that connects with the urethra.

The smooth muscle of the bladder is called the *detrusor muscle.* When the fibers contract, they can increase the pressure of the bladder to 40 to 60 mm Hg and therefore play a major role in emptying the bladder.

The bladder neck (posterior urethra) is composed of detrusor muscle interlaced with a large amount of elastic tissue. The muscle in this area is called the *internal sphincter*; its natural tone keeps the bladder from emptying until the pressure in the main part of the bladder rises above a critical threshold.

Beyond the posterior urethra, the urethra passes through the *urogenital diaphragm*, which contains a layer of muscle called the *external sphincter* of the bladder. This muscle is a voluntary skeletal muscle and can be used consciously to prevent urination even when involuntary controls are attempting to empty the bladder.

Pelvic Nerves Provide the Principal Nervous Supply of the Bladder. Coursing through the pelvic nerves, which connect with the spinal cord through the *sacral plexus,* are both *sensory nerve fibers* and *motor nerve fibers.* The sensory nerve fibers detect the stretch of the bladder wall and initiate reflexes that cause bladder emptying. The motor nerves transmitted to the pelvic nerves are *parasympathetic fibers.*

Micturition Reflex Is a Spinal Cord Reflex

The micturition reflex is a single complete cycle of (1) a progressive and rapid increase in bladder pressure, (2) a period of sustained increase in bladder pressure, and (3) a return of the pressure to the basal tone of the bladder, as follows:

- Sensory signals from the bladder wall stretch receptors are conducted to sacral segments of the spinal cord through the pelvic nerves and then reflexively back to the bladder through the parasympathetic nerves by way of the pelvic nerves.
- Once the micturition reflex is sufficiently powerful, it causes another reflex that passes through the *pudendal nerves* to the external sphincter to inhibit it. If this inhibition is more potent than the voluntary constrictor signals to the external sphincter, urination occurs.
- The micturition reflex is an autonomic spinal cord reflex, but it can be inhibited or facilitated by centers in the brain stem, mainly the *pons,* and several centers in the *cerebral cortex* that are mainly excitatory.

Glomerular Filtration Is the First Step in Urine Formation (p. 312)

The composition of the glomerular filtrate is almost identical to that of plasma except that it has virtually no protein (only about 0.03%). The glomerular filtration rate (GFR) is normally about 125 mL/min, or about 20% of the renal plasma flow; thus the fraction of renal plasma flow that is filtered (*filtration fraction*) averages about 0.2.

The GFR is determined according to the *net filtration pressure* across the glomerular capillaries and the *glomerular capillary filtration coefficient* (Kf), which is the product of the permeability and surface area of the capillaries.

$$GFR = K_f \times \text{Net Filtration Pressure}$$

The net filtration pressure is the sum of hydrostatic and colloid osmotic forces acting across the glomerular capillaries and includes (1) the hydrostatic pressure inside the capillaries—the glomerular hydrostatic pressure (P_G), which is normally about 60 mm Hg and promotes filtration; (2) the hydrostatic pressure in Bowman's capsule outside the capillaries (P_B), which is normally 18 mm Hg and opposes filtration; (3) the colloid osmotic pressure of the glomerular capillary plasma proteins (π_G), which averages 32 mm Hg and opposes filtration; and (4) the colloid osmotic pressure of proteins in Bowman's capsule (π_B), which is near zero and therefore under normal conditions has little effect on filtration.

$$\text{Net Filtration Pressure} = P_G - P_B - \pi_G = 10\,\text{mm Hg}$$

$$GFR = K_f \times (P_G - P_B - \pi_B) = 125\,\text{mL/min}$$

Decreased Glomerular Capillary Filtration Coefficient (K_f) Decreases the GFR. Although changes in K_f have a proportional effect on the GFR, this is not a primary mechanism for physiologic control of the GFR. Nevertheless, in some diseases, such as uncontrolled *hypertension* and *diabetes mellitus*, the GFR is reduced because of increased thickness of the glomerular capillary membrane, which reduces the K_f, or because of severe damage to the capillaries and loss of capillary filtration surface area.

Increased Bowman's Capsule Pressure Decreases the GFR. Changes in Bowman's capsule pressure normally do not control the GFR; however, in certain pathologic states, such as urinary tract obstruction, Bowman's capsule pressure may increase to such a high level that the GFR is reduced. For example, precipitation of calcium or uric acid may lead to "stones" that lodge in the urinary tract, often in the ureter, thereby obstructing urine flow and increasing Bowman's capsule pressure.

Increased Glomerular Capillary Colloid Osmotic Pressure Decreases the GFR. The two factors that influence glomerular capillary colloid osmotic pressure are (1) the arterial colloid osmotic pressure and (2) the fraction of plasma filtered by the glomerular capillaries *(filtration fraction)*. An increase in either the arterial colloid osmotic pressure or the filtration fraction increases the glomerular capillary colloid osmotic pressure. Conversely, a decrease in the arterial plasma colloid osmotic pressure or the filtration fraction reduces the glomerular colloid osmotic pressure. Because the filtration fraction is the GFR/renal plasma flow ratio, a decrease in renal plasma flow increases the filtration fraction. Therefore even with constant glomerular hydrostatic pressure, decreased renal blood flow tends to increase the glomerular colloid osmotic pressure and decrease the GFR.

Increased Glomerular Capillary Hydrostatic Pressure Increases the GFR. Glomerular hydrostatic pressure is determined by three variables, each of which is physiologically regulated:

- *Arterial pressure.* Increased arterial pressure tends to increase the glomerular hydrostatic pressure and the GFR. However, this effect is normally buffered by *autoregulation,* which minimizes the effect of blood pressure on the glomerular hydrostatic pressure.
- *Afferent arteriolar resistance.* Increased resistance of afferent arterioles decreases the glomerular hydrostatic pressure and the GFR.
- *Efferent arteriolar resistance.* Increased efferent arteriolar resistance increases the resistance to outflow of the glomerular capillaries and the glomerular hydrostatic pressure, thereby tending to increase the GFR so long as the increased efferent resistance does not reduce renal blood flow to a great extent. With severe efferent constriction (e.g., more than a three-four fold increase in resistance), the large decrease in renal blood flow more than offsets the increase in glomerular hydrostatic pressure and reduces the GFR.

Glomerular Filtration and Renal Blood Flow Are Controlled by Neurohumoral Systems and Intrarenal Mechanisms *(p. 317)*

The determinants of the GFR that are most variable and subject to physiologic control include the glomerular hydrostatic pressure and glomerular capillary colloid osmotic pressure. These pressures, in turn, are influenced by the sympathetic nervous system, hormones, autacoids (vasoactive substances released in the kidney), and other intrarenal feedback control mechanisms.

Strong Sympathetic Nervous System Activation Decreases GFR. Strong activation of the sympathetic nervous system constricts the renal arterioles and decreases renal blood flow and the GFR. This effect is most important in reducing the GFR during severe, acute disturbances such as those elicited by the defense reaction, brain ischemia, or severe hemorrhage.

Hormones and Autacoids Control the GFR and Renal Blood Flow. Several hormones and autacoids can also influence the GFR and renal blood flow.

- *Norepinephrine and epinephrine,* which are released from the adrenal medulla, constrict afferent and efferent arterioles and decrease the GFR and renal blood flow.
- *Endothelin,* a peptide released from damaged vascular endothelial cells of the kidneys and other tissues, constricts renal arterioles and decreases the GFR and renal blood flow.
- *Angiotensin II* constricts efferent arterioles to a greater extent than afferent arterioles and therefore tends to increase glomerular hydrostatic pressure while decreasing renal blood flow. Increased angiotensin II formation usually occurs with decreased arterial pressure or volume depletion, both of which tend to reduce the GFR. In these instances, increased angiotensin II levels help prevent decreases in the GFR by constricting efferent arterioles.
- *Endothelium-derived nitric oxide* (EDNO) decreases renal vascular resistance and increases the GFR and renal blood flow. EDNO, an autacoid released from vascular endothelial cells throughout the body, is important in preventing excessive vasoconstriction of the kidneys.
- *Prostaglandins* (especially PGE_2 and PGI_2) are not of major importance in the regulation of the GFR and renal blood flow under normal conditions. Prostaglandins, however, may dampen the renal vasoconstrictor

effects of sympathetic nerves or angiotensin II, especially the effects on the afferent arterioles. Blockade of prostaglandin synthesis (e.g., with aspirin and nonsteroidal anti-inflammatory drugs) may therefore cause significant decreases in the GFR and renal blood flow, especially in patients whose extracellular fluid volume is reduced as a result of vomiting, diarrhea, dehydration, or diuretic therapy.

GFR and Renal Blood Flow Are Autoregulated During Changes in Arterial Pressure (p. 319)

In normal kidneys, a fall in arterial pressure to as low as 75 mm Hg or a rise to as high as 160 mm Hg changes the GFR by only a few percentage points; this relative constancy of the GFR and renal blood flow is referred to as *autoregulation.* Although autoregulation of GFR and renal blood flow is not perfect it prevents potentially marked changes in the GFR and therefore in renal excretion of water and solutes that would otherwise occur with changes in blood pressure.

Tubuloglomerular Feedback Is a Key Component of Renal Autoregulation. This feedback has two parts—an afferent arteriolar mechanism and an efferent arteriolar mechanism—both of which depend on the special anatomic arrangement of the *juxtaglomerular complex.* The juxtaglomerular complex consists of *macula densa cells* in the initial portion of the distal tubule and *juxtaglomerular cells* in the walls of the afferent and efferent arterioles. When blood pressure is decreased, delivery of sodium chloride is decreased to the macula densa cells, which are capable of sensing this change. The decrease in sodium chloride concentration at the macula densa, in turn, causes two main effects: (1) a decrease in the resistance of the afferent arterioles, which increases glomerular hydrostatic pressure and the GFR toward normal levels, and (2) an increase in renin release from the juxtaglomerular cells of the afferent and efferent arterioles, which causes increased angiotensin II formation. Angiotensin II then constricts efferent arterioles, increases arterial pressure, and increases glomerular hydrostatic pressure and the GFR toward normal levels.

Myogenic Mechanism Contributes to Autoregulation of Renal Blood Flow and the GFR. This mechanism refers to the intrinsic capability of blood vessels to constrict when blood pressure is increased. The constriction prevents the vessel from being overstretched and, by increasing vascular resistance, helps prevent excessive increases in renal blood flow and the GFR when blood pressure rises. Conversely, with decreased blood pressure, the myogenic mechanism contributes to decreased vascular resistance.

Other Factors That Alter Renal Blood Flow and the GFR

- *A high-protein diet* increases the GFR and renal blood flow in part by stimulating growth of the kidneys and by reducing renal vascular resistance. One mechanism that contributes to the ability of protein to elevate the GFR is tubuloglomerular feedback. A high-protein diet increases the release of amino acids into the blood, which are reabsorbed in the proximal tubule through co-transport with sodium. This in turn causes increased proximal tubule reabsorption of amino acids and sodium, decreased sodium chloride delivery to the macula densa, decreased afferent arteriolar resistance, and increased GFR.

- *Hyperglycemia,* as occurs with uncontrolled diabetes mellitus, may also increase renal blood flow and the GFR through tubuloglomerular feedback because glucose, like amino acids, is co-transported with sodium in the proximal tubule.

- *Glucocorticoids* increase renal blood flow and the GFR by reducing renal vascular resistance.

- *Fever* increases renal blood flow and the GFR by reducing renal vascular resistance.

- *Aging* decreases renal blood flow and the GFR mainly because of a reduction in the number of functional nephrons; renal blood flow and the GFR decrease about 10% during each decade of life after age 40.

CHAPTER 27

Urine Formation by the Kidneys: II. Tubular Reabsorption and Secretion

Renal Tubular Reabsorption and Secretion (p. 323)

After the glomerular filtrate enters the renal tubules, it flows sequentially through the *proximal tubules, loops of Henle, distal tubules, collecting tubules,* and *collecting ducts* before it is excreted as urine. Along this course, some substances are reabsorbed from the tubules into the peritubular capillary blood, whereas others are secreted from the blood into the tubules. The urine that is formed and all of the substances in the urine represent the sum of three basic renal processes.

Urinary Excretion
= Glomerular Filtration − Tubular Reabsorption
+ Tubular Secretion

Tubular Secretion—The Net Movement of Solutes from Peritubular Capillaries into the Tubules

Some substances enter the tubules not only by glomerular filtration but also by secretion from the peritubular capillaries into the tubules via two steps: (1) simple diffusion of the substance from the peritubular capillaries into the renal interstitium and (2) movement of the substance across the tubular epithelium into the lumen through active or passive transport. Substances that are actively secreted into the tubules include *potassium* and *hydrogen ions* as well as certain *organic acids* and *organic bases.*

Reabsorption of Solutes and Water from the Tubules into the Peritubular Capillaries

For a substance to be reabsorbed, it must first be transported across the renal tubular epithelial membrane into the interstitial fluid and then through the peritubular capillary membrane back into the blood. Solutes can be transported either through the cell membranes *(transcellular route)* by active or passive transport or through the junctional spaces between the cells *(paracellular route)* by passive transport; water is transported through and between the epithelial cells by osmosis.

After absorption into the interstitial fluids, water and solutes are transported through the peritubular capillary walls by *ultrafiltration (bulk flow),* which is mediated by hydrostatic and colloid osmotic forces. In contrast to the glomerular capillaries, which filter large amounts of fluid and solutes, the peritubular capillaries have a large reabsorptive force that rapidly moves fluid and solutes from the interstitium into the blood.

Reabsorption Rates for Substances Are Selective and Highly Variable. Some substances that are filtered, such as glucose and amino acids, are almost completely reabsorbed by the tubules, so the urinary excretion rate is essentially zero (Table 27–1).

Most of the ions in the plasma, such as sodium, chloride, and bicarbonate, are also highly reabsorbed from the tubules, but their rates of reabsorption and urinary excretion vary depending on the needs of the body. The metabolic waste products, such as urea and creatinine, are poorly reabsorbed and are excreted in relatively large amounts. Tubular reabsorption is highly selective, allowing the kidneys to regulate excretion of substances independent of one another.

Active Transport Requires Energy and Can Move Solutes against an Electrochemical Gradient. Transport directly coupled to an energy source, such as hydrolysis of adenosine triphosphate (ATP), is termed *primary active transport.* A good example is the *sodium-potassium ATPase pump,* which plays a major role in reabsorption of sodium ions in many parts of the nephron. On the basal and lateral sides of the tubular epithelial cells, the *basolateral membrane* has an extensive sodium-potassium ATPase system that hydrolyzes ATP and uses the released energy to transport sodium ions out of the cell into the interstitium. At the same time, potassium is transported from the interstitium to the inside of the cell. This pumping of sodium out of the cell across the basolateral membrane favors passive diffusion of sodium into the cell across the *luminal membrane* (the side that faces the tubular lumen) and passive diffusion of potassium out of the cell into the tubular lumen.

In certain parts of the nephron there are additional mechanisms for moving large amounts of sodium into the cell. In the proximal tubules, there is an extensive *brush border* on the luminal side of the membrane that multiplies the surface by 20-fold. There also are *sodium carrier proteins* that bind sodium ions on the luminal surface of the membrane and release them inside the cell, providing *facilitated diffusion* of sodium through the membrane into the cell. These sodium carrier

Table 27–1. Filtration, Reabsorption, and Excretion Rates of Various Substances by the Kidneys

Substance	Amount Filtered	Amount Reabsorbed	Amount Excreted	% of Filtered Load Resorbed
Glucose (g/day)	180	180	0	100
Bicarbonate (mmol/day)	4320	4318	2	>99.9
Sodium (mmol/day)	25,560	25,410	150	99.4
Chloride (mmol/day)	19,440	19,260	180	99.1
Urea (g/day)	46.8	23.4	23.4	50
Creatinine (g/day)	1.8	0	1.8	0

proteins are also important for secondary active transport of other substances, such as glucose and amino acids.

Secondary Active Reabsorption of Glucose and Amino Acids Occurs through the Renal Tubular Membrane. During secondary active transport, two or more substances interact with a specific membrane protein and are co-transported together across the membrane. As one of the substances (e.g., sodium) diffuses down its electrochemical gradient, the energy released is used to drive another substance (e.g., glucose) against its electrochemical gradient. Secondary active transport does not require energy directly from ATP or other high-energy phosphate sources; rather, the source of the energy is that liberated by simultaneous facilitated diffusion of another transported substance down its own electrochemical gradient.

Transport Maximums Are Often Displayed for Actively Transported Substances. Many of the nutrients, such as glucose and amino acids, are reabsorbed through secondary active transport with sodium. In most instances, reabsorption of these substances displays a *transport maximum,* which refers to the maximum rate of reabsorption. When the filtered load of these substances exceeds the transport maximum, the excess amount is excreted. The *threshold* is the tubular load at which the transport maximum is exceeded in one or more nephrons, resulting in the appearance of that solute in the urine. The threshold usually occurs at a slightly lower tubular load than the transport maximum because not all nephrons have the same transport maximum and some nephrons excrete glucose before others have reached their transport maximum.

Passive Water Reabsorption by Osmosis Is Coupled to Sodium Reabsorption. When solutes are transported out of the tubule via primary or secondary active transport, their concentrations decrease in the tubule and increase in the interstitium. This creates a concentration difference that causes osmosis of water in the same direction as that in which the solutes are transported— from the tubular lumen to the interstitium. Some parts of the renal tubule, especially the *proximal tubules,* are highly permeable to water, and reabsorption occurs so rapidly that there is only a small concentration gradient across the membrane. In the *ascending loops of Henle,* however, water permeability is always low, so almost no water is reabsorbed despite a large osmotic gradient.

In the *distal tubules, collecting tubules,* and *collecting ducts,* water permeability depends on the presence or absence of *antidiuretic hormone* (ADH). In the presence of ADH, these sections of the renal tubule are highly permeable to water.

Some Solutes Are Reabsorbed by Passive Diffusion. When sodium, a positive ion, is reabsorbed through the tubular cell, negative ions such as *chloride* also tend to diffuse passively through the paracellular pathway (between the cells). Additional reabsorption of chloride also occurs because of a concentration gradient that develops when water is reabsorbed from the tubule by osmosis, thereby concentrating the chloride ions in the tubular lumen.

Noncharged substances, such as *urea,* are also passively reabsorbed from the tubule because osmotic reabsorption of water tends to concentrate these solutes in the tubular lumen, favoring their diffusion into the renal interstitium. Urea and many other waste products do not permeate the tubule nearly as rapidly as water, allowing large amounts of these substances to be excreted in urine.

Reabsorption and Secretion Along Various Parts of the Nephron (p. 329)

Proximal Tubules Have a High Capacity for Reabsorption. Approximately 65% of the filtered load of water, sodium, chloride, potassium, and several other electrolytes is reabsorbed in the proximal tubules. One important function of the proximal tubules therefore is to conserve substances that are needed by the body, such as glucose, amino acids, proteins, water, and electrolytes. In contrast, the proximal tubules are not as permeable to waste products of the body and reabsorb a much smaller percentage of the filtered load of the substances.

The Loop of Henle Has Three Functionally Distinct Segments: Descending Thin Segment, Ascending Thin Segment, and Ascending Thick Segment. The loop of Henle dips into the inner part of the kidney, the renal medulla, and plays an important role in allowing the kidney to form concentrated urine. The *descending thin loop of Henle* is highly permeable to water, which is rapidly reabsorbed from the tubular fluid into the hyperosmotic interstitium (osmolarity rises to 1200–1400 mOsm/L in the inner renal medulla); approximately 20% of the glomerular filtrate volume is reabsorbed in the thin descending loop of Henle, causing the tubular fluid to become hyperosmotic as it moves toward the inner renal medulla.

In the *thin and thick segments of the ascending loop of Henle,* water permeability is virtually zero, but large amounts of sodium, chloride, and potassium are reabsorbed, causing the tubular fluid to become dilute (hypotonic) as it moves back toward the cortex. At the same time, active transport of sodium chloride out of the thick ascending loop of Henle into the interstitium causes a very high concentration of these ions in the interstitial fluid of the renal medulla. As in the proximal tubule, reabsorption of sodium chloride in the loop of Henle is closely linked to activity of the sodium-potassium ATPase pump in the basolateral membrane. In addition, sodium chloride is rapidly transported across the luminal membrane by a *1-sodium, 2-chloride, 1-potassium cotransporter.* About 25% of the filtered loads of sodium, chloride, and potassium are reabsorbed in the loop of Henle, mostly in the thick ascending limb. Considerable amounts of other ions, such as calcium, bicarbonate, and magnesium, are also reabsorbed in the thick ascending loop of Henle.

The thick ascending limb of the loop of Henle is the site of action of the powerful *"loop diuretics"* furosemide (Lasix), ethacrynic acid, and bumetanide, all of which inhibit the 1-sodium, 2-chloride, 1-potassium co-transporter.

The Early Distal Tubule Dilutes the Tubular Fluid. The thick segment of the ascending limb empties into the distal tubule. The first portion of the distal tubule forms part of the *juxtaglomerular complex,* which provides feedback control of the glomerular filtration rate (GFR) and blood flow in the same nephron, as described in Chapter 26. The next early portion of the distal tubule has many of the same characteristics as the ascending loop of Henle and avidly reabsorbs most of the ions; however, it is virtually impermeable to water and urea. For this reason, it is referred to as the *diluting segment;* it also dilutes the tubular fluid. Fluid leaving this part of the nephron usually has an osmolarity of only about 100 mOsm/L.

A *sodium chloride co-transporter* moves sodium chloride from the lumen into the epithelial cells of the early distal tubule. The *thiazide diuretics,* used to treat disorders such as hypertension and heart failure, inhibit the sodium chloride co-transporter.

The Late Distal Tubule and Cortical Collecting Tubule Are Similar. The second half of the distal tubules and the cortical collecting tubules have similar functional characteristics. Anatomically, they are composed of two distinct cell types: the *principal cells,* which absorb sodium and water from the lumen and secrete potassium into the lumen, and the *intercalated cells,* which absorb potassium ions and secrete hydrogen ions into the tubular lumen.

The tubular membranes of both segments are almost completely impermeable to urea, and their permeability to water is controlled by the ADH concentration. With high levels of ADH, these segments are highly permeable to water. The reabsorption of sodium and secretion of potassium by the principal cells are controlled by the hormone *aldosterone.* Secretion of hydrogen ions by the intercalated cells plays an important role in acid-base regulation of the body fluids (discussed later).

The principal cells are the main sites of action of *potassium-sparing diuretics,* including *spironolactone and eplerenone* (antagonists of aldosterone's effects of the mineralocorticoid receptor) and *amiloride* (a sodium channel blocker).

Medullary Collecting Ducts Are the Final Sites for Processing the Urine. Although the medullary collecting ducts reabsorb less than 10% of the filtered water and sodium, they are extremely important when determining the final urine output of water and solutes. Some special characteristics of this tubular segment are as follows:

1. Its permeability to water is controlled by ADH; with high ADH levels, water is rapidly reabsorbed, thereby reducing urine volume and concentrating most solutes in the urine.
2. The medullary collecting duct is highly permeable to urea and there are special *urea transporters* that facilitate urea diffusion across the luminal and basolateral membranes. This allows some of the urea in the tubule to be absorbed into the medullary interstitium and helps to raise the osmolality of the renal medulla, which contributes to the overall ability of the kidneys to form concentrated urine.
3. It secretes hydrogen ions against a large concentration gradient, thereby playing a key role in acid-base regulation.

Regulation of Tubular Reabsorption (p. 334)

Because it is essential to maintain precise balance between tubular reabsorption and glomerular filtration, multiple nervous, hormonal, and local control mechanisms regulate the tubular reabsorption rate as well as the GFR. An important feature of tubular reabsorption is that excretion of water and solutes can be independently regulated, especially through hormonal control.

Glomerulotubular Balance—The Ability of the Tubule to Increase its Reabsorption Rate in Response to a Greater Tubular Load. If the GFR is increased, the absolute rate of tubular reabsorption is increased approximately in proportion to the rise in GFR. Glomerulotubular balance helps prevent overloading of the more distal parts of the renal tubule when the GFR increases; however, glomerulotubular balance does not completely prevent changes in the GFR from altering urinary excretion.

Peritubular Capillary and Renal Interstitial Fluid Physical Forces Influence Tubular Reabsorption. As the glomerular filtrate passes through the renal tubules, more than 99% of the water and most of the solutes are reabsorbed—first into the renal interstitium and then into the peritubular capillaries. Of the fluid that is normally filtered by the glomerular capillaries (125 mL/min), approximately 124 mL/min is reabsorbed into the peritubular capillaries.

Peritubular capillary reabsorption is regulated by hydrostatic and colloid osmotic pressures acting across the capillaries and by the capillary filtration coefficient (K_f), as shown in the following relation:

$$\text{Reabsorption} = K_f \left(P_c - P_{if} - \pi_c + \pi_{if} \right)$$

where P_c is the peritubular capillary hydrostatic pressure, P_{if} is the interstitial fluid hydrostatic pressure, π_c is the colloid osmotic pressure of the peritubular capillary plasma proteins, and π_{if} is the colloid osmotic pressure of proteins in the renal interstitium. The two primary determinants of peritubular capillary reabsorption that are directly influenced by renal hemodynamic changes are the hydrostatic and colloid osmotic pressures of the peritubular capillaries. The peritubular capillary hydrostatic pressure is, in turn, influenced by (1) the arterial pressure and (2) the resistance of the afferent and efferent arterioles (Table 27–2).

Table 27–2. Factors That Can Influence Peritubular Capillary Reabsorption

$\uparrow P_c \rightarrow \downarrow$ Reabsorption
$\downarrow R_A \rightarrow \uparrow P_c$
$\downarrow R_E \rightarrow \uparrow P_c$
$\uparrow$Arterial pressure $\rightarrow \uparrow P_c$
$\uparrow \pi_c \rightarrow \uparrow$Reabsorption
$\uparrow \pi_A \rightarrow \uparrow \pi_c$
$\uparrow$FF $\rightarrow \uparrow \pi_c$
$\uparrow$Capillary filtration coefficient $\rightarrow \uparrow$Reabsorption

π_c, peritubular capillary colloid osmotic pressure; π_A, systemic plasma colloid osmotic pressure; FF, filtration fraction; P_c, peritubular capillary hydrostatic pressure; R_A and R_E, afferent and efferent arteriolar resistances, respectively.

The peritubular capillary colloid osmotic pressure is influenced by (1) the systemic plasma colloid osmotic pressure and (2) the *filtration fraction,* which is the GFR/renal plasma flow ratio. The higher the filtration fraction, the greater is the fraction of plasma that is filtered through the glomerular capillaries; consequently, the more concentrated become the proteins in the plasma that remains behind. An increase in filtration fraction therefore tends to increase the peritubular capillary reabsorption rate.

Increased Arterial Pressure Reduces Tubular Reabsorption. Even small increases in arterial pressure can increase the urinary excretion rates of sodium and water, phenomena referred to as *pressure natriuresis* and *pressure diuresis,* respectively. There are three primary mechanisms by which increased arterial pressure increases urinary excretion:

1. Increased arterial pressure causes slight elevations in renal blood flow and the GFR; in normal kidneys, the GFR and renal blood flow usually change less than 10% between arterial pressures of 75 and 160 mm Hg because of the renal autoregulatory mechanisms discussed in Chapter 26.
2. Increased arterial pressure increases the peritubular capillary hydrostatic pressure, especially in the vasa recta of the renal medulla; this in turn decreases

peritubular capillary reabsorption, which increases back-leakage of sodium into the tubular lumen, thereby decreasing the net sodium and water reabsorption and increasing the urine output.

3. Increased arterial pressure also decreases angiotensin II formation, which greatly decreases sodium reabsorption by the renal tubules (discussed later).

Aldosterone Increases Sodium Reabsorption and Potassium Secretion. Aldosterone, which is secreted by the adrenal cortex, acts on *mineralocorticoid receptors* mainly on the *principal cells* of the cortical collecting tubule to stimulate the sodium-potassium ATPase pump, which increases sodium reabsorption from the tubule and potassium secretion into the tubule. In the absence of aldosterone, as occurs with destruction or malfunction of the adrenals *(Addison's disease)*, there is marked loss of sodium from the body and accumulation of potassium. Conversely, excess aldosterone secretion, as occurs in patients with adrenal tumors *(Conn's syndrome)*, is associated with sodium retention and potassium depletion.

Angiotensin II Increases Sodium and Water Reabsorption. Angiotensin II, the most powerful sodium-retaining hormone of the body, increases sodium and water reabsorption through three main effects:

1. Angiotensin II stimulates aldosterone secretion, which in turn increases sodium reabsorption.

2. Angiotensin II constricts the efferent arterioles, which reduces peritubular capillary hydrostatic pressure and increases filtration fraction by reducing renal blood flow; both of these effects tend to increase the reabsorptive force at the peritubular capillaries and tubular reabsorption of sodium and water.

3. Angiotensin II directly stimulates sodium reabsorption, in most tubular segments.

These multiple actions of angiotensin II cause marked sodium and water retention by the kidneys in circumstances associated with low blood pressure, low extracellular fluid volume, or both, such as during hemorrhage or loss of salt and water from body fluids.

ADH Increases Water Reabsorption. ADH, secreted by the posterior pituitary gland, increases water permeability of the distal tubules, collecting tubules, and collecting ducts. These portions of the nephron then reabsorb water avidly and form highly concentrated urine. These effects help the body conserve water during circumstances such as dehydration, which greatly stimulates ADH secretion. In the absence of ADH, these portions of the nephrons are virtually impermeable to water, causing the kidneys to excrete large amounts of dilute urine.

Atrial Natriuretic Peptide Decreases Sodium and Water Reabsorption. Specific cells of the cardiac atria, when distended as a result of plasma volume expansion, secrete a peptide called *atrial natriuretic peptide*. Greater levels of this peptide inhibit reabsorption of sodium and water by the renal tubules, thereby increasing the excretion of sodium and water.

Parathyroid Hormone Increases Calcium Reabsorption and Decreases Phosphate Reabsorption. Parathyroid hormone is one of the most important calcium- and phosphate-regulating hormones of the body. Its principal action in the kidneys is to increase reabsorption of calcium, especially in the distal tubules. Another action of parathyroid hormone is inhibition of phosphate reabsorption by the proximal tubule.

Sympathetic Nervous System Activation Increases Sodium Reabsorption. Stimulation of the sympathetic nervous system constricts the afferent and efferent arterioles, thereby decreasing the GFR. At the same time, sympathetic activation directly increases sodium reabsorption in the proximal tubule, ascending loop of Henle, and distal tubule while stimulating renin release and angiotensin II formation.

Use of Clearance Methods to Quantify Kidney Function *(p. 340)*

Renal Clearance Is the Volume of Plasma That Is Completely Cleared of a Substance Each Minute. For a given substance X, renal clearance is defined as the ratio of the excretion rate of substance X to its concentration in the plasma, as shown by the following relation:

$$C_X = (U_X \times V)/P_X$$

where C_X is renal clearance in milliliters per minute, $U_X \times V$ is the excretion rate of substance X (U_X is the concentration of X in the urine, and V is urine flow rate in milliliters per minute), and P_X is the plasma concentration of X. Renal clearances can be used to quantify several aspects of kidney functions, including the rates of glomerular filtration, tubular reabsorption, and tubular secretion of various substances.

Renal Clearance of Creatinine or Inulin Can Be Used to Estimate the GFR. *Creatinine,* a byproduct of skeletal muscle metabolism, is filtered at the glomerulus but is not reabsorbed or secreted appreciably by the tubules; therefore the entire 125 mL of plasma that filters into the tubules each minute (GFR) is cleared of creatinine. This means that creatinine clearance is approximately equal to the GFR. For this reason, creatinine clearance is often used as an index of the GFR. An even more accurate measure of GFR is the clearance of *inulin,* a polysaccharide that is not reabsorbed or secreted by the renal tubules.

Renal Clearance of Para-aminohippuric Acid (PAH) Can Be Used to Estimate Renal Plasma Flow. Some substances, such as PAH, are freely filtered and not reabsorbed by the tubules but are secreted into the tubules; therefore, the renal clearance of these substances is greater than the GFR. In fact, about 90% of the plasma flowing through the kidney is completely cleared of PAH, and renal clearance of PAH (C_{PAH}) can be used to estimate the renal plasma flow, as follows:

$$C_{PAH} = (U_{PAH} \times V)/P_{PAH} \cong \text{Renal Plasma Flow}$$

where U_{PAH} and P_{PAH} are urine and plasma concentrations of PAH, respectively, and V is the urine flow rate.

The *filtration fraction* is the GFR/renal plasma flow ratio. If renal plasma flow is 650 mL/min and the GFR is 125 mL/min, the filtration fraction is 125/650, or 0.19.

Tubular Reabsorption or Secretion Can Be Calculated from Renal Clearances. For substances that are completely reabsorbed from the tubules (e.g., amino acids, glucose), the clearance rate is zero because the urinary secretion rate is zero. For substances that are highly reabsorbed (e.g., sodium), the clearance rate is usually less than 1% of the GFR, or less than 1 mL/min. In general, waste products of metabolism, such as urea, are poorly reabsorbed and have relatively high clearance rates.

The tubular reabsorption rate is calculated as the difference between the rate of filtration of the substance (GFR $\times$ P_X) and the urinary excretion rate ($U_X \times V$), as follows:

$$\text{Reabsorption}_X = (\text{GFR} \times P_X) - (U_X \times V)$$

If the excretion rate of a substance is greater than the filtered load, the rate at which it appears in the urine represents the sum of the rate of glomerular filtration plus tubular secretion; the secretion rate is therefore the difference between the rate of urinary excretion of a substance and the rate at which it is filtered, as follows:

$$\text{Secretion}_X = (U_X \times V) - (GFR \times P_X)$$

Urine Concentration and Dilution; Regulation of Extracellular Fluid Osmolarity and Sodium Concentration

To function properly, cells must be bathed in extracellular fluid with a relatively constant concentration of electrolytes and other solutes. The total concentration of solutes in the extracellular fluid (the osmolarity) is determined by the amount of solute divided by the volume of the extracellular fluid. The most abundant solutes in the extracellular fluid are sodium and chloride; to a large extent, extracellular fluid osmolarity is determined by the amounts of extracellular sodium chloride and water, which are determined by the balance between intake and excretion of these substances.

In this chapter, we discuss the mechanisms that permit the kidney to excrete either dilute or concentrated urine and therefore to regulate extracellular fluid sodium concentration and osmolarity. We also discuss the mechanisms that govern fluid intake.

Kidneys Excrete Excess Water by Forming Dilute Urine (p. 345)

When there is excess water in the body, the kidneys can excrete urine with an osmolarity as low as 50 mOsm/L. Conversely, when there is a deficit of water, the kidneys can excrete urine with a concentration as high as 1200 to 1400 mOsm/L. Equally important, the kidneys can excrete a large volume of dilute urine or a small volume of concentrated urine without a major change in the rate of solute excretion.

Antidiuretic Hormone Controls Urine Concentration. When the osmolarity of the body fluids increases above normal, the posterior pituitary gland secretes more antidiuretic hormone (ADH), which increases the permeability of the distal tubules and collecting ducts to water, causing large amounts of water to be reabsorbed and decreasing urine volume without a marked alteration in renal solute excretion.

When there is excess water in the body and the extracellular fluid osmolarity is reduced, the secretion of ADH decreases, thereby reducing the permeability of the distal tubules and collecting ducts to water and causing large amounts of dilute urine to be excreted.

Dilute Urine Is Caused by Decreased ADH and Decreased Water Reabsorption. When the glomerular filtrate is formed, its osmolarity is about the same as that of plasma (300 mOsm/L). As fluid flows through the proximal tubules, solutes and water are reabsorbed in equal proportions and little change in osmolarity occurs. As fluid flows down the descending loop of Henle, water is reabsorbed and tubular fluid reaches equilibrium with the surrounding interstitial fluid, which is extremely hypertonic (osmolarity as high as 1200 to 1400 mOsm/L). In the ascending limb of the loop of Henle, especially the thick segment, sodium, potassium, and chloride are avidly reabsorbed, but because this part of the tubule is impermeable to water, even in the presence of ADH, the tubular fluid becomes more dilute as it flows into the early distal tubule. *Regardless of whether ADH is present, fluid leaving the early distal tubule is hypo-osmotic, with an osmolarity of only about one third that of plasma.*

As the dilute fluid of the early distal tubule passes into the late distal convoluted tubule, cortical collecting ducts, and medullary collecting ducts, there is additional reabsorption of sodium chloride and other solutes. In the absence of ADH the tubule is relatively impermeable to water, and additional reabsorption of solutes causes the tubular fluid to become even more dilute, decreasing its osmolarity to as low as 50 mOsm/L. This failure to reabsorb water and continued reabsorption of solutes lead to a large volume of dilute urine (Fig. 28–1).

Kidneys Conserve Water by Excreting Concentrated Urine (p. 346)

When there is a water deficit in the body and the plasma osmolarity and ADH levels are elevated, the kidneys form concentrated urine by continuing to excrete solutes while increasing water reabsorption and decreasing urine volume. The *two basic requirements for forming concentrated urine* are as follows:

- *A high level of ADH,* which allows the distal tubules and collecting tubules to reabsorb water avidly
- *A high osmolarity of the renal medullary interstitial fluid*

Tubular fluid flowing out of the loop of Henle is normally dilute, with an osmolarity of only about 100 mOsm/L. The medullary interstitium outside the collecting tubules in the renal medulla is normally highly concentrated with sodium and urea owing to the operation of the *countercurrent multiplier,* which

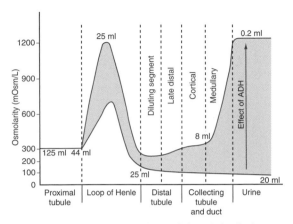

Figure 28–1. Changes in osmolarity of the tubular fluid as it passes through the tubular segments in the presence of high levels of antidiuretic hormone (ADH) and in the absence of ADH. Numerical values indicate the approximate volumes in milliliters per minute or osmolarities in milliosmoles per liter of fluid flowing along the various tubular segments.

depends on the special permeability characteristics of the loop of Henle. As fluid flows into the distal tubules and finally into the collecting tubules and ducts, water is reabsorbed until tubular fluid osmolarity equilibrates with the surrounding medullary interstitial fluid osmolarity. This process leads to highly concentrated urine with an osmolarity of 1200 to 1400 mOsm/L when high ADH levels are present (see Fig. 28–1).

The Countercurrent Multiplier Causes High Osmolarity in the Renal Medulla. For the renal medulla to increase its osmolarity to a range of 1200 to 1400 mOsm/L, the medullary interstitium must accumulate solutes in great excess of water. Once this has occurred, the high osmolarity is maintained by a balanced inflow and outflow of solutes and water in the medulla.

The major factors that contribute to the build-up of solute concentration in the renal medulla are the following:

- Active transport of sodium ions and co-transport of potassium, chloride, and other ions out of the thick ascending limb of the loop of Henle into the medullary interstitium
- Active transport of ions from the collecting ducts into the medullary interstitium

- Facilitated diffusion of large amounts of urea from the inner medullary collecting ducts into the medullary interstitium
- Diffusion of only small amounts of water from the medullary collecting tubules into the interstitium, far less than the reabsorption of solutes into the medullary interstitium, and virtually no water diffusion into the medulla from the ascending loop of Henle

Countercurrent Exchange in the Vasa Recta Preserves the Hyperosmolarity of the Renal Medulla. There are two special features of the *vasa recta* (which carry blood flow to the renal medulla) that help preserve the high solute concentrations:

1. *Vasa recta blood flow is low,* accounting for only 1% to 2% of the total renal blood flow. This sluggish flow is sufficient to supply the metabolic needs of the tissues and helps minimize solute loss from the medullary interstitium.
2. *The vasa recta serve as countercurrent exchangers,* minimizing washout of solutes from the medullary interstitium. This countercurrent exchange feature is due to the U shape of the vasa recta capillaries.

As blood descends into the medulla, it becomes progressively more concentrated because the vasa recta capillaries are highly permeable to water and solutes. However, as blood ascends back toward the cortex, it becomes progressively less concentrated as solutes diffuse back out into the medullary interstitium and water moves into the vasa recta. Although there is a large amount of fluid and solute exchange across the vasa recta, there is little net loss of solutes from the interstitial fluid.

Quantifying the Renal Urine Concentration and Dilution with "Free-Water" and Osmolar Clearances *(p. 354)*

When urine is dilute, water is excreted in excess of solutes. Conversely, when urine is concentrated, solutes are excreted in excess of water. The rate at which solutes are cleared from the blood can be expressed as the *osmolar clearance* (C_{osm}); this is a measurement of the volume of plasma cleared of solutes each minute:

$$C_{osm} = (U_{osm} \times V)/P_{osm}$$

where U_{osm} is the urine osmolarity, V is the urine flow rate, and P_{osm} is the plasma osmolarity.

The relative rates at which solutes in water are excreted can be assessed using the concept of *free-water clearance* (C_{H_2O}), which is defined as the difference between water excretion (urine flow rate) and osmolar clearance.

$$C_{H_2O} = V - C_{osm} = V - (U_{osm} \times V)/P_{osm}$$

The rate of free-water clearance is the rate at which solute-free water is excreted by the kidneys. When free-water clearance is *positive*, excess water is being excreted by the kidneys; when free-water clearance is *negative*, excess solutes are being removed from blood by the kidneys and water is being conserved.

Disorders of Urinary Concentrating Ability *(p. 354)*

Impaired ability of the kidneys to concentrate urine can occur with one or more of the following abnormalities:

- *Decreased secretion of the ADH,* which is referred to as *"central" diabetes insipidus.* This results in an inability to produce or release ADH from the posterior pituitary resulting from head injuries, infections, or congenital abnormalities.
- *Inability of the kidneys to respond to ADH,* a condition called *"nephrogenic" diabetes insipidus.* This abnormality can be caused by failure of the countercurrent mechanism to form a hyperosmotic renal medullary interstitium or by failure of the distal and collecting tubules and collecting ducts to respond to ADH. Many *renal diseases can impair the concentrating mechanism,* especially those that damage the renal medulla. In addition, *impaired functioning of the loop of Henle,* as occurs with diuretics that inhibit electrolyte reabsorption in that segment, can compromise urine-concentrating ability. Marked *increases in renal medullary blood flow* can "wash out" some of the solutes in the renal medulla and reduce the maximal concentrating ability. No matter how much ADH is present, maximal urine concentration is limited by the degree of hyperosmolarity of the medullary interstitium.

Also, certain drugs, such as lithium (used to treat manic-depressive disorders) and tetracyclines (antibiotics used to treat infections), can impair the ability of the distal nephron segments to respond to ADH.

Control of Extracellular Fluid Osmolarity and Sodium Concentration *(p. 355)*

The regulation of extracellular fluid osmolarity and sodium concentration are closely linked because sodium is the most abundant cation in the extracellular compartment. Plasma sodium concentration is normally regulated within close limits of 140 to 145 mEq/L, with an average concentration of about 142 mEq/L. Osmolarity averages about 300 mOsm/L (about 282 mOsm/L when corrected for interionic attraction) and seldom changes more than 2% to 3%.

Although multiple mechanisms control the amount of sodium and water excreted by the kidneys, two primary systems are particularly involved in regulating the concentration of sodium and the osmolarity of extracellular fluid: (1) the osmoreceptor-ADH feedback system and (2) the thirst mechanism.

Osmoreceptor-ADH Feedback System

When osmolarity (plasma sodium concentration) increases above normal, the osmoreceptor-ADH feedback system operates as follows:

- Increased extracellular fluid osmolarity stimulates *osmoreceptor cells* in the anterior hypothalamus, near the supraoptic nuclei, to send signals that are relayed to the posterior pituitary gland.
- Action potentials conducted to the posterior pituitary stimulate release of ADH, which is stored in secretory granules in the nerve endings.
- ADH, which is transported in blood to the kidneys, increases water permeability of the late distal tubules, cortical collecting tubules, and medullary collecting ducts.
- Increased water permeability in the distal nephron segments causes increased water reabsorption and excretion of a small volume of concentrated urine. This causes dilution of solutes in extracellular fluid, thereby correcting the initial excessively concentrated extracellular fluid.

The opposite sequence of events occurs when extracellular fluid becomes too dilute (hypo-osmotic).

ADH Is Synthesized in the Supraoptic and Paraventricular Nuclei of the Hypothalamus and Released from the Posterior Pituitary. The hypothalamus contains two types of large neuron that synthesize ADH: about five sixths of the ADH is synthesized in the *supraoptic nuclei* and about one sixth in the *paraventricular nuclei.* Both nuclei have axonal extensions to the posterior pituitary. Once ADH is synthesized, it is transported down the axons or the neurons that terminate in the posterior pituitary.

Secretion of ADH in response to an osmotic stimulus is rapid, so plasma ADH levels can increase several-fold within minutes, providing a rapid means of altering renal excretion of water.

Cardiovascular Reflex Stimulation of ADH Release by Decreased Arterial Pressure, Decreased Blood Volume, or Both. ADH release is also controlled by cardiovascular reflexes, including the *arterial baroreceptor reflex* and the *cardiopulmonary reflex,* both of which were discussed in Chapter 18. Afferent stimuli carried by the *vagus* and *glossopharyngeal nerves* synapse with nuclei of the tractus solitarius; and projections from these nuclei relay signals to the hypothalamic nuclei that control ADH synthesis and secretion. Whenever blood pressure and blood volume are reduced, such as occurs during hemorrhage, increased ADH secretion through these reflex pathways causes increased fluid reabsorption by the kidneys, helping to restore blood pressure and blood volume toward normal levels.

Although the usual day-to-day regulation of ADH secretion is effected mainly by changes in plasma osmolarity, large changes in blood volume, such as occur during hemorrhage, also elicit marked increases in ADH levels.

Other Stimuli Cause ADH Secretion. The various factors that can increase or decrease ADH secretion are summarized in Table 28–1.

Table 28–1. Regulation of ADH Secretion

Increase ADH	Decrease ADH
↑Plasma osmolarity	↓Plasma osmolarity
↓Blood volume	↑Blood volume
↓Blood pressure	↑Blood pressure
Nausea	—
Hypoxia	—
Drugs	Drugs
Morphine	Alcohol
Nicotine	Clonidine (antihypertensive drug)
Cyclophosphamide	Haloperidol (dopamine blocker)

Importance of Thirst in Controlling Extracellular Fluid Osmolarity and Sodium Concentration (p. 357)

The kidneys minimize fluid loss through the osmoreceptor-ADH feedback system; however, adequate fluid intake is necessary to counterbalance fluid losses that normally occur through sweating and breathing and through the intestinal tract. Fluid intake is regulated by the thirst mechanism, which together with the osmoreceptor-ADH mechanism maintains precise control of extracellular fluid osmolarity and sodium concentration.

Many of the stimuli involved in controlling ADH secretion also increase thirst, the conscious desire for water (Table 28–2). Two of the most important stimuli for thirst are increased extracellular fluid osmolarity and decreased extracellular fluid volume and arterial pressure. A third important stimulus for thirst is *angiotensin II*. Because angiotensin II is also stimulated by low blood volume and low blood pressure, its effect on thirst as well as its actions on the kidneys to decrease fluid excretion help restore blood volume and blood pressure toward normal.

Other factors that influence water intake include dryness of the mouth and mucous membranes of the esophagus and the degree of gastric distention. These stimuli to the gastrointestinal tract are relatively short-lived, and the desire to drink is completely satisfied only when plasma osmolarity, blood volume, or both return to normal.

The ADH and Thirst Mechanisms Operate Together to Control Extracellular Osmolarity. Normally, these two mechanisms work in parallel to regulate extracellular fluid osmolarity and sodium concentration precisely, despite the constant challenge of dehydration. Even with additional challenges, such as high salt intake, these feedback mechanisms are able to keep plasma osmolarity

Table 28–2.   Control of Thirst

Increase Thirst	Decrease Thirst
↑Plasma osmolarity	↓Plasma osmolarity
↓Blood volume	↑Blood volume
↓Blood pressure	↑Blood pressure
↑Plasma angiotensin II	↓Plasma angiotensin II
Dryness of mouth	Gastric distention

reasonably constant. When either the ADH or thirst mechanism fails, the other ordinarily can still keep extracellular osmolarity and sodium concentration relatively constant, so long as there is sufficient fluid intake to balance the daily obligatory urine volume and water losses caused by respiration, sweating, and gastrointestinal losses. If both the ADH and thirst mechanisms fail simultaneously, however, neither sodium concentration nor osmolarity can be adequately controlled. In the absence of these mechanisms, there are no other feedback mechanisms in the body capable of precisely regulating plasma osmolarity.

Angiotensin II and Aldosterone Do Not Normally Play a Major Role in Controlling Extracellular Osmolarity and Sodium *Concentration*. As discussed in Chapter 27, angiotensin II and aldosterone are the two most important hormonal regulators of renal tubular sodium reabsorption. Despite the importance of these hormones in regulating sodium *excretion*, they do not have a major effect on plasma sodium *concentration* for two reasons:

1. Angiotensin II and aldosterone increase both sodium and water reabsorption by the renal tubules, leading to greater extracellular fluid volume and sodium *quantity* but little change in sodium *concentration*.
2. So long as the ADH and thirst mechanisms are functional, any tendency toward increased plasma sodium concentration is compensated for by increased water intake or increased ADH secretion, which tends to dilute the extracellular fluid back toward normal.

Under the extreme conditions associated with the complete loss of aldosterone secretion resulting from adrenalectomy or Addison's disease, there is a tremendous loss of sodium by the kidneys, which can lead to decreased plasma sodium concentration. One of the reasons is that large losses of sodium are accompanied by severe volume depletion and decreased blood pressure, which can activate the thirst mechanism and lead to further dilution of plasma sodium concentration even though increased water intake helps minimize decreased body fluid volumes. There are extreme conditions during which plasma sodium concentration may change significantly, even with a functional ADH-thirst mechanism. Even so, the ADH-thirst mechanism is by far the most powerful feedback system in the body for controlling extracellular fluid osmolarity and sodium concentration.

CHAPTER 29

Renal Regulation of Potassium, Calcium, Phosphate, and Magnesium; Integration of Renal Mechanisms for Control of Blood Volume and Extracellular Fluid Volume

Regulation of Extracellular Fluid Potassium Concentration and Potassium Excretion
(p. 361)

Extracellular fluid potassium concentration normally is regulated precisely at about 4.2 mEq/L, seldom rising or falling more than ±0.3 mEq/L. A special difficulty in regulating potassium concentration is the fact that about 98% of the total body potassium is contained in the cells and only 2% in the extracellular fluid. Failure to rapidly rid the extracellular fluid of the potassium ingested each day could result in life-threatening *hyperkalemia* (increased plasma potassium concentration). A small loss of potassium from the extracellular fluid could cause severe *hypokalemia* in the absence of rapid compensatory responses.

Internal Potassium Distribution Is Regulated. After ingestion of a large meal, the rise in extracellular fluid potassium concentration would be lethal if the ingested potassium did not move rapidly into the cells. For example, absorption of 40 mmol of potassium (the amount contained in a meal rich in vegetables and fruit) into an extracellular fluid volume of 14 L would increase the plasma potassium concentration by about 2.9 mmol/L if all the potassium remained in the extracellular compartment. Fortunately, most of the ingested potassium rapidly moves into the cells until the kidneys can, over time, eliminate the excess. Table 29–1 summarizes some of the factors that can influence the distribution of potassium between the intra- and extracellular compartments.

The most important hormone that increases cell potassium uptake after a meal is *insulin.* In people who have insulin deficiency resulting from diabetes mellitus, the rise in plasma potassium concentration after eating a meal is much greater than normal.

Increased potassium intake also stimulates secretion of *aldosterone*, which increases cell potassium uptake. Excess aldosterone secretion, as occurs in Conn's syndrome, is almost invariably associated with hypokalemia,

Table 29–1. Factors That Can Alter Potassium Distribution between the Intracellular and Extracellular Fluid

Factors That Shift K$^+$ into Cells (Decrease Extracellular K$^+$)	Factors That Shift K$^+$ Out of Cells (Increase Extracellular K$^+$)
Insulin	Insulin deficiency (diabetes mellitus)
Aldosterone	Aldosterone deficiency (Addison's disease)
β-adrenergic stimulation	β-adrenergic blockade Cell lysis
Alkalosis	Strenuous exercise Increased extracellular fluid osmolarity Acidosis

due in part to movement of extracellular potassium into the cells. Conversely, patients with deficient aldosterone production (Addison's disease) often have significant hyperkalemia resulting from accumulation of potassium in the extracellular space as well as to renal retention of potassium.

Metabolic *acidosis* increases the extracellular potassium concentration in part by causing loss of potassium from the cells, whereas *metabolic alkalosis* decreases the extracellular fluid potassium concentration.

Cell injury can cause release of large amounts of potassium from the cells into the extracellular compartment. This can cause significant hyperkalemia if large amounts of tissue are destroyed, as occurs with severe muscle injury or red blood cell lysis.

Strenuous exercise can cause hyperkalemia by releasing potassium from skeletal muscle.

Increased extracellular fluid osmolarity causes cell dehydration, which in turn raises the intracellular potassium concentration and promotes diffusion of potassium from the cells to the extracellular fluid.

Daily Variations in Potassium Excretion Are Controlled Mainly by Changes in Secretion in Distal and Collecting Tubules. Maintaining potassium balance depends primarily on renal excretion because the amount of potassium in the feces is normally about

5% to 10% of the potassium intake. Renal potassium excretion is determined by the sum of three processes: (1) the rate of potassium filtration [the glomerular filtration rate (GFR) multiplied by the plasma potassium concentration]; (2) the rate of potassium reabsorption by the tubules; and (3) the rate of potassium secretion by the tubules. About 65% of the filtered potassium is reabsorbed in the proximal tubule and another 25% to 30% in the loop of Henle.

The normal day-to-day variation of potassium excretion, however, is regulated mainly by secretion in the distal and collecting tubules rather than by changes in glomerular filtration or tubular reabsorption. Potassium is sometimes reabsorbed in these tubular segments (e.g., during potassium depletion), and at other times it is secreted in large amounts depending on the needs of the body. With high potassium intake, the required extra excretion of potassium is achieved almost entirely through increased secretion of potassium in the distal and collecting tubules.

Potassium Secretion Occurs in the *Principal Cells* of the Late Distal Tubules and Cortical Collecting Tubules. Secretion of potassium from the peritubular capillary blood into the lumen of the distal and collecting tubules is a three-step process involving (1) passive diffusion of potassium from blood to the renal interstitium, (2) active transport of potassium from interstitium into tubular cells by the sodium-potassium ATPase pump at the basolateral membrane, and (3) passive diffusion of potassium from the cell interior to the tubular fluid. The primary factors that control potassium secretion by the principal cells include the following:

- *Increased extracellular potassium concentration, which increases potassium secretion.* The mechanisms for this effect include stimulation of the sodium-potassium ATPase pump, an increase in the potassium gradient from the interstitial fluid to the tubular lumen, and the effect of a higher potassium concentration to stimulate aldosterone secretion, which further stimulates potassium secretion.

- *Increased aldosterone concentration, which increases potassium secretion.* This effect is mediated through multiple mechanisms, including stimulation of the sodium-potassium ATPase pump and increased permeability of the luminal membrane for potassium.

- *Increased tubular flow rate, which increases potassium secretion.* The mechanism for the effect of a high volume flow rate is as follows: When potassium is secreted into the tubular fluid, the luminal concentration of potassium increases, thereby reducing the driving force for potassium diffusion into the tubule. With increased tubular flow rate, however, the secreted potassium is continuously flushed down the tubule, and the rise in tubular potassium concentration is minimized, thereby increasing the net potassium secretion.

- *Acute increases in hydrogen ion concentration (acidosis), which decrease potassium secretion.* The mechanism for this effect is inhibition of the sodium-potassium ATPase pump by the elevated hydrogen ion concentration.

Aldosterone Is the Primary Hormonal Mechanism for Feedback Control of Extracellular Fluid Potassium Ion Concentration. There is direct feedback by which aldosterone and extracellular fluid potassium ion concentration are linked. This feedback mechanism operates as follows: Whenever the extracellular fluid potassium concentration increases above normal, aldosterone secretion is stimulated, which increases renal excretion of potassium, returning the extracellular potassium concentration toward normal. The opposite changes take place when the potassium concentration is too low.

Acute Acidosis Decreases Potassium Secretion. Acute increases in hydrogen ion concentration of the extracellular fluid (acidosis) reduce potassium secretion, whereas decreased hydrogen ion concentration (alkalosis) increases potassium secretion. Increased hydrogen ion concentration inhibits potassium secretion is by reducing the activity of the sodium-potassium ATPase pump.

Control of Renal Calcium Excretion and Extracellular Calcium Ion Concentration (p. 367)

As with other substances, the intake of calcium must be balanced with the net loss of calcium over the long term. Unlike ions such as sodium and chloride, however, a large share of calcium excretion occurs in the feces. Only about 10% of the ingested calcium normally is reabsorbed in the intestinal tract, with the remainder excreted in the feces. Most of the calcium in the body (99%) is stored in the bones, with only about 1% in the intracellular fluid and 0.1% in the extracellular fluid. Bones therefore act as large reservoirs for storing calcium and as sources of calcium when the extracellular fluid calcium concentration tends to decrease *(hypocalcemia)*.

Parathyroid Hormone (PTH) Is an Important Regulator of Bone Uptake and Release of Calcium

Decreased extracellular fluid calcium concentration promotes increased secretion of PTH, which acts directly on bones to increase the *resorption* of bone salts (release of bone salts from the bones) and therefore release of large amounts of calcium into the extracellular fluid. When the calcium ion concentration is elevated *(hypercalcemia)*, PTH secretion decreases, and the excess calcium is deposited in the bones.

The bones, however, do not have an inexhaustible supply of calcium. Over the long term, the intake of calcium must be balanced with calcium excretion by the gastrointestinal tract and kidneys. The most important regulator of calcium reabsorption at both of these sites is PTH; thus PTH regulates the plasma calcium concentration through three main effects: (1) stimulating bone resorption; (2) stimulating activation of vitamin D, which increases intestinal absorption of calcium; and (3) directly increasing renal tubular calcium reabsorption. This is discussed in more detail in Chapter 79.

PTH Reduces Renal Calcium Excretion. Calcium is not secreted by the renal tubules, and its excretion rate is therefore determined by the rate of calcium filtration and tubular reabsorption. One of the primary controllers of renal tubular calcium reabsorption is PTH. With increased levels of PTH, there is increased calcium reabsorption through the thick ascending loop of Henle and distal tubule, which reduces urinary excretion of calcium. Conversely, decreased PTH promotes calcium excretion by reducing reabsorption in the loop of Henle and distal tubules.

Greater plasma phosphate concentration stimulates PTH, which increases calcium reabsorption by the renal tubules and decreases calcium excretion.

Calcium reabsorption is also stimulated by *metabolic acidosis* and inhibited by *metabolic alkalosis.*

Integration of Renal Mechanisms for Control of Extracellular Fluid Volume *(p. 370)*

When discussing control of extracellular fluid volume, we must consider factors that regulate the amount of sodium chloride in extracellular fluid because the sodium chloride content of the extracellular fluid usually parallels the extracellular fluid volume, provided the antidiuretic hormone (ADH)-thirst mechanisms are operative. In most cases, the burden of extracellular volume regulation is placed on the kidneys, which must adapt their excretion to match varying intakes of salt and water.

Sodium Excretion Is Precisely Matched with Sodium Intake Under Steady-State Conditions. An important consideration for overall control of sodium excretion—or excretion of any electrolyte—is that under steady-state conditions a person must excrete almost precisely the amount of sodium ingested. Even with disturbances that cause major changes in renal excretion of sodium, the balance between intake and excretion is usually restored within a few days.

Sodium Excretion Is Controlled by Altering Glomerular Filtration or Tubular Reabsorption Rates. The kidney alters sodium and water excretion by changing the rate of filtration, the rate of tubular reabsorption, or both, as follows:

$$\text{Excretion} = \text{Glomerular Filtration} - \text{Tubular Reabsorption}$$

As discussed previously, glomerular filtration and tubular reabsorption are both regulated by multiple factors, including hormones, sympathetic activity, and arterial pressure. Normally, the GFR is about 180 L/day, tubular reabsorption is 178.5 L/day, and urine excretion is 1.5 L/day. Small changes in either the GFR or tubular reabsorption have the potential to cause large changes in renal excretion.

Tubular reabsorption and GFR are usually regulated precisely, so excretion by the kidneys can be exactly matched to the intake of water and electrolytes. Even with disturbances that alter the GFR or tubular reabsorption, changes in urinary excretion are minimized by various buffering mechanisms. Two intrarenal buffering mechanisms are (1) *glomerulotubular balance*, which allows the renal tubules to increase their reabsorption rates in response to increased GFR and filtered sodium load, and (2) *macula densa feedback*, in which increased sodium chloride delivery to the distal tubules, resulting from an increased GFR or decreased proximal or loop of Henle sodium reabsorption, causes afferent arteriolar constriction and decreased GFR.

Because neither of these two intrarenal feedback mechanisms operates perfectly to restore urine output to normal, changes in the GFR or tubular reabsorption can lead to significant changes in sodium and water excretion. When this happens, *systemic feedback mechanisms* come into play—such as changes in blood pressure and changes in various hormones—that eventually return sodium excretion to equal intake.

Importance of Pressure Natriuresis and Pressure Diuresis for Maintaining Body Sodium and Fluid Balance *(p. 371)*

One of the most powerful mechanisms for controlling blood volume and extracellular fluid volume and for maintaining sodium and fluid balance is the effect of blood pressure on sodium and water excretion (*pressure natriuresis* and *pressure diuresis,* respectively). As discussed in Chapter 19, this feedback between the kidneys and circulation also plays a dominant role in long-term blood pressure regulation.

Pressure diuresis refers to the effect of increased arterial pressure to increase urinary volume excretion, whereas pressure natriuresis refers to the increased sodium excretion that occurs with increased arterial pressure. Because pressure diuresis and natriuresis usually occur in parallel, we often refer to these mechanisms simply as *pressure natriuresis.*

Pressure Natriuresis Is a Key Component of the *Renal–Body Fluid Feedback Mechanism.* During changes in sodium and fluid intake, this mechanism helps maintain fluid balance and minimizes changes in blood volume, extracellular fluid volume, and arterial pressure as follows:

1. An increase in fluid intake (assuming that sodium accompanies the fluid) above the level of urine output causes a temporary accumulation of fluid in the body and a small increase in blood volume and extracellular fluid volume.

2. An increase in blood volume increases the mean circulatory filling pressure and cardiac output.

3. An increase in cardiac output increases the arterial pressure, which increases urine output by way of pressure natriuresis. The steepness of the normal pressure natriuresis relation ensures that only a slight increase in blood pressure is required to increase urinary excretion several-fold.

4. An increase in fluid excretion balances the greater intake, and further accumulation of fluid is prevented.

The renal–body fluid feedback mechanism prevents continuous accumulation of salt and water in the body during increased salt and water intake. So long as kidney function is normal and pressure natriuresis is operating effectively, large increases in salt and water intake can be accommodated with only slight increases in blood volume, extracellular fluid volume, and arterial pressure. The opposite sequence of events occurs when fluid intake falls below normal.

As discussed later, there are nervous and hormonal systems, in addition to intrarenal mechanisms, that can raise salt and water excretion to match increased intake even without measurable increases in arterial pressure in many persons. Some individuals, however, are more "salt sensitive" and have significant increases in arterial pressure with even moderate increases in sodium intake. When blood pressure does rise, pressure natriuresis provides a critical means of maintaining balance between sodium intake and urinary sodium excretion.

Distribution of Extracellular Fluid Between the Interstitial Spaces and Vascular System (p. 373)

Ingested fluid and salt initially enter the blood but rapidly become distributed between the interstitial spaces and the plasma. Blood volume and extracellular fluid volume usually are controlled simultaneously and in parallel. There are conditions, however, that can markedly alter the distribution of extracellular fluid between the interstitial spaces and blood.

As discussed in Chapter 25, the principal factors that can cause loss of fluid from the plasma into the interstitial spaces (edema) include (1) increased capillary hydrostatic pressure, (2) decreased plasma colloid osmotic pressure, (3) increased permeability of the capillaries, and (4) obstruction of the lymphatic vessels.

Nervous and Hormonal Factors Increase the Effectiveness of Renal–Body Fluid Feedback (p. 373)

Nervous and hormonal mechanisms act in concert with pressure natriuresis to minimize the changes in blood volume, extracellular fluid volume, and arterial pressure that occur in response to day-to-day challenges. Abnormal kidney function or abnormal nervous and hormonal factors that influence the kidneys, however, can lead to serious changes in blood pressure and body fluid volumes (discussed later).

Sympathetic Nervous System Control of Renal Excretion by Arterial Baroreceptor and Low-Pressure Stretch Receptor Reflexes. The kidneys receive extensive sympathetic innervation, and under some conditions changes in sympathetic activity can alter renal sodium and water excretion and the extracellular fluid volume. For example, when blood volume is reduced by hemorrhage, reflex activation of the sympathetic nervous system occurs because of decreased pressure in the pulmonary blood vessels and other low-pressure regions of the thorax and because of low arterial pressure. The increased sympathetic activity in turn has several effects by which to reduce sodium and water excretion: (1) renal vasoconstriction, which decreases the GFR; (2) increased tubular reabsorption of salt and water; and (3) stimulation of renin release and increased formation of angiotensin II and aldosterone, both of which further elevate tubular reabsorption. All of these mechanisms together play an important role in the rapid restitution of the blood volume that occurs during acute conditions associated with reduced blood volume, low arterial pressure, or both.

Reflex decreases in renal sympathetic activity may contribute to rapid elimination of excess fluid in the circulation after ingestion of a meal that contains large amounts of salt and water.

Angiotensin II Is a Powerful Controller of Renal Excretion. When sodium intake is increased above normal, renin secretion decreases and causes reduced angiotensin II formation. Reduced angiotensin II levels have several effects on the kidney that decrease tubular sodium reabsorption (see Chapter 27). Conversely, when sodium intake is reduced, increased levels of angiotensin cause sodium and water retention and oppose decreases in arterial pressure that would otherwise occur. Changes in the activity of the renin-angiotensin system act as powerful amplifiers of the pressure natriuresis mechanism for maintaining stable blood pressure and body fluid volumes.

Although angiotensin II is one of the most powerful sodium- and water-retaining hormones in the body, *neither a decrease nor an increase in circulating angiotensin II has a large effect on extracellular fluid volume or blood volume in persons with an otherwise normal cardiovascular system.* The reason for this is that with large increases in angiotensin II levels, such as occurs with a renin-secreting tumor in the kidney, there is only transient sodium and water retention, which elevates the arterial pressure; this quickly increases kidney output of sodium and water, thereby overcoming the sodium-retaining effects of angiotensin II and reestablishing a balance between intake and output of sodium at a higher arterial pressure.

Conversely, *blockade of angiotensin II formation* with drugs, such as converting enzyme inhibitors and angiotensin II antagonists, greatly increases the ability of the kidneys to excrete salt and water but does not cause a major change in extracellular fluid volume. After blockade of angiotensin II, there is a transient increase in sodium and water excretion, but this reduces the arterial pressure, which helps re-establish the sodium balance. This effect of angiotensin II blockers has proved to be important for lowering blood pressure in hypertensive patients.

Aldosterone Has a Major Role in Controlling Renal Sodium Excretion. The function of aldosterone in regulating sodium balance is closely related to that described for angiotensin II; with decreased sodium intake, the increased angiotensin II levels stimulate aldosterone secretion, which contributes to decreased urinary sodium excretion and the maintenance of sodium balance. Conversely, with high sodium intake, suppression of aldosterone formation decreases tubular sodium reabsorption, allowing the kidneys to secrete large amounts of sodium. Changes in aldosterone formation also help the pressure natriuresis mechanism maintain sodium balance during variations in sodium intake.

However, *when there is excess aldosterone formation, as occurs in patients with tumors of the adrenal gland, the increased sodium reabsorption and decreased sodium excretion usually last only a few days,* and the extracellular fluid volume increases by only about 10% to 15%, causing increased arterial pressure. When the arterial pressure rises sufficiently, the kidneys "escape" from sodium and water retention (because of pressure natriuresis) and thereafter excrete amounts of sodium equal to the daily intake, despite continued high levels of aldosterone.

ADH Controls Renal Water Excretion. As explained previously, ADH plays an important role in allowing the kidneys to form a small volume of concentrated urine while excreting normal amounts of sodium. This effect is especially important during water deprivation. Conversely, when there is excess extracellular fluid volume, decreased ADH levels reduce reabsorption of water by the kidneys and help rid the body of excess volume.

Excessive levels of ADH, however, rarely cause large increases in arterial pressure or extracellular fluid volume. Infusion of large amounts of ADH into animals initially increases the extracellular fluid volume by only 10% to 15%. As the arterial pressure rises in response to this increased volume, much of the excess volume is excreted because of pressure diuresis; after several days, the blood volume and extracellular fluid volume are elevated by no more than 5% to 10%, and the arterial pressure is elevated by less than 10 mm Hg. High levels of ADH do not cause major increases in body fluid volume or arterial pressure, although *high ADH levels can cause severe reductions in the extracellular sodium ion concentration.*

Integrated Responses to Changes in Sodium Intake *(p. 376)*

Integration of the various control systems that regulate sodium and fluid excretion can be summarized by examining the homeostatic responses to increases in dietary sodium intake. As sodium intake is increased, sodium output initially lags behind intake. This causes slight increases in the cumulative sodium balance and the extracellular fluid volume. It is mainly the small increase in extracellular fluid volume that triggers various mechanisms in the body to increase the amount of sodium excretion. These mechanisms are as follows:

- *Activation of low-pressure receptor reflexes* that originate from the stretch receptors of the right atrium and pulmonary blood vessels. These reflexes inhibit sympathetic activity and angiotensin II formation, both of which tend to decrease tubular sodium reabsorption.

- *Increased secretion from the cardiac atria of atrial natriuretic peptide* (ANP), which reduces renal tubular sodium reabsorption.

- *Suppression of angiotensin II formation,* caused by increased arterial pressure and extracellular volume expansion, decreases tubular sodium reabsorption by eliminating the normal effect of angiotensin II to increase sodium reabsorption. In addition, decreased angiotensin II reduces aldosterone secretion, further reducing sodium reabsorption.

- *A small increase in arterial pressure,* which promotes sodium excretion through *pressure natriuresis.* If the nervous, hormonal, and intrarenal mechanisms are operating effectively, measurable increases in blood pressure may not occur even with large increases in sodium intake.

The combined activation of natriuretic systems and suppression of sodium- and water-retaining systems leads to increased excretion of sodium when sodium intake is increased. The opposite changes take place when sodium intake is reduced below normal levels.

Conditions That Cause Large Increases in Blood Volume and Extracellular Fluid Volume *(p. 376)*

Despite the powerful regulatory mechanisms that maintain blood volume and extracellular fluid volume at reasonably constant levels, there are abnormal conditions that can cause large increases in both of these variables. Almost all of these conditions result from circulatory abnormalities, including the following:

- *Heart diseases.* With congestive heart failure the blood volume may increase by 10% to 15%, and the extracellular fluid volume sometimes increases by 200% or more. Fluid retention by the kidneys helps return the arterial pressure and cardiac output toward normal if the heart failure is not too severe. If the heart is greatly weakened, however, the arterial pressure cannot increase sufficiently to restore urine output to normal. When this occurs, the kidneys retain a high volume of urine until the person develops severe circulatory congestion and eventually dies of edema, especially pulmonary edema.
- *Increased capacity of the circulation.* Any condition that increases vascular capacity also causes the blood volume to increase and fill this extra capacity. Examples of conditions associated with increased vascular capacity include *pregnancy* (resulting from increased vascular capacity of the uterus, placenta, and other enlarged organs) and *varicose veins,* which in severe cases may hold as much as an extra liter of blood.

Conditions That Cause Large Increases in Extracellular Fluid Volume but with Normal Blood Volume (p. 377)

There are several pathophysiologic conditions in which the extracellular fluid volume becomes markedly increased but the blood volume remains normal or even slightly decreased. These conditions are usually initiated by leakage of fluid and protein into the interstitium, which tends to decrease the blood volume. The kidneys' response to these conditions is similar to the response after hemorrhage—the kidneys retain salt and water in an attempt to restore the blood volume toward normal. Two examples are as follows:

• *Nephrotic syndrome*, characterized by a loss of plasma proteins in urine, reduces the plasma colloid osmotic pressure and causes the capillaries throughout the body to filter large amounts of fluid; this in turn causes edema and decreased plasma volume.

• *Liver cirrhosis*, characterized by decreased synthesis of plasma proteins by the liver. A sequence of events occurs during cirrhosis of the liver similar to that seen with nephrotic syndrome, except that with liver cirrhosis the decreased plasma protein concentration results from destruction of the liver cells, rendering them unable to synthesize enough plasma proteins. Cirrhosis is also associated with fibrous tissue in the liver structures, which greatly impedes the flow of portal blood through the liver. This elevates the capillary pressure throughout the portal circulation and contributes to leakage of fluid and proteins into the peritoneal cavity, a condition called *ascites.*

CHAPTER 30

Acid-Base Regulation

Hydrogen Ion (H^+) Concentration Is Precisely Regulated. The H^+ concentration in the extracellular fluid is maintained at a very low level, averaging 0.00000004 Eq/L (40 nEq/L). Normal variations are only about 3 to 5 nEq/L. Because the hydrogen ion concentration in extracellular fluid is extremely low and because these small numbers are difficult with which to work, the H^+ concentration is usually expressed as pH units. The pH is the logarithm of the reciprocal of H^+ concentration, expressed as equivalents per liter:

$$pH = \log \frac{1}{[H^+]} = -\log[H^+]$$

Arterial blood has a normal pH of 7.4, whereas the pH of venous blood and interstitial fluids is about 7.35. A person is considered to have *acidosis* when the arterial pH falls significantly below 7.4 and to have *alkalosis* when the pH rises above 7.4. The lower limit of pH at which a person can live for more than a few hours is about 6.8, and the upper limit is about 8.0.

Defenses against Changes in Hydrogen Ion Concentration: Buffers, Lungs, and Kidneys (p. 380)

The body has three primary lines of defense against changes in hydrogen ion concentration in the body fluids:

- *The chemical acid-base buffer systems of the body fluids,* which immediately combine with acid or base to prevent excessive changes in hydrogen ion concentration.
- *The respiratory system,* which regulates the removal of carbon dioxide (CO_2) and therefore carbonic acid (H_2CO_3) from the extracellular fluid. This mechanism operates within seconds to minutes and acts as a second line of defense.
- *The kidneys,* which excrete either alkaline or acidic urine, thereby adjusting the extracellular fluid hydrogen ion concentration toward normal during alkalosis or acidosis. This mechanism operates slowly but powerfully over a period of hours or several days to regulate the acid-base balance.

Buffering of Hydrogen Ions in the Body Fluids (p. 380)

A *buffer* is any substance that can reversibly bind H^+. The general form of a buffering reaction is as follows:

$$\text{Buffer} + H^+ \rightleftharpoons H\,\text{Buffer}$$

In this example, free H^+ combines with the buffer to form a weak acid (H buffer). When the H^+ concentration increases the reaction is forced to the right and more H^+ binds to the buffer for as long as available buffer is present. When the H^+ concentration decreases, the reaction shifts toward the left, and H^+ is released from the buffer.

Among the most important buffer systems in the body are *proteins* in the cells and, to a lesser extent, proteins in the plasma and interstitial fluids. The *phosphate buffer system* ($HPO_4^{2-}/H_2PO_4^-$) is not a major buffer in the extracellular fluid but is important as an intracellular buffer and as a buffer in renal tubular fluid. The most important extracellular fluid buffer is the *bicarbonate buffer system* (HCO_3^-/Pco_2), primarily because the components of the system, CO_2 and HCO_3^-, are closely regulated by the lungs and kidneys, respectively.

Bicarbonate Buffer System

The bicarbonate buffer system consists of a water solution that has two main ingredients: a weak acid, H_2CO_3, and a bicarbonate salt such as $NaHCO_3$. H_2CO_3 is formed in the body through the reaction of CO_2 with H_2O:

$$CO_2 + H_2O \underset{}{\overset{\text{Carbonic Anhydrase}}{\rightleftharpoons}} H_2CO_3$$

H_2CO_3 ionizes to form small amounts of H^+ and HCO_3^-:

$$H_2CO_3 \rightleftharpoons H^+ + HCO_3^-$$

The second component of the system, bicarbonate salt, occurs mainly as sodium bicarbonate ($NaHCO_3$) in the extracellular fluid. $NaHCO_3$ ionizes almost completely to form HCO_3^- and Na^+:

$$NaHCO_3 \rightleftharpoons Na^+ + HCO_3^-$$

Putting the entire system together, we have the following:

$$CO_2 + H_2O \rightleftharpoons H_2CO_3 \rightleftharpoons H^+ + \underbrace{HCO_3^-}_{+\ Na^+}$$

When a strong acid is added to this buffer solution, the increased hydrogen ions are buffered by HCO_3^-:

$$\uparrow H^+ + HCO_3^- \rightarrow H_2CO_3 \rightarrow CO_2 + H_2O$$

The opposite reaction takes place when a strong base, such as sodium hydroxide (NaOH), is added to a bicarbonate buffer solution:

$$NaOH + H_2CO_3 \rightarrow NaHCO_3 + H_2O$$

In this case, the OH^- from the NaOH combines with H_2CO_3 to form additional HCO_3^-. The weak base $NaHCO_3$ replaces the strong base NaOH. At the same time, the concentration of H_2CO_3 decreases (because it reacts with NaOH), causing more CO_2 to combine with H_2O to replace the H_2CO_3:

$$CO_2 + H_2O \rightarrow H_2CO_3 \rightarrow \uparrow HCO_3^- + H^+$$
$$+ \qquad\qquad +$$
$$NaOH \qquad\quad Na^+$$

The net result is a tendency for the CO_2 levels to decrease, but the reduced CO_2 in the blood inhibits respiration and therefore decreases the rate of CO_2 expiration. The rise in blood HCO_3^- is compensated for by the rise in renal excretion of HCO_3^-.

The Henderson-Hasselbalch Equation Gives the Relation of Bicarbonate and Carbon Dioxide to pH. The following is the Henderson-Hasselbalch equation:

$$pH = 6.1 + \log \frac{HCO_3^-}{0.03 \times Pco_2}$$

In this equation, CO_2 represents the acidic element because it combines with water to form H_2CO_3, and HCO_3^- represents the basic element. HCO_3^- is expressed as millimoles per liter, and Pco_2 is expressed as millimeters of mercury. The greater the Pco_2, the lower is the pH; the greater the HCO_3^-, the higher is the pH.

When disturbances of acid-base balance result from primary changes in extracellular HCO_3^-, they are referred to as *metabolic* acid-base disorders. Acidosis caused by a primary decrease in HCO_3^- concentration is termed *metabolic acidosis*, whereas alkalosis caused by a primary increase in HCO_3^- concentration is called *metabolic alkalosis*. Acidosis caused by an increase in P_{CO_2} is called *respiratory acidosis*, whereas alkalosis caused by a decrease in P_{CO_2} is called *respiratory alkalosis*.

Respiratory Regulation of Acid-Base Balance (*p. 384*)

Because the lungs expel CO_2 from the body, rapid ventilation by the lungs decreases the concentration of CO_2 in the blood, which in turn decreases the carbonic acid (H_2CO_3) and H^+ concentrations in the blood. Conversely, a decrease in pulmonary ventilation increases CO_2 and H^+ concentrations in the blood.

Increased Hydrogen Ion Concentration Stimulates Pulmonary Ventilation. Not only does the pulmonary ventilation rate influence the H^+ concentration by changing the P_{CO_2} of the body fluids, increased H^+ concentration markedly stimulates pulmonary ventilation. As pH decreases from the normal value of 7.4 to the strongly acidic value of 7.0, pulmonary ventilation increases to four to five times the normal rate. This in turn reduces the P_{CO_2} of blood and returns the H^+ concentration back toward normal. Conversely, if the pH increases above normal, the respiration becomes depressed, and the H^+ concentration increases toward normal. The respiratory system can return the H^+ concentration and pH to about two thirds of normal within a few minutes after a sudden disturbance of acid-base balance.

Abnormalities of Respiration Can Cause Acid-Base Disturbances. Impairment of lung function, such as in severe *emphysema*, decreases the ability of the lungs to eliminate CO_2; this causes a build-up of CO_2 in the extracellular fluid and a tendency toward *respiratory acidosis*. The ability to respond to metabolic acidosis is impaired because the compensatory reductions in P_{CO_2} that would normally occur because of increased ventilation are blunted. Conversely, overventilation (rare) causes a reduction in P_{CO_2} and a tendency toward *respiratory alkalosis*.

Renal Control of Acid-Base Balance (*p. 385*)

The kidneys control the acid-base balance by excreting either acidic urine, which reduces the amount of acid in extracellular fluid, or basic urine, which removes base from the extracellular fluid.

The overall mechanism by which the kidneys excrete acidic or basic urine is as follows: A large quantity of HCO_3^- is filtered continuously into the tubules; if HCO_3^- is excreted into the urine, base is removed from the blood. A large quantity of H^+ is also secreted into the tubular lumen, thus removing acid from the blood. If more H^+ is secreted than HCO_3^- is filtered, there is a net loss of acid from the extracellular fluid. Conversely, if more HCO_3^- is filtered than H^+ is secreted, there is a net loss of base. In addition to secretion of H^+ and reabsorption of filtered HCO_3^-, the kidneys can generate new HCO_3^- from reactions that take place in the renal tubule. *The kidneys regulate extracellular fluid H^+ concentrations through three basic mechanisms:* (1) secretion of H^+, (2) reabsorption of filtered HCO_3^-, and (3) production of new HCO_3^-.

Secretion of Hydrogen Ions and Reabsorption of Bicarbonate Ions by the Renal Tubules

Hydrogen ion secretion and bicarbonate reabsorption occur in virtually all parts of the tubules except the descending and ascending thin limbs of the loop of Henle. Bicarbonate is not reabsorbed directly by the tubules; instead, it is reabsorbed as a result of the reaction of secreted hydrogen ions with filtered bicarbonate ions in the tubular fluid under the influence of carbonic anhydrase in the tubular epithelium. For each HCO_3^- reabsorbed, there must be a H^+ secreted.

H^+ Is Secreted into the Tubular Fluid by Sodium–Hydrogen Countertransport in the Proximal Tubule, the Thick Ascending Segment of the Loop of Henle, and the Distal Tubule *(Fig. 30–1).* The secreted H^+ is consumed by reaction with HCO_3^-, forming H_2CO_3, which dissociates into CO_2 and H_2O. The CO_2 diffuses into the cell and is used to re-form H_2CO_3 and eventually HCO_3^-, which is reabsorbed across the basolateral membranes of the tubules.

Normally, more than 99% of the filtered HCO_3^- is reabsorbed by the renal tubules, with about 95% of the reabsorption occurring in the proximal tubules, loops of Henle, and early distal tubules.

In the Late Distal and Collecting Tubules, H^+ is Secreted by Primary Active Transport. The same basic mechanisms, however, are used for HCO_3^- reabsorption in the late distal and collecting tubule as used in the other tubular segments. Although the total amount of H^+

Figure 30–1. Cellular mechanisms for (1) active secretion of hydrogen ions into the renal tubule; (2) tubular reabsorption of bicarbonate by combination with hydrogen ions to form carbonic acid, which dissociates to form carbon dioxide and water; and (3) sodium ion reabsorption in exchange for the hydrogen ions secreted. This pattern of hydrogen ion secretion occurs in the proximal tubule, the thick ascending segment of the loop of Henle, and the early distal tubule.

secreted in the late distal tubules and collecting ducts is not large, these segments are capable of increasing the H^+ concentration as much as 900-fold, which reduces the pH of the tubular fluid to about 4.5, the lower limit of pH that can be achieved in normal kidneys.

Bicarbonate Ions Are "Titrated" Against Hydrogen Ions in the Tubules. Under normal conditions, the rate of tubular H^+ secretion is about 4400 mEq/day, and the rate of filtration of HCO_3^- is about 4320 mEq/day. The quantities of these two ions entering the tubules are almost equal, and they combine with each other to form CO_2 and H_2O; HCO_3^- and H^+ normally "titrate" each other in the tubules.

The titration process is not exact because there is usually a slight excess of H^+ in the tubules to be secreted into the urine. The excess H^+ (about 80 mEq/day) rids the body of nonvolatile acids produced by metabolism. Most of the H^+ is not excreted as free hydrogen ions but, rather, in combination with other urinary buffers, especially phosphate and ammonia.

With Alkalosis, There Is an Excess of Bicarbonate Ions Over Hydrogen Ions in the Urine. Because the HCO_3^- cannot be reabsorbed unless it reacts with H^+, the excess HCO_3^- is left in the urine and is eventually excreted, which helps correct the alkalosis.

With Acidosis, There Is an Excess of Hydrogen Ions Over Bicarbonate Ions in the Urine. This causes complete reabsorption of the filtered HCO_3^-, and the excess H^+ passes into the urine after combining with buffers in the tubules such as phosphate and ammonia. Thus the basic mechanism by which the kidneys correct for acidosis or alkalosis is incomplete titration of H^+ against HCO_3^-, leaving one to pass into the urine and therefore to be removed from the extracellular fluid.

Combination of Excess Hydrogen Ions with Phosphate and Ammonia Buffers in the Tubules—A Mechanism for Generating "New" Bicarbonate Ions (p. 388)

When H^+ is secreted in excess of HCO_3^- filtered into the tubular fluid, only a small part of the excess H can be excreted in the urine in ionic form (H^+); the minimum urine pH is about 4.5, corresponding to an H^+ concentration of $10^{-4.5}$ mEq/L, or 0.03 mEq/L.

Excretion of large amounts of H^+ (more than 500 mEq/day in severe acidosis) in the urine is accomplished primarily by combining H^+ with buffers in the tubular fluid. The two most important buffers are phosphate buffer and ammonia buffer. For each H^+ secreted that combines with a nonbicarbonate buffer, a new HCO_3^- is formed in the renal tubular cells and added to the body fluids.

Urinary Phosphate Buffer Carries Excess Hydrogen Ions into the Urine and Generates New Bicarbonate. The phosphate buffer system is composed of HPO_4^{2-} and $H_2PO_4^-$. The H^+ remaining in the renal tubule in excess of that which reacts with HCO_3^- can react with HPO_4^{2-} to form $H_2PO_4^-$, which can be excreted as a sodium salt (NaH_2PO_4). For each H^+ excreted with phosphate buffer, a new HCO_3^- is generated in the renal tubule and reabsorbed. The HCO_3^- generated in the tubular cell represents a net gain of HCO_3^- by the blood rather than merely a replacement of filtered HCO_3^-.

Under normal conditions, about 75% of the filtered phosphate is reabsorbed, and only about 30 to 40 mEq/day is available for buffering the H^+; therefore much of the buffering of excess H^+ in the tubular fluid in the presence of severe acidosis occurs through the ammonia buffer system.

Ammonia Is the Most Important Urinary Buffer in Chronic Acidosis. The ammonia buffer system is composed of ammonia (NH_3) and ammonia ion (NH_4^+). Ammonia ion is synthesized from *glutamine,* which is actively transported into the cells of the proximal tubules, thick ascending limbs in the loop of Henle, and distal tubules. Once inside the cell, each molecule of glutamine is metabolized to form two NH_4^+ and two HCO_3^-. The NH_4^+ is secreted into the tubular lumen in exchange for sodium, and the HCO_3^- moves across the basolateral membrane along with the reabsorbed sodium ion. For each molecule of glutamine metabolized, two NH_4^+ are secreted into the urine and two HCO_3^- are reabsorbed into the blood. *The HCO_3^- generated by this process constitutes new bicarbonate added to the blood.*

One of the most important features of the renal ammonia buffer system is that *renal glutamine metabolism is markedly stimulated by acidosis,* thereby increasing the formation of NH_4^+ and new HCO_3^- to be used for hydrogen ion buffering.

Quantifying Renal Tubular Acid Secretion (*p. 389*)

- The total rate of hydrogen secretion can be calculated as follows:

H^+ Secretion Rate $= HCO_3^-$ Reabsorption Rate

  $+$ Titratable Acid Excretion Rate

  $+ NH_4^+$ Excretion Rate

- This assumes that almost all the H^+ secreted either combines with HCO_3^-, which is reabsorbed, or is excreted with phosphate (titratable acid) or ammonia buffer.

- *The net acid excretion rate* is calculated as follows:

  Net Acid Excretion Rate

  $=$ Urinary Titratable Acid Excretion Rate

  $+ NH_4^+$ Excretion Rate

  $- HCO_3^-$ Excretion Rate

The reason we subtract HCO_3^- excretion is that loss of HCO_3^- is the same as adding H^+ to the blood. With acidosis, the net acid excretion rate increases markedly, thereby removing acid from the blood. The net acid excretion rate also equals the rate of a new bicarbonate addition to the blood. *With acidosis, there is a net addition of bicarbonate back to the blood as more NH_4^+ and urinary titratable acid are excreted.* With alkalosis, titratable acid and NH_4^+ excretion drop to zero, whereas HCO_3^- excretion increases. *With alkalosis, there is a negative net acid secretion.*

Renal Tubular Hydrogen Ion Secretion Is Stimulated by Increases in Pco_2 and Extracellular $[H^+]$. With alkalosis, tubular secretion of H^+ decreases to a level that is too low to achieve complete HCO_3^- reabsorption, enabling the kidneys to increase HCO_3^- excretion. With acidosis, tubular H^+ secretion is sufficient to reabsorb all the filtered HCO_3^- and the excess H^+ is excreted as NH_4^+ and titratable acid, thereby contributing large amounts of new HCO_3^- to the blood.

The two most important stimuli for increasing H^+ secretion by the tubules in acidosis are (1) an increase in the Pco_2 of the extracellular fluid in respiratory acidosis and (2) an increase in hydrogen ion concentration of the extracellular fluid (decreased pH) in respiratory and metabolic acidosis.

Renal Correction of Acidosis—Increased Excretion of Hydrogen Ions and Addition of New Bicarbonate Ions to the Extracellular Fluid *(p. 391)*

The condition of acidosis occurs when the arterial pH falls below 7.4. If the decrease in pH is caused by a decrease in HCO_3^-, the condition is referred to as *metabolic acidosis,* whereas a decrease in pH caused by an increase in Pco_2 is referred to as *respiratory acidosis.*

Regardless of whether the acidosis is respiratory or metabolic, both conditions cause a decrease in the HCO_3^-/H^+ ratio in renal tubular fluid. This results in an excess of H^+ in the renal tubules, causing complete reabsorption of HCO_3^- and leaving still additional H^+ available to combine with the urinary buffers NH_4^+ and HPO_4^{2-}. In acidosis, the kidneys reabsorb all of the filtered HCO_3^- and contribute new bicarbonate through the formation of NH_4^+ and titratable acid.

Metabolic Acidosis Results from Decreased Bicarbonate in Extracellular Fluids. The decreased extracellular fluid HCO_3^- concentration causes a decrease in glomerular filtration of HCO_3^-. The compensatory responses include stimulation of respiration, which eliminates CO_2 and returns the pH toward normal. At the same time, renal compensation increases reabsorption of HCO_3^- and excretion of titratable acid and NH_4^+, which leads to the formation of new HCO_3^- and return of the pH toward normal.

Some of the primary causes of metabolic acidosis are as follows:

- *Decreased renal tubular secretion of hydrogen ion or decreased reabsorption of bicarbonate.* This can occur as a result of a condition called *renal tubular acidosis,* in which the kidneys are unable to secrete adequate amounts of H^+. As a result, large amounts of HCO_3^- are lost in the urine, causing a continued state of metabolic acidosis. *Chronic renal failure,* which occurs when kidney function declines markedly and H^+ is not adequately secreted by the tubules, also causes build-up of acids in body fluids.
- *Formation of excess metabolic acids in the body.* An example is the metabolic acidosis that occurs with *diabetes mellitus* in which large amounts of acetoacetic acid are formed from metabolism of fats.
- *Ingestion of excess metabolic acids.* This can occur, for example, with ingestion of certain drugs, such as *acetylsalicylic acid (aspirin)* and *methyl alcohol,* which are metabolized to form formic acid.
- *Excessive loss of base from the body fluids.* This most commonly occurs with severe *diarrhea* in which large amounts of gastrointestinal secretions, containing bicarbonate, are lost from the body.

Respiratory Acidosis Is Caused by Decreased Ventilation, which Increases Pco_2. A decrease in the pulmonary ventilation rate increases the Pco_2 of the extracellular fluid, causing a rise in H_2CO_3, H^+ concentration, and respiratory acidosis. As compensation, the increased Pco_2 stimulates H^+ secretion by the renal tubules, causing increased HCO_3^- reabsorption. The excess H^+ remaining in the tubular cells combines with buffers, especially ammonia, which leads to the generation of new HCO_4^-, which is added back to the blood. These changes help return the plasma pH toward normal.

Common causes of respiratory acidosis are pathologic conditions that damage the respiratory centers or the ability of the lungs to eliminate CO_2 effectively.

For example, damage to the respiratory center in the medulla oblongata can cause respiratory acidosis. Obstruction of the passages of the respiratory tract, pneumonia, decreased pulmonary surface area, or any factor that interferes with the exchange of gases between the blood and alveolar membrane can cause respiratory acidosis.

Renal Correction of Alkalosis—Decreased Tubular Secretion of Hydrogen Ions and Increased Excretion of Bicarbonate Ions (p. 391)

Alkalosis occurs when the arterial pH rises above 7.4. If the increase in pH results mainly from an increase in plasma HCO_3^-, it is called *metabolic alkalosis,* whereas alkalosis caused by a decrease in Pco_2 is called *respiratory alkalosis.*

The compensatory responses to alkalosis are basically opposite those of acidosis. With alkalosis, the HCO_3^-/CO_2 ratio in the extracellular fluid increases, causing an increase in pH (a decrease in H^+ concentration). Regardless of whether the alkalosis is caused by metabolic or respiratory abnormalities, there still is an increase in the HCO_3^-/H^+ ratio in renal tubular fluid. The net effect is an excess of HCO_3^- that cannot be reabsorbed from the tubules and therefore is excreted in the urine. With alkalosis, HCO_3^- is removed from the extracellular fluid through renal excretion, which has the same effect as adding H^+ to the extracellular fluid.

Metabolic Alkalosis Results from Increased HCO_3^- in Extracellular Fluid. This causes an increase in the filtered load of HCO_3^-, which in turn results in an excess of HCO_3 over H^+ in the renal tubular fluid. The excess HCO_3^- in the tubular fluid fails to be reabsorbed because it does not have sufficient H^+ with which to react and therefore is excreted in the urine. With metabolic alkalosis, the primary compensations are increased renal excretion of HCO_3^- and a decreased ventilation rate, which increases the Pco_2.

Metabolic alkalosis is not nearly as common as metabolic acidosis, but some of the main causes are as follows:

• *Excess aldosterone secretion.* This promotes excessive reabsorption of sodium ions and at the same time stimulates secretion of H^+ by the intercalated cells of the collecting tubules. It leads to increased secretion of H^+

Table 30–1. Characteristics of Primary Acid-Base Disturbances

Disorder	pH	H$^+$	Pco$_2$	HCO$_3^-$
Respiratory acidosis	↓	↑	⇑	↑
Respiratory alkalosis	↑	↓	⇓	↓
Metabolic acidosis	↓	↑	↓	⇓
Metabolic alkalosis	↑	↓	↑	⇑

The primary event is indicated by the double arrow (⇑ or ⇓). Note that respiratory acid-base disorders are initiated by an increase or a decrease in Pco$_2$, whereas metabolic disorders are initiated by an increase or decrease in HCO$_3^-$.

by the kidneys, excessive production of HCO$_3^-$ by the kidney, and therefore metabolic alkalosis.

- *Vomiting of gastric contents.* Vomiting the gastric contents alone, without vomiting lower gastrointestinal contents, causes loss of HCl secreted by the stomach mucosa. The net result is a loss of acid from the extracellular fluid and the development of metabolic alkalosis.
- *Ingestion of alkaline drugs.* One of the most common causes of metabolic alkalosis is ingestion of drugs such as sodium bicarbonate for the treatment of gastritis or peptic ulcer.

Respiratory Alkalosis Is Caused by Increased Ventilation, which Decreases Pco$_2$. Respiratory alkalosis is rarely due to physical pathologic conditions; however, a *psychoneurosis* occasionally causes overbreathing to the extent that a person becomes alkalotic. A physiological respiratory alkalosis occurs when a person ascends to a *high altitude.* The low oxygen content of the air stimulates respiration, which causes excessive loss of CO$_2$ and the development of mild respiratory alkalosis. The primary compensations are the chemical buffers of the body fluids and the ability of the kidneys to increase HCO$_3^-$ excretion.

Table 30–1 shows the various acid-base disturbances and the characteristic changes in pH, hydrogen ion concentration, Pco$_2$, and bicarbonate ion concentration.

CHAPTER 31

Diuretics, Kidney Diseases

Diuretics and Their Mechanisms of Action (p. 397)

A Diuretic Increases the Rate of Urine Volume Output. Many diuretics also increase urinary excretion of solutes, especially sodium and chloride, as well as urine volume. Most of the diuretics used clinically act primarily by decreasing the rate of sodium chloride reabsorption in the renal tubules, which in turn causes natriuresis (increased sodium excretion) and diuresis (increased water output).

The most common clinical use of diuretics is to reduce extracellular fluid volume in diseases associated with edema and hypertension.

Balance between Salt and Water Intake and Renal Output Occurs during Chronic Diuretic Therapy. Some diuretics can increase urine output by more than 20-fold within a few minutes after they are administered; however, the effect of diuretics on renal output of salt and water subsides within a few days owing to activation of compensatory mechanisms initiated by decreased extracellular fluid volume. For example, reduced extracellular fluid volume decreases the arterial pressure and glomerular filtration rate (GFR) and increases renin secretion and angiotensin II formation. All these responses eventually override the effect of a diuretic on urine output so in the steady state urine output becomes equal to intake—but only after a reduction in extracellular fluid volume has occurred.

There are many diuretics available for clinical use, and they have different mechanisms of action and therefore inhibit tubular reabsorption at different sites along the renal nephron. The general classes of diuretics and their mechanisms of action are shown in Table 31–1.

Kidney Diseases (p. 399)

Severe kidney disease can be divided into two main categories: (1) *acute renal failure,* in which the kidneys abruptly stop working entirely, or almost entirely, but may eventually recover nearly normal function and (2) *chronic renal failure,* in which there is progressive loss of function of nephrons that gradually decreases overall kidney function. Within these two general categories, there are many specific kidney diseases that can affect

Table 31-1. Classes of Diuretics, Mechanisms of Action, and Tubular Sites of Action

Class	Example	Mechanism of Action	Tubular Site of Action
Osmotic diuretics	Mannitol	Inhibits water and solute reabsorption by increasing the osmolarity of tubular fluid	Mainly proximal tubule
Loop diuretics	Furosemide	Inhibits Na^+–K^+–Cl^- co-transport in luminal membrane	Thick ascending loop of Henle
Thiazide diuretics	Chlorothiazide	Inhibits Na^+–Cl^- co-transport in luminal membrane	Early distal tubules
Carbonic anhydrase inhibitors	Acetazolamide	Inhibits H^+ secretion and HCO_3^- reabsorption, which reduces Na^+ reabsorption	Proximal tubules
Mineralocorticoid receptor antagonists	Spironolactone	Inhibits action of aldosterone on tubular receptor, decreases Na^+ reabsorption, and decreases K^+ secretion	Collecting tubules
Sodium channel blockers	Amiloride	Blocks entry of Na^- into sodium channels of luminal membrane, decreases Na^+ reabsorption, and decreases K^+ secretion	Collecting tubules

the blood vessels, glomeruli, tubules, renal interstitium, and parts of the urinary tract outside the kidney. In this chapter, we discuss physiological abnormalities that occur in a few of the most important types of kidney diseases.

Diseases of the kidneys are among the most important causes of death and disability in many countries throughout the world. For example, in 2009, more than 26 million adults in the United States were estimated to have chronic kidney disease, and many more millions of people have acute renal failure or less severe forms of kidney dysfunction.

Acute Renal Failure

There are three main categories of acute renal failure.

Prerenal Acute Failure Is Caused by Decreased Blood Supply to the Kidneys. This can be a consequence of heart failure, which reduces cardiac output and blood pressure, or conditions associated with diminished blood volume, such as severe hemorrhage. When blood flow to the kidney falls to less than 20% of normal, the renal cells start to become hypoxic. Further decreases in flow, if prolonged, cause damage or death to the renal cells. If the acute renal failure is not corrected, this type of failure can evolve into *intrarenal acute renal failure.*

Intrarenal Acute Renal Failure Results from Abnormalities in the Kidney Itself, Including Those That Affect the Blood Vessels, Glomeruli, or Tubules. *Acute glomerulonephritis* is a type of intrarenal acute renal failure caused by an abnormal immune reaction that causes inflammation of the glomeruli. The acute inflammation usually subsides within about 2 weeks, although in some patients many of the glomeruli are destroyed beyond repair. In a small percentage of patients, continued renal deterioration leads to progressive *chronic renal failure* (discussed next).

Other causes of intrarenal acute renal failure include acute *tubular necrosis,* which is caused by severe renal ischemia or toxins and medications that damage the tubular epithelial cells. If the damage is not too severe, some regeneration of the tubular epithelial cells can occur, and renal function can be restored.

Postrenal Acute Renal Failure Is Caused by Obstruction of the Urinary Collecting System Anywhere from the Calyces to the Outflow from the Bladder. Important causes of obstruction of the urinary tract are *kidney stones,* which are caused by precipitation of calcium, urate, or cysteine.

Chronic Renal Failure: Irreversible Decrease in the Number of Functional Nephrons (p. 401)

Serious clinical symptoms of chronic renal failure often do not occur until the number of functional nephrons falls to at least 70% below normal. The maintenance of normal plasma concentrations of electrolytes and normal body fluid volumes occurs at the expense of systemic compensations, such as hypertension, which over the long term can lead to additional clinical problems.

Chronic renal failure, like acute renal failure, can occur because of disorders of the blood vessels, glomeruli, tubules, renal interstitium, and lower urinary tract. Despite the wide variety of diseases that can cause chronic renal failure, the end result is essentially the same—a decrease in the number of functional nephrons.

Chronic Renal Failure May Initiate a Vicious Circle That Leads to End-Stage Renal Disease. In some cases, an initial insult to the kidney leads to progressive deterioration of renal function and further loss of nephrons to the point at which to survive a person must be placed on dialysis treatment or must undergo transplantation with a functional kidney. This condition is referred to as *end-stage renal disease.*

The causes of this progressive injury are not known, but some investigators believe that thay may be related in part to increased pressure or stretch in the remaining glomeruli that results from adaptive vasodilatation or increased blood pressure. The increased pressure and stretch of arterioles and glomeruli are believed eventually to cause *sclerosis* (replacement of normal tissue with fibrous tissue) of these vessels. These sclerotic lesions eventually obliterate the glomerulus, leading to further reduction in kidney function and a slowly progressing vicious circle that terminates in end-stage renal disease. Among the most common causes of end-stage renal disease are *diabetes mellitus* and *hypertension,* which together account for more than 70% of all cases of chronic renal failure.

Some of the general causes of chronic renal failure are as follows:

- *Injured renal blood vessels.* Some of the most common causes of renal vascular injury are *atherosclerosis* of the large renal arteries, *fibromuscular hyperplasia* of one or more of the large arteries, and *nephrosclerosis,* a condition caused by sclerotic lesions of the smaller vessels and glomeruli that is often a result of hypertension or diabetes mellitus.

- *Injured glomeruli.* One example is *chronic glomerulonephritis*, which can be the result of several diseases that cause inflammation and damage to the glomerular capillaries. In contrast to the acute form of this disease, chronic glomerulonephritis is a slowly progressive disease that may lead to irreversible kidney failure. It may be a primary kidney disease, occurring after acute glomerulonephritis, or it may be secondary to a systemic disease, such as *lupus erythematosus.*

- *Injured renal interstitium.* Primary or secondary disease of the renal interstitium is referred to as *interstitial nephritis.* This can result from vascular, glomerular, or tubular damage that destroys individual nephrons, or it can involve primary damage to the renal interstitium caused by poisons, drugs, or bacterial infections. Renal interstitial injury caused by bacterial infection is called *pyelonephritis.* This infection can result from bacteria that reach the kidneys through the bloodstream or, more commonly, ascension from the lower urinary tract through the ureters to the kidney. With long-standing pyelonephritis, invasion of the kidneys by bacteria not only causes damage to the renal interstitium but also results in progressive damage to the renal tubules, glomeruli, and other structures, eventually leading to loss of functional nephrons.

Nephron Function in Chronic Renal Failure *(p. 404)*

The Loss of Functional Nephrons Requires Surviving Nephrons to Excrete More Water and Solutes. The kidneys normally filter about 180 L of fluid each day at the glomerular capillaries and then transform this filtrate to approximately 1.5 L of urine as the fluid flows along successive nephron segments. Regardless of the number of functional nephrons, the kidneys must excrete the same volume of urine (if intake is constant) to maintain fluid balance. The loss of functional nephrons therefore requires the surviving nephrons to excrete extra amounts of water and solutes to prevent serious accumulation of these substances in the body fluids. This is achieved by increasing the GFR or decreasing the tubular reabsorption rate in the surviving nephrons. These adaptations allow water and electrolyte balances to be maintained with little change in extracellular volume or electrolyte composition, even in patients who have lost as much as 70% of their nephrons.

In contrast to the electrolytes, many of the waste products of metabolism, such as urea and creatinine, accumulate almost in proportion to the number of nephrons that have been destroyed. These substances are not avidly reabsorbed by the renal tubules, and their excretion rate depends largely on the rate of glomerular filtration. If the GFR decreases, these substances accumulate in the body transiently, increasing the plasma concentration until the filtered load (GFR × plasma concentration) and the excretion rate (urine concentration × urine volume) return to normal, which is the same rate at which the substance is either ingested or produced in the body.

Some substances, such as phosphate, urate, and hydrogen ions, are maintained near normal until the GFR falls below 20% to 30% of normal. Plasma concentrations rise, thereafter, but not in proportion to the decline in the GFR (Figure 31–1). In the case of sodium and chloride ions, their plasma concentrations are maintained virtually constant even with severe decreases in GFR (see curve C of Figure 31–1). This is accomplished by greatly decreasing tubular reabsorption of these electrolytes.

Effects of Renal Failure on the Body Fluids—Uremia (p. 406)

The effect of renal failure on the body's fluids depends on the food and water intake and the degree of kidney function impairment. Assuming that intake remains relatively constant, important effects of renal failure include the following:

- *Water retention and development of edema.*
- *An increase in extracellular fluid urea (uremia) and other nonprotein nitrogens (azotemia).* The nonprotein nitrogens include urea, uric acid, creatinine, and a few less important compounds. These, in general, are the end products of protein metabolism.
- *Acidosis.* This results from failure of the kidneys to rid the body of normal acidic products. The buffers of the body fluids can normally buffer 500 to 1000 millimoles of acid without lethal increases in the extracellular hydrogen ion concentration. Each day, however, the body normally produces about 50 to 80 millimoles more metabolic acid than metabolic

Figure 31–1. Representative patterns of adaptation for different types of solutes in chronic renal failure. Curve A shows the approximate changes in the plasma concentrations of solutes such as creatinine and urea that are filtered and poorly reabsorbed. Curve B shows the approximate concentrations for solutes such as phosphate, urate, and hydrogen ion. Curve C shows the approximate concentrations for solutes such as sodium and chloride.

alkali. Complete renal failure therefore leads to severe accumulation of acid in the blood within a few days.
• *Anemia.* If the kidneys are seriously damaged, they are unable to form adequate amounts of erythropoietin, which stimulates bone marrow to produce red blood cells.
• *Osteomalacia.* With prolonged kidney failure, inadequate amounts of the active form of vitamin D are produced, causing decreased intestinal absorption of calcium and decreased availability of calcium to the bones. These conditions lead to osteomalacia, in which the bones are partially absorbed and become greatly weakened. Another important cause of demineralization of the bones in chronic renal failure

is the *rise in serum phosphate concentration* that occurs because of the decreased GFR. The higher serum phosphate level increases binding of phosphate with calcium in the plasma, decreasing the serum ionized calcium, which in turn stimulates *parathyroid hormone* secretion, increasing the release of calcium from bones and further demineralization.

VI

Blood Cells, Immunity, and Blood Coagulation

CHAPTER 32

Red Blood Cells, Anemia, and Polycythemia

A major function of red blood cells is to transport hemoglobin, which in turn carries oxygen from the lungs to the tissues. Normal red blood cells are biconcave discs, although the shapes can change markedly as the cells pass through the capillaries. The normal red blood cell has a great excess of cell membrane relative to the quantity of material it contains. Deformation of the cell does not stretch the membrane and consequently does not rupture the cell. The average number of red blood cells per cubic millimeter is 5,200,000 ± 300,000 in men and 4,700,000 ± 300,000 in women.

Red Blood Cells Have the Ability to Concentrate Hemoglobin. In normal individuals, the percentage of hemoglobin is almost always near the maximum level in each cell (about 34 g/dL). The blood contains an average of 15 g of hemoglobin per 100 mL (16 g in men and 14 g in women). Each gram of pure hemoglobin is capable of combining with approximately 1.34 mL of oxygen. In a healthy person, more than 20 mL of oxygen can be carried in combination with the hemoglobin in each 100 mL of blood.

Genesis of Blood Cells. All circulating blood cells are derived from *pluripotential hemopoietic stem cells*. The pluripotential cells differentiate to form the peripheral blood cells. As these cells reproduce, a portion is exactly like the original pluripotential cells. These cells are retained in the bone marrow to maintain a constant supply. The early offspring of the stem cells cannot be recognized as different types of blood cell even though they already have been committed to a particular cell line; these cells are called *committed stem cells*. Different committed stem cells produce different colonies of specific types of blood cells.

The growth and reproduction of the various stem cells are controlled by multiple proteins called *growth inducers*, which promote growth, but not differentiation, of the cells. This is the function of another set of proteins, called *differentiation inducers*. Each of these inducers causes one type of stem cell to differentiate one or more steps toward the final type of adult blood cell. The formation of growth inducers and differentiation inducers is controlled by factors outside the bone marrow. In the case of red blood cells, exposure of the body to a low level of oxygen for a long period induces growth, differentiation, and production of greatly increased numbers of erythrocytes.

Regulation of Red Blood Cell Production— The Role of Erythropoietin (p. 416)

The total mass of red blood cells in the circulatory system is regulated within narrow limits. Any condition that causes the quantity of oxygen that is transported in the tissues to decrease ordinarily increases the rate of red blood cell production. The principal factor that stimulates red blood cell production is the circulating hormone *erythropoietin.* In a normal individual, about 90% of erythropoietin is formed in the kidneys, with the remainder formed mainly in the liver. The structure in the kidney in which the erythropoietin is formed is not known. Some studies suggest that erythropoietin is secreted by fibroblast-like interstitial cells surrounding the tubules in the cortex and outer medulla where much of the kidney's oxygen consumption occurs. Other cells including the renal epithelial cells themselves also secrete erythropoietin in response to hypoxia (Fig. 32–1).

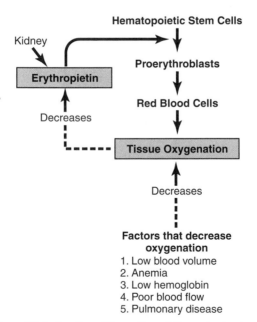

Figure 32–1. Function of the erythropoietin mechanism to increase production of red blood cells when tissue oxygenation decreases.

When both kidneys are surgically removed or destroyed by renal disease, the individual invariably becomes extremely anemic because the amount of erythropoietin formed in nonrenal tissues is sufficient to cause only one third to one half as many red blood cells to be formed as are needed by the body.

Vitamin B_{12} and Folic Acid Are Important for the Final Maturation of Red Blood Cells. Both vitamin B_{12} and folic acid are essential to the synthesis of DNA. The lack of either of these vitamins results in a diminished quantity of DNA and, consequently, failure of nuclear maturation and division. In addition to failure to proliferate, the red blood cells become larger than normal, developing into *megaloblasts.* These cells have irregular shapes and flimsy cell membranes; they are capable of carrying oxygen normally, but their fragility causes them to have a short life span—one half to one third that of normal. Vitamin B_{12} or folic acid deficiency therefore causes *maturation failure* during the process of erythropoiesis.

A common cause of maturation failure is an inability to absorb vitamin B_{12} from the gastrointestinal tract. This often occurs in persons with *pernicious anemia,* a disease in which the basic abnormality is atrophic gastric mucosa. The parietal cells of the gastric gland secrete a glycoprotein called *intrinsic factor,* which combines with vitamin B_{12} to make it available for absorption by the gut. The intrinsic factor binds tightly with vitamin B_{12} and protects the vitamin from digestion by the gastrointestinal enzymes. The intrinsic factor-vitamin B_{12} complex binds to specific receptor sites on the brush border membranes of mucosal cells of the ileum. Vitamin B_{12} is then transported into the blood via the process of pinocytosis. A lack of intrinsic factor causes loss of much of the vitamin resulting from enzyme action in the gut and failure of absorption.

Formation of Hemoglobin *(p. 417)*

Synthesis of hemoglobin begins when the red blood cell is in the proerythroblast stage and continues into the reticulocyte stage, at which point the cell leaves the bone marrow and passes into the bloodstream. During the formation of hemoglobin, the *heme* molecule combines with a long polypeptide chain called a *globin* to form a subunit of hemoglobin called a *hemoglobin chain.* Four hemoglobin chains bind together loosely to form the entire hemoglobin molecule.

The most important feature of the hemoglobin molecule is its ability to bind loosely and reversibly with oxygen. The oxygen atom binds loosely with one of the so-called coordination bonds of the iron atom in hemoglobin. When bound to the iron heme, oxygen is carried as molecular oxygen, composed of two oxygen atoms. Oxygen is released into the tissue fluids in the form of dissolved molecular oxygen rather than as ionic oxygen.

Iron Metabolism *(p. 418)*

Iron is important for the formation of hemoglobin, myoglobin, and other substances, such as the cytochromes, cytochrome oxidase, peroxidase, and catalase. The total average quantity of iron in the body is about 4 to 5 g. About 65% of this amount is in the form of hemoglobin. About 4% is in the form of myoglobin, 1% is in the form of the various heme compounds that promote intracellular oxidation, 0.1% is combined with the protein *transferrin* in the blood plasma, and 15% to 30% is stored mainly in the reticuloendothelial system and liver parenchymal cells, principally in the form of *ferritin*.

Iron Is Transported and Stored. When iron is absorbed from the small intestine it immediately combines with a β-globulin called *apotransferrin,* to form *transferrin,* which is transported in the plasma. This iron is loosely bound. Excess iron in the blood is deposited in liver hepatocytes and in reticuloendothelial cells of the bone marrow. Once inside the cell's cytoplasm, iron combines with the protein *apoferritin* to form *ferritin.* Varying quantities of iron can combine in clusters of iron radicals in the ferritin.

When the quantity of iron in the plasma decreases to less than normal, iron is removed from ferritin quite easily and transported by transferrin in the plasma to the portions of the body where it is needed. A unique characteristic of the transferrin molecule is its ability to bind strongly with receptors in the cell membranes of the erythroblasts and bone marrow. Transferrin is ingested via endocytosis into the erythroblasts along with the bound iron. Transferrin delivers the iron directly to the mitochondria, where heme is synthesized.

When red blood cells have reached the end of their life span and are destroyed, the hemoglobin released is ingested by cells of the monocyte-macrophage system. The free iron that is liberated can be stored in the ferritin pool or reused for formation of hemoglobin.

Anemias *(p. 420)*

Anemia means a deficiency of red blood cells and can be caused by rapid loss of red blood cells or slow production of red blood cells.

- *Blood loss anemia* occurs after significant hemorrhage. The body is able to replace the plasma within 1 to 3 days; however, the concentration of red blood cells remains low. After significant hemorrhage, a period of 3 to 4 weeks is required to return the number of red blood cells to normal levels.

- *Aplastic anemia* is the result of nonfunctioning bone marrow, which may be due to exposure to gamma radiation for cancer treatment or toxic chemicals such as insecticides or benzene in gasoline. Autoimmune disorders such as lupus erythematosus result in an immune system attack on the healthy cells of the bone marrow, which destroys stem cells and may lead to aplastic anemia. Individuals with severe aplastic anemia usually die unless they are treated with blood transfusions or bone marrow transplants.

- *Megaloblastic anemia* is the result of a lack of vitamin B_{12}, folic acid, or intrinsic factor. Lack of these substances leads to slow reproduction of the erythrocytes in the bone marrow. As a result, these erythrocytes grow into large, odd-shaped cells called *megaloblasts.*

- *Hemolytic anemia* is the result of fragile red blood cells that rupture as they pass through the capillaries. With hemolytic anemia, the number of red blood cells that form is normal or in excess of normal; however, because these cells are extremely fragile, their life span is very short. *Sickle cell anemia* is a type of hemolytic anemia caused by an abnormal composition of the globin chains of hemoglobin. When this abnormal hemoglobin is exposed to low concentrations of oxygen, it precipitates into long crystals inside the red blood cell. This causes the cell to have an abnormal sickle shape and to be extremely fragile.

Polycythemia *(p. 421)*

Polycythemia is a condition in which the number of red blood cells in the circulation increases owing to hypoxia or genetic aberration. Individuals who live at high altitudes have *physiologic polycythemia* as a result of the thin atmosphere. Polycythemia can also occur in individuals with cardiac failure because of decreased delivery of oxygen to the tissues.

Polycythemia vera is a genetic aberration in the hemocytoblastic cell line. The blast cells continue to produce red blood cells even though too many blood cells are present in the circulation. The hematocrit can rise to 60% to 70%.

Polycythemia greatly increases the viscosity of the blood; as a result, blood flow through the vessels is often sluggish.

CHAPTER 33

Resistance of the Body to Infection: I. Leukocytes, Granulocytes, the Monocyte-Macrophage System, and Inflammation

Our bodies have a special system for combating the various infectious and toxic agents to which we are continuously exposed. The leukocytes (white blood cells) are the mobile units of the protective system of the body. They are formed in the bone marrow and lymph tissue and transported in the blood to areas of inflammation to provide a rapid and potent defense against any infectious agent that might be present. Five types of leukocytes are normally found in the blood; the normal percentages are as follows:

- Polymorphonuclear neutrophils—62.0%
- Polymorphonuclear eosinophils—2.3%
- Polymorphonuclear basophils—0.4%
- Monocytes—5.3%
- Lymphocytes—30.0%

The three types of polymorphonuclear cell have a granular appearance and are called *granulocytes*, or *"polys."* The granulocytes and monocytes protect the body against invading organisms by ingesting them via the process of *phagocytosis.* The lymphocytes function mainly in connection with the immune system to attach to specific invading organisms and destroy them.

Genesis of White Blood Cells. Two lineages of white blood cells are formed from the *pluripotential hemopoietic stem cells:* the *myelocytic lineage* and the *lymphocytic lineage.* Granulocytes and monocytes are the products of the myelocytic lineage, whereas lymphocytes are the products of the lymphocytic lineage. Granulocytes and monocytes are formed only in the bone marrow. Lymphocytes are produced mainly in the various lymphoid organs, including the lymph glands, spleen, and thymus.

The Life Span of White Blood Cells Varies. The main reason white blood cells are present in the blood is for transportation from the bone marrow or lymphoid tissue to areas of the body where they are needed. The life span of granulocytes released from the bone marrow is normally 4 to 5 hours in the circulating blood and an additional 4 to 5 days in the tissues. When there is serious tissue infection, the total life span is often shortened to only a few hours because the granulocytes proceed rapidly to the infected area, perform their function, and in the process are destroyed.

The monocytes also have a short transit time of 10 to 12 hours before they enter the tissues. Once in the tissues, they swell to a much larger size to become *tissue macrophages,* in which form they can live for months unless they are destroyed while performing phagocytic functions.

Lymphocytes enter the circulatory system continuously along with the drainage of lymph from the lymph nodes. After a few hours, they pass back into the tissue via diapedesis and re-enter the lymph to return to the blood again and again; thus there is continuous circulation of lymphocytes throughout the tissue. The lymphocytes have a life span of months or even years depending on the need of the body for these cells.

Neutrophils and Macrophages Defend against Infections *(p. 425)*

It is mainly the neutrophils and monocytes that attack and destroy invading bacteria, viruses, and other injurious agents. The neutrophils are mature cells that can attack and destroy bacteria and viruses in the circulating blood. The blood monocytes are immature cells that have little ability to fight infectious agents. Once they enter the tissue, they mature into tissue macrophages that are extremely capable of combating disease agents. Both the neutrophils and macrophages move through the tissues via ameboid motion when stimulated by products formed in inflamed areas. This attraction of the neutrophils and macrophages to the inflamed area is called *chemotaxis.*

One of the Most Important Functions of the Neutrophils and Macrophages Is Phagocytosis. For obvious reasons, phagocytosis is highly selective. Certain physical characteristics increase the chance for phagocytosis. Most natural structures in the tissue have smooth surfaces that resist phagocytosis; if the surface is rough, the likelihood of phagocytosis is increased. Most naturally occurring substances in the body have protective protein coats that repel phagocytes. Dead tissues and most foreign particles often have no protective coat, which makes them subject to phagocytosis. The body also has specific means of recognizing certain foreign materials to which antibodies adhere; the binding of antibodies to foreign particles enhances phagocytosis.

Once a foreign particle has been phagocytized, lysosomes and other cytoplasmic granules immediately come in contact with the phagocytic vesicles and dump digestive enzymes and bactericidal agents into the vesicle.

Inflammation: Role of Neutrophils and Macrophages *(p. 428)*

When tissue injury occurs, multiple substances are released that cause secondary changes in the tissue. These substances increase local blood flow and the permeability of the capillaries, which cause large quantities of fluid to leak into the interstitial spaces, the migration of large numbers of granulocytes and monocytes into the tissues, and local swelling.

One of the first results of inflammation is to "wall off" the area of injury from the remaining tissues. The tissue spaces and lymphatics in the inflamed area are blocked by fibrinogen clots, so fluid barely flows through these spaces. This walling-off procedure delays the spread of bacteria or toxic products. The intensity of the inflammatory process is usually proportional to the degree of tissue injury. Staphylococci that invade the tissue liberate extremely lethal cellular toxins, which is followed by the rapid development of inflammation. Staphylococcal infections are characteristically walled off rapidly. By comparison, streptococci do not cause such intense local tissue destruction, so the walling off develops slowly. As a result, streptococci have a far greater tendency to spread through the body and cause death than do staphylococci, even though staphylococci are far more destructive to the tissues.

Macrophage and Neutrophil Response During Inflammation *(p. 428)*

The Tissue Macrophage Is the First Line of Defense against Invading Organisms. Within minutes after inflammation begins, the macrophages present in the tissues immediately begin their phagocytic actions. Many sessile macrophages break loose from their attachments and become mobile in response to *chemotactic factors.* These macrophages migrate to the area of inflammation and contribute their activity.

Neutrophil Invasion of the Inflamed Tissue Is a Second Line of Defense. During the first hour or so after inflammation begins, large numbers of neutrophils invade the inflamed area as a result of products in the inflamed tissue that attract these cells and cause chemotaxis toward that area.

Within a few hours after the onset of severe acute inflammation, the number of neutrophils increases by as many as four- to fivefold. This *neutrophilia* is caused by inflammatory products that are transported in the blood to the bone marrow, where neutrophils from the marrow capillaries are mobilized and move into the circulating blood. This process results in more neutrophils being made available to the inflamed tissue area.

A Second Macrophage Invasion of the Inflamed Tissue Is the Third Line of Defense. Along with the invasion of neutrophils, monocytes from the blood enter the inflamed tissue and enlarge to become macrophages. The number of monocytes in the circulating blood is low, and the storage pool of monocytes in the bone marrow is much less than that of the neutrophils. The build-up of macrophages in inflamed tissue is much slower than that of neutrophils. After several days to several weeks, the macrophages become the dominant phagocytic cell in the inflamed area because of the increased bone marrow production of monocytes.

The Fourth Line of Defense is the Greatly Increased Production of Both Granulocytes and Monocytes by Bone Marrow. This process results from stimulation of the granulocytic and monocytic progenitor cells of the marrow; it takes 3 to 4 days for the newly formed granulocytes and monocytes to reach the stage of leaving the marrow area.

Many Factors Are Involved in the Feedback Control of the Macrophage and Neutrophil Response. More than two dozen factors have been implicated in controlling the macrophage-neutrophil response to inflammation. Five factors are thought to play a dominant role:

1. Tumor necrosis factor (TNF)
2. Interleukin-1 (IL-1)
3. Granulocyte-monocyte colony-stimulating factor (GM-CSF)
4. Granulocyte colony-stimulating factor (G-CSF)
5. Monocyte colony-stimulating factor (M-CSF)

These five factors are formed by activated macrophages and T cells in the inflamed tissues. The main instruments of the increased production of granulocytes and monocytes by bone marrow are the three colony-stimulating factors; the combination of TNF, IL-1, and colony-stimulating factors provides a powerful feedback mechanism that begins with tissue inflammation and proceeds to the formation of defensive white blood cells and removal of the cause as well as the inflammation.

Formation of Pus. When the neutrophils and macrophages engulf large numbers of bacteria and necrotic tissue, essentially all the neutrophils and many of the macrophages eventually die. The combination of various portions of necrotic tissue, dead neutrophils, dead macrophages, and tissue fluid is commonly known as *pus*. When the infection has been suppressed, the dead cells and necrotic tissue in the pus gradually autolyze over a period of days and are absorbed into the surrounding tissues until most of the evidence of the tissue damage is gone.

Eosinophils Are Produced in Large Numbers in Persons with Parasitic Infections. Most parasites are too large to be phagocytized. The eosinophils attach themselves to the surface of the parasites and release substances such as hydrolytic enzymes, reactive forms of oxygen, and larvicidal polypeptides called *major basic proteins*, which then kill many of the invading parasites.

The eosinophils normally constitute about 2% of all the blood leukocytes. In addition to combating parasitic infections, eosinophils have a propensity to collect in tissues in which allergic reactions have occurred. The migration of the eosinophils to inflamed allergic tissue results from the release of eosinophil chemotactic factor from mast cells and basophils. The eosinophils are believed to detoxify some of the inflammation-inducing substances released by the mast cells and basophils and destroy allergen-antibody complexes, thus preventing spread of the inflammatory process.

Basophils Are Circulating Mast Cells. Mast cells and basophils liberate heparin into the blood, which prevents blood coagulation. These cells release histamine as well as smaller quantities of bradykinin and serotonin, which contribute to the inflammation process. The mast cells and basophils play an important role in some allergic reactions. The immunoglobulin E (IgE) class of antibodies (those responsible for allergic reactions) has a propensity to become attached to mast cells and basophils. The resulting attachment of the allergic antigen to the IgE antibody causes the mast cells or basophils to rupture and release exceedingly large quantities of histamine, bradykinin, serotonin, heparin, slow-reacting substance of anaphylaxis, and lysosomal enzymes. These substances in turn cause the local vascular and tissue reactions that are characteristic of allergic manifestation.

The Leukemias *(p. 431)*

The leukemias are divided into two general types: *lymphogenous* and *myelogenous.* The lymphogenous leukemias are caused by uncontrolled cancerous production of lymphoid cells, which usually begins in a lymph node or other lymphogenous tissue and then spreads to other areas of the body. The myelogenous leukemias begin by cancerous production of young myelogenous cells in the bone marrow and then spread throughout the body; thus white blood cells are produced by many extramedullary organs. Leukemic cells are usually nonfunctional, so they cannot provide the usual protection against infection that is associated with white blood cells.

Almost all leukemias spread to the spleen, lymph nodes, liver, and other regions that have a rich vascular supply regardless of whether the origin of the leukemia is in the bone marrow or lymph nodes. The rapidly growing cells invade the surrounding tissues, using the metabolic elements of these tissues, and subsequently cause tissue destruction via metabolic starvation.

CHAPTER 34

Resistance of the Body to Infection: II. Immunity and Allergy Innate Immunity

Innate and Acquired Immunity

Immunity is the ability to resist almost all types of organisms or toxins that damage tissues of the body. Most organisms have *innate immunity,* which consists of general actions such as phagocytosis of bacteria, destruction of pathogens by acidic secretions, digestive enzymes in the gastrointestinal tract, resistance of the skin to invasion, and certain chemicals in the blood that attach to foreign organisms or toxins and destroy them. *Acquired immunity* is the ability to develop extremely powerful protective mechanisms against specific invading agents such as lethal bacteria, viruses, toxins, and even foreign tissues from other organisms.

Acquired Immunity Is Initiated by Antigens. Two basic types of acquired immunity occur in the body. *Humoral immunity,* or *B-cell immunity,* involves the development of circulating antibodies that are capable of attacking an invading agent. *Cell-mediated immunity,* or *T-cell immunity,* is achieved through the formation of large numbers of activated lymphocytes that are specifically designed to destroy the foreign agent.

Because acquired immunity does not occur until after invasion by a foreign organism or toxin, the body must have some mechanism for recognizing the invasion. Each invading organism or toxin usually contains one or more specific chemical compounds that are different from all other compounds; these compounds are called *antigens,* and they initiate the development of acquired immunity.

For a substance to be antigenic, it usually must have a molecular weight of at least 8000 kD. The process of antigenicity depends on the regular occurrence on the surface of the large molecules of molecular groups called *epitopes;* proteins and large polysaccharides are almost always antigenic because they contain this type of stereochemical characteristic.

Lymphocytes Are Responsible for Acquired Immunity. Lymphocytes are found in the lymph nodes and in special lymphoid tissue such as the spleen, submucosal areas of the gastrointestinal tract, and bone marrow. Lymphoid tissue is distributed advantageously in the body to intercept invading organisms and toxins before the invaders can become widespread.

There are two populations of lymphocytes, both of which are derived from *pluripotent hemopoietic stem cells* that differentiate to form lymphocytes. One population of lymphocytes is processed in the thymus gland; these are called *T lymphocytes* and are responsible for cell-mediated immunity. Another population of lymphocytes is processed in the liver during mid fetal life and in the bone marrow during late fetal life and after birth; these are called *B lymphocytes* and are responsible for humoral immunity.

The Thymus Gland Preprocesses T Lymphocytes. Lymphocytes divide rapidly and develop extreme diversity for reacting against various specific antigens in the thymus gland. The processed T cells leave the thymus and spread to lymphoid tissues throughout the body. Most of the preprocessing of the T lymphocytes in the thymus occurs shortly before and after birth. Removal of the thymus gland after this time diminishes but does not eliminate the T-lymphocyte system. Removal of the thymus several months before birth, however, prevents the development of all cell-mediated immunity.

The Liver and Bone Marrow Preprocess the B Lymphocytes. Much less is known about the details or processing of B lymphocytes. In humans, B lymphocytes are known to be preprocessed in the liver during mid fetal life and in bone marrow during late fetal life and after birth. B lymphocytes differ from T lymphocytes; they actively secrete antibodies, which are large protein molecules capable of combining with and destroying substances. B lymphocytes have a greater diversity than T lymphocytes, forming millions, perhaps even billions, of antibodies with different specific reactivities. After processing, B lymphocytes migrate to lymphoid tissues throughout the body, where they lodge in locations near the T-lymphocyte areas.

When a specific antigen comes in contact with the T and B lymphocytes in the lymphoid tissue, a set of T and B lymphocytes becomes activated to form *activated T cells* and *activated B cells,* which subsequently form antibodies. The activated T cells and newly formed antibodies react specifically with the antigen that initiated their development and inactivate or destroy the antigen.

A Preformed Repertoire of Lymphocytes Awaits Activation by an Antigen. There are millions of types of preformed T and B lymphocytes that are capable of responding to the appropriate antigen. Each of these preformed lymphocytes is capable of forming only one type of antibody or one type of T cell with a single type of specificity. Once the specific lymphocyte is activated by its antigen, it reproduces wildly, forming tremendous numbers of duplicate lymphocytes. If the lymphocyte is a B lymphocyte, the progeny eventually secrete antibodies that circulate throughout the body. If the lymphocyte is a T lymphocyte, its progeny develop into *sensitized T cells* that are released into the blood, where they circulate through the tissue fluids throughout the body and back into the lymph. Each set of lymphocytes capable of forming one specific antibody or activated T cell is called a *clone of lymphocytes.* The lymphocytes in each clone are identical, and all are derived from one progenitor lymphocyte of a specific type.

Specific Attributes of the B-Lymphocyte System—Humoral Immunity and the Antibodies *(p. 437)*

On entry of a foreign antigen, the macrophages in the lymphoid tissue phagocytize the antigen and present it to adjacent B lymphocytes. The previously dormant B lymphocytes specific for the antigen immediately enlarge and eventually become *antibody secreting plasma cells.* The plasma cells produce γ-globulin antibodies, which are secreted into the lymph and carried to the circulating blood.

The Formation of "Memory" Cells Enhances the Immune Response to Subsequent Antigen Exposure. Some of the B lymphocytes formed during activation of the specific clone do not form plasma cells but, instead, form new B lymphocytes similar to those of the original clone. This causes the population of the specifically activated clone to become greatly enhanced. These B lymphocytes circulate throughout the body and inhabit all the lymphoid tissue but remain immunologically dormant until activated again by a new quantity of the same antigen. The cells of the expanded clone of lymphocytes are called *memory cells.* Subsequent exposure to the same antigen causes a more rapid and potent antibody response because of the increased number of lymphocytes in the specific clone. The increased potency and duration of the secondary response are the reasons why *vaccination* is usually accomplished through injection of antigen in multiple doses with periods of several weeks or months between injections.

Antibodies Are γ-Globulin Proteins Called *Immunoglobulins*. All immunoglobulins are composed of combinations of light and heavy polypeptide chains. Each light and heavy chain has a *variable portion* and a *constant portion*. The variable portion is different for each specific antibody; it is this portion that attaches to a particular type of antigen. The constant portion determines other properties of the antibody, such as diffusibility, adherence to structures in tissues, and attachment to the complement complex. There are five general classes of antibodies, each with a specific function: IgM, IgA, IgG, IgD, and IgE. The IgG class is the largest and constitutes about 75% of the antibodies of a normal person.

Antibodies Act by Directly Attacking the Invader or Activating the Complement System, Which Subsequently Destroys the Invading Organism. The antibodies can inactivate the invading agent directly in one of the following ways:

- *Agglutination,* in which multiple large particles with antigens on their surfaces, such as bacteria or red blood cells, are bound together in a clump
- *Precipitation,* in which the molecular complex of soluble antigens and antibodies becomes so large that it is rendered insoluble
- *Neutralization,* in which the antibodies cover the toxic sites of the antigenic agent
- *Lysis,* in which antibodies are occasionally capable of causing rupture of an invading cell by directly attacking the cell membranes

Although antibodies have some direct effects in the destruction of the invaders, most of the protection afforded by antibodies derives from the amplifying effects of the complement system.

The Complement System Is Activated by the Antigen-Antibody Reaction. *Complement* is a collective term used to describe a system of proteins normally present in the plasma that can be activated by the antigen-antibody reaction. When an antibody binds with an antigen, a specific reactive site on the *constant* portion of the antibody becomes uncovered, or activated. This activated antibody site binds directly with the C1 molecule of the complement system, setting in motion a *cascade* of sequential reactions. When complement is activated, multiple end products are formed. Several of these end products help destroy the invading organism or neutralize a toxin.

Complement can stimulate phagocytosis by both neutrophils and macrophages, cause rupture of the cell membranes of bacteria or other invading organisms, promote agglutination, attack the structure of viruses, promote chemotaxis of neutrophils and macrophages, and induce the release of histamine by mast cells and basophils, promoting vasodilation and leakage of plasma, which in turn promote the inflammatory process. Activation of complement by an antigen-antibody reaction is called the *classical pathway.*

Special Attributes of the T-Lymphocyte System—Activated T Cells and Cell-Mediated Immunity *(p. 439)*

When macrophages present a specific antigen, T lymphocytes of the specific lymphoid clone proliferate, causing large numbers of activated T cells to be released in the same way antibodies are released by the activated B cells. These activated T cells pass into the circulation and are distributed throughout the body, where they circulate for months or even years. *T-lymphocyte memory cells* are formed in the same way that B memory cells are formed in the antibody system; on subsequent exposure to the same antigen, the release of activated T cells occurs far more rapidly and much more powerfully than during the first response.

Antigens bind with *receptor molecules* on the surface of the T cells in the same way they bind with antibodies. These receptor molecules are composed of a variable unit similar to the variable portion of the humoral antibody, but the stem section of the receptor molecule is firmly bound to the cell membrane.

Antigen-Presenting Cells, Major Histocompatibility Complex (MHC) Proteins, and Antigen Receptors on the T Lymphocyte. T-cell responses are extremely antigen-specific, like the antibody responses of B cells, and are as important as antibodies for defending against infection. Whereas B lymphocytes recognize intact antigens, T lymphocytes respond to antigens only when they are bound to specific molecules called MHC proteins on the surface of an *antigen-presenting cell* (Figure 34–1).

There are three major types of antigen-presenting cells: macrophages, B lymphocytes, and dendritic cells.

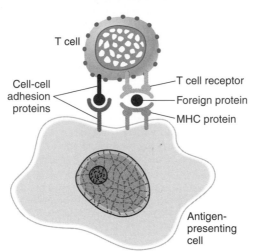

Figure 34–1. Activation of T cells requires the interaction of T-cell receptors with an antigen (foreign protein) that is transported to the surface of the antigen-presenting cell by a major histocompatibility complex (MHC) protein. Cell-to-cell adhesion proteins enable the T cell to bind to the antigen-presenting cell long enough to become activated.

Dendritic cells are located throughout the body and are most effective in presenting antigens to T cells.

The MHC proteins bind peptide fragments of the antigen proteins degraded inside the antigen-presenting cell and then transport them to the cell surface. There are two types of MHC protein: *MHC I* and *MCH II.* MHC I proteins present antigens to cytotoxic T cells, and MHC II proteins present antigens to helper T cells. Antigens on the surface of the antigen-presenting cell bind with receptor molecules on the surface of the T cell in the same way they bind with plasma antibodies.

Several Types of T Cells and Their Different Functions *(p. 440)*

The three major groups of T cells are *helper T cells, cytotoxic T cells,* and *suppressor T cells.* The function of each of these cell types is quite distinct.

Helper T Cells Are the Most Numerous Type of T Cell in the Body. Helper T cells serve as regulators of virtually all immune functions. This task is accomplished through the formation of a series of protein mediators called *lymphokines,* which act on other cells of the immune system and bone marrow. Helper T cells secrete *interleukins* 2 through 6, *granulocyte-monocyte colony stimulating factor,* and *interferon-γ.* In the absence of the lymphokines produced by the helper T cells, the remainder of the immune system is almost paralyzed. It is the helper T cells that are inactivated or destroyed by the *human immunodeficiency virus (acquired immunodeficiency syndrome),* which leaves the body almost totally unprotected against infectious disease.

Helper T cells perform the following functions:

- *Stimulate growth and proliferation of cytotoxic and suppressor T cells* through the actions of interleukins 2, 4, and 5
- *Stimulate B cell growth and differentiation to form plasma cells and antibodies* mainly through the actions of interleukins 4, 5, and 6
- *Activate the macrophage system*
- *Stimulate helper T cells themselves.* Interleukin-2 has a direct positive feedback effect of stimulating activation of the helper T cell, which acts as an amplifier to enhance the cellular immune response

Cytotoxic T Cells Are Capable of Killing Microorganisms through a Direct Attack. For this reason, they are also called *killer cells.* Surface receptors on the cytotoxic T cells cause them to bind tightly to those organisms or cells that contain their binding-specific antigen. After binding, the cytotoxic T cells secrete *hole-forming proteins,* called *perforins,* which literally punch large holes in the membrane of the attacked cells. These holes disrupt the osmotic equilibrium of the cells, leading to cell death. Cytotoxic T cells are especially important for destroying cells infected by viruses, cancer cells, or transplanted organ cells.

Suppressor T Cells Suppress the Functions of both Cytotoxic and Helper T Cells. It is believed that these suppressor functions serve the purpose of regulating the activities of the other cells so excessive immune reactions that might severely damage the body do not occur.

Tolerance of the Acquired Immunity System to Ones Own Tissues—Role of Preprocessing in the Thymus and Bone Marrow *(p. 442)*

The immune system normally recognizes a person's own tissue as being completely distinct from that of invading organisms. It is believed that most of the phenomenon of *tolerance* develops during the processing of T lymphocytes in the thymus and B lymphocytes in the bone marrow. The mechanism of tolerance induction is not completely understood; however, it is thought that continuous exposure to self-antigen in the fetus causes the self-reacting T and B lymphocytes to be destroyed.

Failure of the tolerance mechanism leads to autoimmune diseases in which the immune system attacks the tissues of the body, such as *rheumatic fever,* in which the body becomes immunized against the tissues of the joints and valves of the heart; *glomerulonephritis,* in which the body becomes immunized against the basement membrane of the glomeruli; *myasthenia gravis,* in which the body becomes immunized against the acetylcholine receptor proteins of the neuromuscular junction; and *lupus erythematosus,* in which the body becomes immunized against many tissues.

Allergy and Hypersensitivity *(p. 443)*

An important but undesirable side effect of immunity is the development of *allergy* or other types of *immune hypersensitivity.* Allergy can be caused by activated T cells and can cause skin eruptions, edema, or asthmatic attacks in response to certain chemicals or drugs. In some individuals, a resin in the poison ivy plant induces the formation of activated helper and cytotoxic T cells that diffuse into the skin and elicit a cell-mediated characteristic type of immune reaction to this plant.

Some allergies are caused by IgE antibodies. These antibodies are called *reagins,* or *sensitizing antibodies,* to distinguish them from the more common IgG antibodies. A special characteristic of IgE antibodies is their ability to bind strongly with mast cells and basophils, causing the release of multiple substances that induce vasodilation, increased capillary permeability, and attraction of neutrophils and eosinophils. *Hives, hay fever,* and *asthma* can result from this mechanism.

CHAPTER 35

Blood Types; Transfusion; Tissue and Organ Transplantation

O-A-B Blood Types *(p. 445)*

The antigens *type A* and *type B* occur on the surfaces of red blood cells in a large proportion of the population. These antigens, or *agglutinogens,* cause blood transfusion reactions. It is on the basis of the presence or absence of the agglutinogens on the red blood cells that blood is grouped for the purpose of transfusion. When neither A nor B agglutinogen is present, the blood group is *type O.* When only the type A agglutinogen is present, the blood group is *type A.* When only type B agglutinogen is present, the blood group is *type B.* When both type A and B agglutinogens are present, the blood group is *type AB.*

When type A agglutinogen is not present on a person's red blood cells, antibodies known as *anti-A agglutinins* develop in the plasma. When type B agglutinogen is not present on the red blood cells, antibodies known as *anti-B agglutinins* develop in the plasma. Type O blood contains both anti-A and anti-B agglutinins, and type A blood contains type A agglutinogens and anti-B agglutinins. Type B blood contains type B agglutinogens and anti-A agglutinins; type AB blood contains both type A and B agglutinogens but no agglutinins.

The agglutinins are γ-globulins of the IgM and IgG immunoglobulin subclasses. The origin of the agglutinins in individuals who do not have the antigenic substance in their blood seems to be entry into the body of small numbers of group A and group B antigens in food and through contact with bacteria.

When bloods are mismatched so anti-A or anti-B plasma agglutinins are mixed with red blood cells containing A or B agglutinogens, the red blood cells agglutinate into clumps. These clumps can plug small blood vessels throughout the circulatory system. In some cases, the antibodies induce lysis of red blood cells through activation of the complement system.

One of the most lethal effects of transfusion reactions is renal failure. The excess hemoglobin from the hemolyzed red blood cells leaks through the glomerular membranes into the renal tubules. Reabsorption of water from the tubules causes the hemoglobin concentration to rise, resulting in hemoglobin precipitation and subsequent blockade of the tubules.

Rh Blood Types (p. 447)

The Rh system is another important factor during blood transfusion. In the Rh system, spontaneous occurrence of agglutinins almost never happens; instead, the individual must first be exposed to an Rh antigen, usually through transfusion of blood or pregnancy. When red blood cells containing Rh factor are injected into a person without the factor, anti-Rh agglutinins develop and reach a maximum concentration within about 2 to 4 months. On multiple exposures to the Rh factor, the Rh-negative person eventually becomes strongly sensitized to it. The mismatch of Rh factor blood leads to agglutination and hemolysis.

Erythroblastosis fetalis is a disease of fetuses and newborn infants characterized by progressive agglutination and subsequent phagocytosis of red blood cells. In a typical case, the mother is Rh-negative and the father is Rh-positive. If the baby has inherited the Rh-positive antigen from the father and the mother has developed anti-Rh agglutinins in response to this antigen, these agglutinins can diffuse through the placenta into the fetal circulation and cause red blood cell agglutination.

Transplantation of Tissues and Organs (p. 449)

An *autograft* is the transplantation of tissues or whole organs from one part of the body to another. An *isograft* is the transplantation of an organ from one identical twin to another. An *allograft* is the transplantation of an organ from one human being to another. A *xenograft* is the transplantation of an organ from one species to another.

In the case of autografts and isografts, all cells in the transplanted organ contain virtually the same antigens and survive indefinitely if provided with an adequate blood supply. In the case of allografts and xenografts, immune reactions almost always occur. These reactions cause the cells in the graft to die within 1 to 5 weeks after transplantation unless specific therapy is given to prevent the immune reaction. When the tissues are properly "typed" and are similar between donor and recipient for their cellular antigens, successful long-term allograft survival can occur. Simultaneous drug therapy is needed to minimize the immune reactions.

Tissue Typing Is Performed to Identify the Human Leukocyte Antigen (HLA) Complex of Antigens. The most important antigens in graft rejection comprise a complex called the *HLA antigens.* Only six of these antigens are ever present on the cell surface of any one person, but there are more than 150 types of HLA antigens; this number represents more than a trillion possible combinations. As a consequence, it is virtually impossible for two individuals, with the exception of identical twins, to have the same six HLA antigens.

The HLA antigens occur on white blood cells as well as on the cells of tissues. Some of the HLA antigens are not severely antigenic; therefore a precise match of antigens between donor and recipient is not essential for allograft survival, but the best results occur in those with the closest possible match between donor and recipient.

Prevention of graft rejection can be accomplished by suppressing the immune system with (1) *glucocorticoid hormones;* (2) various drugs toxic to the lymphoid system, such as *azathioprine;* or (3) *cyclosporine,* which has a specific inhibitory effect on the formation of helper T cells. This drug is especially efficacious in blocking the T-cell–mediated rejection reaction.

CHAPTER 36

Hemostasis and Blood Coagulation

The term *hemostasis* means prevention of blood loss. Whenever a vessel is severed or ruptured, hemostasis is achieved through (1) vascular spasm, (2) formation of a platelet plug, (3) formation of a blood clot as a result of blood coagulation, and (4) eventual growth of fibrous tissue to close the rupture permanently.

- *Trauma to the blood vessel causes the wall of the blood vessel to constrict.* The constriction results from nervous reflexes, local myogenic spasms, and local humoral factors released from the traumatized tissue and blood platelets, such as the vasoconstrictor substance *thromboxane A_2*.

- *A platelet plug can fill a small hole in a blood vessel.* When platelets come in contact with a damaged vascular surface, they begin to swell and assume irregular forms; release granules containing multiple factors, which increase the adherence of the platelets (i.e., adenosine diphosphate); and form thromboxane A_2. The adenosine diphosphate and thromboxane act on nearby platelets to activate them, so they adhere to the originally activated platelets, forming a platelet plug.

- *Formation of the blood clot is the third mechanism for hemostasis.* Clot formation begins to develop within 15 to 20 seconds if the trauma to the vascular wall has been severe and within 1 to 2 minutes if the trauma has been minor. Within 3 to 6 minutes after rupture of a vessel, the entire opening or the broken end of the vessel is filled with the clot (if the vessel opening was not too large). After 20 minutes to 1 hour, the clot retracts, closing the vessel further. Once a blood clot has formed, it is invaded by fibroblasts, which subsequently form connective tissue throughout the clot.

Mechanism of Blood Coagulation *(p. 453)*

Blood coagulation takes place in three essential steps:

- A complex of substances called *prothrombin activator* is formed in response to rupture of or damage to the blood vessel.
- Prothrombin activator catalyzes the conversion of *prothrombin* to *thrombin.*
- The thrombin acts as an enzyme to convert *fibrinogen* to *fibrin threads* that enmesh platelets, blood cells, and plasma to form the clot.

Prothrombin Is Converted to Thrombin. Prothrombin is an unstable plasma protein that can easily split into smaller compounds, one of which is thrombin. Prothrombin is produced continuously by the liver. If the liver fails to produce prothrombin, within 24 hours the concentration in the plasma falls too low to provide normal blood coagulation. *Vitamin K is required by the liver for normal activation of prothrombin;* therefore either the lack of vitamin K or the presence of liver disease prevents normal prothrombin formation and results in bleeding tendencies.

Fibrinogen Is Converted to Fibrin, and a Clot Forms. Fibrinogen is a high-molecular-weight protein formed in the liver. Because of its large molecular size, little fibrinogen normally leaks through the capillary pores into the interstitial fluid. Thrombin is an enzyme that acts on the fibrinogen molecule to remove four low-molecular-weight peptides to form a molecule of *fibrin monomer.* The fibrin monomer molecule polymerizes with other fibrin monomer molecules to form the long fibrin threads that produce the reticulum of the clot. The newly formed fibrin reticulum is strengthened by a substance called *fibrin-stabilizing factor,* which normally is present in small amounts in plasma. This substance is also released from platelets entrapped in the clot. Fibrin-stabilizing factor, an enzyme, causes covalent bonding between the fibrin monomer molecules and adjacent fibrin threads, thereby strengthening the fibrin meshwork.

During the Initiation of Coagulation, Prothrombin Activator Is Formed in Two Basic Ways. (1) via the *extrinsic pathway,* which begins with trauma to the vascular wall and surrounding tissue, and (2) via the *intrinsic pathway,* which begins in the blood itself. Both pathways involve a series of β-globulin plasma proteins. These blood clotting factors are proteolytic enzymes that induce the successive cascading reactions of the clotting process.

- *The extrinsic mechanism* for initiating the formation of prothrombin activator begins with trauma to the vascular wall or extravascular tissues and occurs according to the following three steps:

  1. *Release of tissue thromboplastin.* Traumatized tissue releases a complex of several factors called tissue thromboplastin; these factors include phospholipids from the membranes of the traumatized tissue and a lipoprotein complex that functions as a proteolytic enzyme.

2. *Activation of factor X to form activated factor X.*
The lipoprotein complex of tissue thromboplastin
complexes with *blood coagulation factor VII* and
in the presence of tissue phospholipids and calcium ions acts enzymatically on factor X to form
activated factor X.

3. *Effect of activated factor X to form prothrombin
activator.* The activated factor X immediately forms
a complex with the tissue phospholipid released as
part of the tissue thromboplastin and with *factor V*
to form a complex called prothrombin activator.
Within a few seconds this splits prothrombin to form
thrombin, and the clotting process proceeds as previously described. Activated factor X is the protease
that causes splitting of prothrombin to thrombin.

- *The intrinsic mechanism* for initiating the formation
of prothrombin activator begins with trauma to the
blood or exposure of the blood to collagen in the
traumatized vascular wall. This occurs via the following cascade of reactions:

  1. *Activation of factor XII and release of platelet
phospholipids.* Through trauma, factor XII is activated to form a proteolytic enzyme called *activated
factor XII.* Simultaneously, the blood trauma damages
blood platelets, which causes the release of platelet
phospholipids containing a lipoprotein called *platelet
factor III,* which plays a role in subsequent clotting
reactions.

  2. *Activation of factor XI.* The activated factor XII
acts enzymatically on factor XI to activate factor
XI. This second step in the intrinsic pathway
requires high-molecular-weight *kininogen.*

  3. *Activation of factor IX by activated factor XI.*
The activated factor XI then acts enzymatically
on factor IX to activate it.

  4. *Activation of factor X.* The activated factor IX, acting in concert with factor VIII and with platelet
phospholipids and factor III from the traumatized
platelets, activates factor X. When either factor
VIII or platelets are in short supply, this step is
deficient. Factor VIII is the factor that is missing
in the person who has *classic hemophilia.* Platelets
are the clotting factor lacking in the bleeding disease called *thrombocytopenia.*

  5. *Activation of activated factor X to form prothrombin activator.* This step in the intrinsic pathway is

the same as the last step in the extrinsic pathway (i.e., activated factor X combines with factor V and platelets or tissue phospholipids to form the complex called prothrombin activator). The prothrombin activator in turn initiates cleavage of prothrombin to form thrombin, thereby setting into motion the final clotting process.

Calcium Ions Are Required for Blood Clotting. Except for the first two steps in the intrinsic pathway, calcium ions are required for promotion of all the reactions; in the absence of calcium ions, blood clotting does not occur. Fortunately, the calcium ion concentration rarely falls sufficiently low to affect the kinetics of blood clotting significantly. When blood is removed, it can be prevented from clotting by reducing the calcium ion concentration below the threshold level for clotting. This can be accomplished through either deionization of the calcium via reaction with substances such as a *citrate ion* or precipitation of the calcium with substances such as an *oxalate ion.*

Prevention of Blood Clotting in the Normal Vascular System—Intravascular Anticoagulants *(p. 456)*

The most important factors for the prevention of clotting in the normal vascular system are (1) the *smoothness of the endothelium,* which prevents contact activation of the intrinsic clotting system; (2) a *layer of glycocalyx in the endothelium,* which repels the clotting factors and platelets; and (3) a *protein bound with the endothelial membrane* (called *thrombomodulin*), which binds thrombin. The thrombomodulin-thrombin complex also activates a plasma protein called *protein C,* which inactivates activated factors V and VIII. When the endothelial wall is damaged, its smoothness and its glycocalyx-thrombomodulin layer are lost, which activates factor XII and platelets and initiates the intrinsic pathway of clotting.

Agents that remove thrombin from blood, such as the fibrin threads that form during the process of clotting and an α-globulin called *antithrombin III,* are the most important anticoagulants in the blood. Thrombin becomes absorbed to the fibrin threads as they develop; this prevents the spread of thrombin into the remaining blood and prevents excessive spread of the clot. The thrombin that does not adsorb to the fibrin threads combines with antithrombin III, which inactivates the thrombin.

Heparin. In the presence of excess heparin, removal of thrombin from the circulation is almost instantaneous. *Mast cells* located in the pericapillary connective tissue throughout the body and the *basophils* of the blood produce heparin. These cells continually secrete small amounts of heparin that diffuse into the circulatory system.

Lysis of Blood Clots—Plasmin. *Plasminogen* is a plasma protein that when activated becomes a substance called *plasmin,* a proteolytic enzyme that resembles trypsin. Plasmin digests the fibrin threads as well as other clotting factors. Plasminogen becomes trapped in the clot along with other plasma proteins.

The injured tissues and vascular endothelium slowly release a powerful activator called *tissue plasminogen activator* (t-PA), which converts plasminogen to plasmin and removes the clot. Plasmin not only destroys fibrin fibers but also functions as a proteolytic enzyme to digest fibrinogen and a number of other clotting factors. Small amounts of plasmin are continuously formed in the blood. The blood also contains another factor, α_2-*antiplasmin,* which binds with plasmin and causes inactivation; the rate of plasmin formation must rise above a certain critical level before it becomes effective.

Conditions That Cause Excessive Bleeding in Human Beings (p. 457)

Excessive bleeding can result from a deficiency of vitamin K, from hemophilia, or from thrombocytopenia (platelet deficiency). Vitamin K is necessary for the formation of five important clotting factors: *prothrombin, factor VII, factor IX, factor X,* and *protein C.* In the absence of vitamin K, insufficiency of these coagulation factors can lead to a serious bleeding tendency.

Hemophilia Is Caused by a Deficiency of Factor VIII or IX and Occurs Almost Exclusively in Males. *Hemophilia A,* or *classic hemophilia,* is caused by a deficiency of factor VIII and accounts for about 85% of cases. The other 15% of cases of hemophilia are the result of a deficiency of factor IX. Both of these factors are transmitted genetically via the female chromosome as a recessive trait; women almost never have hemophilia because at least one of their two X chromosomes has the appropriate genes.

Thrombocytopenia Is a Deficiency of Platelets in the Circulatory System. People with thrombocytopenia have a tendency to bleed from small vessels or capillaries. As a result, small punctate hemorrhages occur throughout the body tissues. The skin of such a person displays many small, purplish blotches, giving the disease the name *thrombocytopenic purpura.*

Thromboembolic Conditions in the Human Beings *(p. 459)*

An abnormal clot that develops in a blood vessel is called a *thrombus.* An *embolus* is a free-flowing thrombus. Emboli generally do not stop flowing until they come to a narrow point in the circulatory system. Thromboembolic conditions in human beings are usually the result of a roughened endothelial surface or sluggish blood flow. The rough endothelium can initiate the clotting process. When blood flow is too slow, the concentration of procoagulant factors often rises high enough in a local area to initiate clotting.

Anticoagulants for Clinical Use *(p. 459)*

- *Heparin* is extracted from several animal tissues and can be prepared in almost pure form. It increases the effectiveness of *antithrombin III.* The action of heparin in the body is almost instantaneous, and at normal dosages (0.5 to 1.0 mg/kg) it can increase the clotting time from about 6 minutes to 30 minutes or longer. If too much heparin is given, a substance called *protamine* can be administered, which combines electrostatically with heparin to cause its inactivation.
- *Coumarins* such as *warfarin* cause the plasma levels of prothrombin and factors VIII, IX, and X to fall. Warfarin causes this effect by competing with vitamin K for reactive sites in the enzymatic processes for the formation of prothrombin and the other three clotting factors.

VII

Respiration

CHAPTER 37

Pulmonary Ventilation

The respiratory system supplies oxygen to the tissues and removes carbon dioxide. The major functional events of respiration include (1) pulmonary ventilation, which is the movement of air in and out of the alveoli; (2) diffusion of oxygen and carbon dioxide between the blood and alveoli; (3) transport of oxygen and carbon dioxide to and from the peripheral tissues; and (4) regulation of respiration. This chapter provides a discussion of pulmonary ventilation.

Mechanics of Pulmonary Ventilation *(p. 465)*

Muscles That Cause Lung Expansion and Contraction

Lung Volume Increases and Decreases as the Thoracic Cavity Expands and Contracts. Any time the length or thickness of the thoracic cavity increases or decreases, simultaneous changes in lung volume occur.

- *Normal quiet breathing* is accomplished with the diaphragm. During inspiration, contraction of the diaphragm pulls the lower surfaces of the lungs downward. During expiration, the diaphragm relaxes, and the elastic recoil of the lungs, chest wall, and abdominal structures compresses the lungs.
- During *heavy breathing,* the elastic forces are not sufficiently powerful to cause rapid expiration. The extra force is achieved mainly through contraction of the abdominal muscles, which pushes the abdominal contents upward against the diaphragm.

Raising and Lowering the Rib Cage Causes the Lungs to Expand and Contract. When the rib cage is elevated, the ribs project almost directly forward so the sternum also moves forward and away from the spine, increasing the anteroposterior thickness of the chest.

- *Muscles that raise the rib cage are muscles of inspiration.* Contraction of the external intercostals causes the ribs to move upward and forward in a "bucket handle" motion. Accessory muscles include the sternocleidomastoid muscles, the anterior serrati, and the scaleni.
- *Muscles that depress the rib cage are muscles of expiration,* including the internal intercostals and the abdominal recti. Other abdominal muscles compress the abdominal contents upward toward the diaphragm.

Movement of Air In and Out of the Lungs and the Pressures That Cause the Movement (p. 465)

Pleural Pressure Is the Pressure of the Fluid in the Space between the Lung Pleura and Chest Wall Pleura. The normal pleural pressure at the beginning of inspiration is about −5 cm of water, which is the amount of suction required to hold the lungs at their resting volume. During inspiration, expansion of the chest cage pulls the surface of the lungs with still greater force and creates a still more negative pressure, averaging about −7.5 cm of water.

Alveolar Pressure Is the Air Pressure Inside the Lung Alveoli. When the glottis is open and there is no movement of air, the pressures in all parts of the respiratory tree are equal to the atmospheric pressure, which is considered to be 0 cm of water.

- *During inspiration,* the pressure in the alveoli decreases to about −1 cm of water, which is sufficient to move about 0.5 L of air into the lungs within the 2 seconds required for inspiration.
- *During expiration,* opposite changes occur: The alveolar pressure rises to about +1 cm of water, which forces the 0.5 L of inspired air out of the lungs during the 2 to 3 seconds of expiration.

Lung Compliance Is the Change in Lung Volume for each Unit Change in Transpulmonary Pressure. Transpulmonary pressure is the difference between the alveolar and pleural pressures. The normal total compliance of both lungs together in the average adult is about 200 mL/cm of water. Compliance is dependent on the following elastic forces:

- *Elastic forces of the lung tissues* are determined mainly by the elastin and collagen fibers.
- *Elastic forces caused by surface tension* in the alveoli account for about two thirds of the total elastic forces in normal lungs.

Surfactant, Surface Tension, and Collapse of the Lungs (p. 467)

Water Molecules Are Attracted to One Another. The water surface lining the alveoli attempts to contract as the water molecules pull toward one another. This attempts to force air out of the alveoli, causing the alveoli to attempt to collapse. The net effect is to cause an elastic contractile force of the entire lung, called the *surface tension elastic force.*

Surfactant Reduces the Work of Breathing (Increases Compliance) by Decreasing Alveolar Surface Tension. Surfactant is secreted by type II alveolar epithelial cells. Its most important component is phospholipid dipalmitoylphosphatidylcholine. The presence of surfactant on the alveolar surface reduces the surface tension to one twelfth to one half of the surface tension of a pure water surface.

Smaller Alveoli Have a Greater Tendency to Collapse. Note from the following formula (Law of Laplace) that the collapse pressure generated in the alveoli is inversely related to the radius of the alveolus. This means that the smaller the alveolus the greater is the collapse pressure:

$$\text{Pressure} = (2 \times \text{Surface Tension})/\text{Radius}$$

Surfactant, "Interdependence," and Lung Fibrous Tissue Are Important for "Stabilizing" the Size of the Alveoli. If some of the alveoli were small and others were large, theoretically the smaller alveoli would tend to collapse and cause expansion of the larger alveoli. This instability of alveoli does not occur normally for the following reasons:

- *Interdependence.* The adjacent alveoli, alveolar ducts, and other air spaces tend to support each other in such a way that a large alveolus usually cannot exist adjacent to a small alveolus because they share common septal walls.
- *Fibrous tissue.* The lung is constructed of about 50,000 functional units, each of which contains one or a few alveolar ducts and their associated alveoli. All of them are surrounded by fibrous septa that act as additional supports.
- *Surfactant.* Surfactant reduces surface tension, allowing the interdependence phenomenon and fibrous tissue to overcome the surface tension effects. As an alveolus becomes smaller, the surfactant molecules on the alveolar surface are squeezed together, increasing their concentration and thereby reducing the surface tension still further.

Pulmonary Volumes and Capacities (p. 469)

Most pulmonary volumes and capacities can be measured with a spirometer. The total lung capacity, functional residual capacity, and residual volume cannot be measured with a spirometer. Figure 37–1 shows a

Figure 37–1. Respiratory excursions during normal breathing and during maximum inspiration and maximum expiration.

recording for successive breath cycles at various depths of inspiration and expiration. The recording was made using an apparatus called a *spirometer.*

The Pulmonary Volumes Added Together Equal the Maximum Volume to Which the Lungs Can Be Expanded. The four pulmonary *volumes* are listed on the left in Figure 37–1.

- *Tidal volume* (VT) is the volume of air (about 500 mL) inspired and expired with each normal breath.
- *Inspiratory reserve volume* (IRV) is the extra volume of air (about 3000 mL) that can be inspired over and above the normal tidal volume.
- *Expiratory reserve volume* (ERV) is the extra amount of air (about 1100 mL) that can be expired by forceful expiration after the end of a normal tidal expiration.
- *Residual volume* (RV) is the volume of air (about 1200 mL) remaining in the lungs after the most forceful expiration.

Pulmonary Capacities Are Combinations of Two or More Pulmonary Volumes. The pulmonary capacities are listed in Figure 37–1 and can be described as follows:

- *Inspiratory capacity* (IC) equals the tidal volume plus the inspiratory reserve volume. This is the amount of air (about 3500 mL) a person can breathe beginning at the normal expiratory level and distending the lungs to the maximum amount.

- *Functional residual capacity* (FRC) equals the expiratory reserve volume plus the residual volume. This is the amount of air that remains in the lungs at the end of a normal expiration (about 2300 mL).

- *Vital capacity* (VC) equals the inspiratory reserve volume plus the tidal volume plus the expiratory reserve volume. This is the maximum amount of air a person can expel from the lungs after first filling the lungs to their maximum extent and then expiring to the maximum extent (about 4600 mL).

- *Total lung capacity* (TLC) is the maximum volume to which the lungs can be expanded with the greatest possible inspiratory effort (about 5800 mL); it is equal to the vital capacity plus the residual volume.

Minute Respiratory Volume and Alveolar Ventilation *(p. 471)*

The Minute Respiratory Volume Is the Total Amount of New Air That Is Moved Into the Respiratory Passages Each Minute. It is equal to the tidal volume multiplied by the respiratory rate. The normal tidal volume is about 500 mL, and the normal respiratory rate is about 12 breaths per minute; therefore the minute respiratory volume normally averages about 6 L/min.

Alveolar Ventilation Is the Rate at which New Air Reaches the Gas Exchange Areas of the Lungs. During inspiration, some of the air never reaches the gas exchange areas but, instead, fills respiratory passages; this air is called *dead space air.* Because alveolar ventilation is the total volume of new air that enters the alveoli, it is equal to the respiratory rate multiplied by the amount of new air that enters the alveoli with each breath:

$$\dot{V}_A = Freq \cdot (V_T - V_D)$$

where $\dot{V}_A$ is the volume of alveolar ventilation per minute, Freq is the frequency of respiration per minute, V_T is the tidal volume, and V_D is the dead space volume. Thus with a normal tidal volume of 500 mL, a normal dead space of 150 mL, and a respiratory rate of 12 breaths per minute, alveolar ventilation equals 12 × (500 − 150), or 4200 mL/min.

There Are Three Types of Dead Space Air

- *Anatomical dead space* is the air in the conducting airways that does not engage in gas exchange.

- *Alveolar dead space* is the air in the gas exchange portions of the lung that cannot engage in gas exchange; it is nearly zero in normal individuals.
- *Physiological dead space* is the sum of the anatomic dead space and the alveolar dead space (i.e., the total dead space air).

Functions of the Respiratory Passageways (p. 472)

Trachea, Bronchi, and Bronchioles

Air Is Distributed to the Lungs by Way of the Trachea, Bronchi, and Bronchioles. The trachea is the first-generation passageway, and two main right and left bronchi are the second-generation passageways. Each division thereafter is an additional generation. There are between 20 and 25 generations before the air reaches the alveoli.

The Walls of the Bronchi and Bronchioles Are Muscular. The walls are composed mainly of smooth muscle in all areas of the trachea and bronchi not occupied by cartilage plates. The walls of the bronchioles are almost entirely smooth muscle, except for the most terminal bronchioles (respiratory bronchioles), which have only a few smooth muscle fibers. Many obstructive diseases of the lung result from narrowing of the smaller bronchi and bronchioles, often because of excessive contraction of the smooth muscle itself.

The Greatest Resistance to Air Flow Occurs in the Larger Bronchi, Not in the Small, Terminal Bronchioles. The reason for this high resistance is that there are relatively few bronchi in comparison with about 65,000 parallel terminal bronchioles, each of which pass only a minute amount of air. However, under disease conditions, the smaller bronchioles often play a greater role in determining air flow resistance for two reasons: (1) they are easily occluded because of their small size and (2) they constrict easily because they have a greater proportion of smooth muscle fibers in their walls.

Epinephrine and Norepinephrine Cause Dilation of the Bronchiole Tree. Direct control of the bronchioles by sympathetic nerve fibers is relatively weak because few of these fibers penetrate as far as the central portions of the lung. The bronchial tree, however, is exposed to circulating norepinephrine and epinephrine released from the adrenal gland medullae. Both of these hormones, especially epinephrine because of its greater stimulation of β-*adrenergic receptors,* cause dilation of the bronchial tree.

The Parasympathetic Nervous System Constricts the Bronchioles. A few parasympathetic nerve fibers derived from the vagus nerve penetrate the lung parenchyma. These nerves secrete acetylcholine, which causes mild to moderate constriction of the bronchioles. When a disease process such as asthma has already caused some constriction, parasympathetic nervous stimulation often worsens the condition. When this occurs, administration of drugs that block the effects of acetylcholine, such as atropine, can sometimes be used to relax the respiratory passages sufficiently to relieve the obstruction.

Mucus Lining the Respiratory Passageways; Action of Cilia to Clear the Passageways *(p. 473)*

All the Respiratory Passages Are Kept Moist with a Layer of Mucus. The mucus is secreted in part by individual goblet cells in the epithelial lining of the passages and in part by small submucosal glands. In addition to keeping the surfaces moist, the mucus traps small particles from the inspired air. The mucus itself is removed from the passages by the actions of ciliated epithelial cells.

The Entire Surface of the Respiratory Passages Is Lined with Ciliated Epithelium. Included in these passageways are the nose and lower passages down as far as the terminal bronchioles. The cilia beat continually, and the direction of their "power stroke" is toward the pharynx (i.e., the cilia in the lungs beat upward, whereas those in the nose beat downward). This continual beating causes the coat of mucus to flow toward the pharynx. The mucus and its entrapped particles are then swallowed or coughed to the exterior.

CHAPTER 38

Pulmonary Circulation, Pulmonary Edema, Pleural Fluid

Special problems related to pulmonary hemodynamics have important implications for gas exchange in the lungs. The present discussion is concerned specifically with these features of the pulmonary circulation.

Physiologic Anatomy of the Pulmonary Circulatory System (p. 477)

The Lung Has Three Circulations: Pulmonary, Bronchial, and Lymphatic

- *Pulmonary circulation.* The pulmonary artery is thin-walled and distensible, giving the pulmonary arterial tree large compliance. This large compliance allows the pulmonary arteries to accommodate about two thirds of the stroke volume of the right ventricle. The pulmonary veins have distensibility characteristics similar to those of the veins in the systemic circulation.
- *Bronchial circulation.* Bronchial blood flow amounts to about 1% to 2% of the total cardiac output. Oxygenated blood in the bronchial arteries supplies the connective tissue, septa, and large and small bronchi of the lungs. Because the bronchial blood empties into the pulmonary veins and bypasses the right heart, the right ventricular output is about 1% to 2% less than the left ventricular output.
- *Lymphatic circulation.* Lymphatics are found in all the supportive tissues of the lungs. Particulate matter entering the alveoli is removed by way of lymphatic channels; plasma proteins leaking from the lung capillaries are also removed from the lung tissues, helping prevent edema.

Pressures in the Pulmonary System (p. 477)

Blood Pressures in the Pulmonary Circulation Are Low Compared with Those in the Systemic Circulation

- *Pulmonary artery pressure.* In the normal human being, the average systolic pulmonary arterial pressure is about 25 mm Hg, the diastolic pulmonary arterial pressure is about 8 mm Hg, and the mean pulmonary arterial pressure is about 15 mm Hg.

- *Pulmonary capillary pressure.* The mean pulmonary capillary pressure has been estimated through indirect means to be about 7 mm Hg.
- *Left atrial and pulmonary venous pressures.* The mean pressure in the left atrium and the major pulmonary veins averages about 2 mm Hg in the recumbent human being.

The Left Atrial Pressure Can Be Estimated by Measuring the Pulmonary Wedge Pressure. Direct measurement of left atrial pressure is difficult because it requires passing a catheter retrograde through the left ventricle. The *pulmonary wedge pressure* can be measured by floating a balloon-tipped catheter through the right heart and pulmonary artery until the catheter wedges tightly in a smaller branch of the artery. Because all blood flow has been stopped in the blood vessels extending from the plugged artery, an almost direct connection is made through the pulmonary capillaries with the blood in the pulmonary veins. The wedge pressure is usually only 2 to 3 mm Hg higher than the left atrial pressure. Wedge pressure measurements are used often for studying changes in left atrial pressure in persons with various types of heart failure.

Blood Volume of the Lungs *(p. 478)*

The Lungs Provide an Important Blood Reservoir. The pulmonary blood volume is about 450 mL, or about 9% of the total blood volume. Under various physiological and pathological conditions, the quantity of blood in the lungs can vary from as little as one-half to two times normal.

Blood Shifts between the Pulmonary and Systemic Circulatory Systems as a Result of Cardiac Pathology. Left heart failure, mitral stenosis, or mitral regurgitation causes blood to dam up in the pulmonary circulation, greatly increasing pulmonary vascular pressures and volumes. Because the volume of the systemic circulation is about nine times that of the pulmonary system, a shift of blood from one system to the other affects the pulmonary system greatly but usually has only mild effects on the systemic circulation.

Blood Flow through the Lungs and Its Distribution *(p. 479)*

Pulmonary Blood Flow Is Nearly Equal to Cardiac Output. Under most conditions, the pulmonary vessels act as passive, distensible tubes that enlarge with increasing pressure and narrow with decreasing pressure. Blood is distributed to the segments of the lungs in which the alveoli are best oxygenated. This is achieved via the following mechanism.

Pulmonary Blood Flow Distribution Is Controlled by Alveolar Oxygen. When the alveolar oxygen concentration decreases below normal, the adjacent blood vessels constrict. This is opposite to the effect normally observed in systemic vessels. This vasoconstrictor effect of a low oxygen level distributes blood flow away from poorly ventilated alveoli.

The Autonomic Nervous System Does Not Have a Major Function in Normal Control of Pulmonary Vascular Resistance. However, sympathetic stimulation has a significant effect in constricting the large pulmonary capacitative vessels, especially the veins. This constriction of large pulmonary veins provides a means by which sympathetic stimulation can displace much of the extra blood in the lungs into other segments of the circulation when needed to combat low blood pressure.

Effect of Hydrostatic Pressure Gradients in the Lungs on Regional Pulmonary Blood Flow (p. 479)

In the normal adult, the distance between the apex and base of the lungs is about 30 cm, which creates a 23 mm Hg difference in blood pressure. This pressure gradient has a marked effect on blood flow in the various regions of the lung.

Hydrostatic Pressure Gradients in the Lung Create Three Zones of Pulmonary Blood Flow. Under normal and various pathologic lung conditions, any one of three possible zones of pulmonary blood flow can be found:

- *Zone 1 (top of the lung)* has no blood flow because the capillary pressure never rises higher than the alveolar pressure. In this zone, alveolar pressure > artery pressure > venous pressure; thus the capillaries are pressed flat. Zone 1 does not occur during normal conditions; it can occur when pulmonary artery pressure is decreased following hemorrhage and when alveolar pressure is increased during positive-pressure ventilation.

- *Zone 2 (middle of the lung)* has an intermittent blood flow that occurs during systole (when the arterial pressure is greater than the alveolar pressure) but not during diastole (when the arterial pressure is less than the alveolar pressure). Zone 2 blood flow is thus determined by the difference between arterial and alveolar pressures.

• *Zone 3 (bottom of the lung)* has a high, continuous blood flow because the capillary pressure remains greater than the alveolar pressure during the entire cardiac cycle.

Pulmonary Vascular Resistance Decreases During Heavy Exercise. During exercise the blood flow through the lungs increases fourfold to sevenfold. This extra flow is accommodated in the lungs in two ways: (1) by increasing the number of open capillaries, sometimes as much as threefold, and (2) by distending the capillaries and increasing the flow through each capillary by more than twofold. In the normal person, these two changes together decrease the pulmonary vascular resistance so much that the pulmonary arterial pressure rises very little, even during maximum exercise.

Pulmonary Capillary Fluid Dynamics (p. 481)

The alveolar walls are lined with so many capillaries that the capillaries almost touch one another; therefore, the capillary blood flows in the alveolar walls as a "sheet" rather than through individual vessels.

Capillary Exchange of Fluid in the Lungs; Pulmonary Interstitial Fluid Dynamics (p. 481)

The Dynamics of Fluid Exchange through the Lung Capillaries Are Qualitatively the Same as Those for Peripheral Tissues. Quantitatively, however, there are several important differences:

• *Pulmonary capillary pressure* is low (about 7 mm Hg) compared with a higher functional capillary pressure in the peripheral tissues (about 17 mm Hg).

• *Interstitial fluid pressure* is slightly more negative than in the peripheral subcutaneous tissue; values range from about −5 to −8 mm Hg.

• *Capillary permeability* is high, allowing extra amounts of protein to leak from the capillaries; therefore, the interstitial fluid colloid osmotic pressure is also high, averaging about 14 mm Hg, compared with an average of less than 7 mm Hg in many peripheral tissues.

• *The alveolar walls are thin.* The alveolar epithelium covering the alveolar surfaces is so weak it ruptures when the interstitial pressure becomes greater than atmospheric pressure (i.e., more than 0 mm Hg), which allows dumping of fluid from the interstitial spaces into the alveoli.

The Mean Filtration Pressure at the Pulmonary Capillaries Is +1 mm Hg. This value is derived as follows:

- *Total outward force (29 mm Hg).* Forces tending to cause movement of fluid out of the capillaries include the capillary pressure (7 mm Hg), interstitial fluid colloid osmotic pressure (14 mm Hg), and interstitial fluid pressure (−8 mm Hg).
- *Total inward force (28 mm Hg).* Only the plasma colloid pressure (28 mm Hg) tends to cause absorption of fluid into the capillaries.
- *Net mean filtration pressure (+1 mm Hg).* Because the total outward force (29 mm Hg) is slightly greater than the total inward force (28 mm Hg), the net mean filtration pressure is slightly positive (29 − 28 = +1 mm Hg). This net filtration pressure causes a continual loss of fluid from the capillaries.

Pulmonary Edema *(p. 482)*

Pulmonary Edema Develops in the Same Way Peripheral Edema Does. The most common causes of pulmonary edema are as follows:

- *Left-sided heart failure* or mitral valvular disease causes a great increase in pulmonary capillary pressure with subsequent flooding of the interstitial spaces and alveoli.
- *Damage to the pulmonary capillary membrane* caused by infections or breathing of noxious substances produces rapid leakage of plasma proteins and fluid out of the capillaries.

When the Pulmonary Interstitial Fluid Volume Increases by More than 50%, Fluid Pours into the Alveoli. Therefore, except in the mildest cases of pulmonary edema, the edema fluid enters the alveoli.

Acute Safety Factors Tend to Prevent Edema in the Lungs. All the following factors must be overcome before edema can occur: (1) normal negativity of the interstitial fluid pressure, (2) lymphatic pumping of fluid out of the interstitial spaces, and (3) decreased colloid osmotic pressure of the interstitial fluid caused by "washout" resulting from increased loss of fluid from the pulmonary capillaries.

The Pulmonary Capillary Pressure Normally Must Rise to Equal the Plasma Colloid Osmotic Pressure before Significant Pulmonary Edema Occurs. In the human being, who normally has a plasma colloid osmotic pressure of 28 mm Hg, the pulmonary capillary pressure must rise from the normal level of 7 mm Hg to more than 28 mm Hg to cause pulmonary edema, giving an acute safety factor against pulmonary edema of about 21 mm Hg.

The Lymphatic System Provides a Chronic Safety Factor against Pulmonary Edema. The lymph vessels can expand greatly and proliferate over a period of several weeks to months, increasing their ability to carry fluid away from the interstitial spaces by perhaps as much as 10-fold. In a patient with chronic mitral stenosis, a pulmonary capillary pressure of 40 to 45 mm Hg has been measured without the development of significant pulmonary edema.

Lethal Pulmonary Edema Can Occur within Hours. When the pulmonary capillary pressure does rise even slightly above the safety factor level, lethal pulmonary edema can occur within minutes to hours. With acute left-sided heart failure, in which the pulmonary capillary pressure occasionally rises to 50 mm Hg, death often ensues within less than 30 minutes from the onset of acute pulmonary edema.

Fluid in the Pleural Cavity (p. 483)

The Lungs Slide Back and Forth in the Pleural Cavity as They Expand and Contract During Normal Breathing. Small amounts of interstitial fluid transudate continually across the pleural membranes into the pleural space. These fluids contain proteins, which give the pleural fluid a mucoid character, allowing easy slippage of the moving lungs. The total amount of fluid in the pleural cavities is only a few milliliters. The pleural space—the space between the parietal and visceral pleurae—is called a potential space because it normally is so narrow it is not obviously a physical space.

Pleural Effusion—The Collection of Large Amounts of Free Fluid in the Pleural Space—Is Analogous to Edema Fluid in the Tissues. The possible causes of effusion are the following:

- *Blockage of lymphatic drainage* from the pleural cavity allows excess fluid to accumulate.

- *Cardiac failure* causes excessively high peripheral and pulmonary capillary pressures, leading to excessive transudation of fluid into the pleural cavity.
- *Decreased plasma colloid osmotic pressure* allows excessive transudation of fluid from the capillaries.
- *Increased capillary permeability* caused by infection or any other source of inflammation of the pleural surfaces allows rapid dumping of both plasma proteins and fluid into the pleural cavity.

CHAPTER 39

Physical Principles of Gas Exchange; Diffusion of Oxygen and Carbon Dioxide through the Respiratory Membrane

The diffusion of oxygen from alveoli into pulmonary blood and diffusion of carbon dioxide in the opposite direction occur through random molecular motion of the gaseous molecules. The rate at which the respiratory gases diffuse is a much more complicated problem, requiring a deeper understanding of the physics of diffusion and gas exchange.

Physics of Gas Diffusion and Gas Partial Pressures (p. 485)

Respiratory Gases Diffuse from Areas of High Partial Pressure to Areas of Low Partial Pressure. The rate of diffusion of the respiratory gases (oxygen, nitrogen, carbon dioxide) is directly proportional to the pressure caused by each gas alone, which is called the *partial pressure* of the gas. Partial pressures are used to express the concentrations of gases because it is the pressures that cause the gases to move via diffusion from one part of the body to another. The partial pressures of oxygen, carbon dioxide, and nitrogen are designated P_{O_2}, P_{CO_2}, and P_{N_2}, respectively.

The Partial Pressure of a Gas Is Calculated by Multiplying its Fractional Concentration by the Total Pressure Exerted by all Gases. Air has a composition of about 79% nitrogen and about 21% oxygen. The total pressure at sea level (atmospheric pressure) averages 760 mm Hg; therefore 79% of the 760 mm Hg is caused by nitrogen (about 600 mm Hg) and 21% by oxygen (about 160 mm Hg). The partial pressure of nitrogen in the mixture is 600 mm Hg, and the partial pressure of oxygen is 160 mm Hg; the total pressure is 760 mm Hg, the sum of the individual partial pressures.

The Partial Pressure of a Gas in a Solution Is Determined Not Only by Its Concentration but Also by Its Solubility Coefficient. Some molecules, especially carbon dioxide, are physically or chemically attracted to water molecules, which allows far more of them to become dissolved without a build-up of excess pressure in the solution. The relation between gas concentration and gas solubility in determining the partial pressure of a gas is expressed by Henry's law:

$$\text{Pressure} = \frac{\text{Concentration of Dissolved Gas}}{\text{Solubility Coefficient}}$$

The Vapor Pressure of Water at Body Temperature Is 47 mm Hg. When air enters the respiratory passageways, water evaporates from the surfaces and humidifies the air. The pressure the water molecules exert to escape from the surface is the vapor pressure of the water, which is 47 mm Hg at body temperature. Once the gas mixture has become fully humidified, the partial pressure of the water vapor in the gas mixture is also 47 mm Hg. This partial pressure is designated P_{H_2O}.

Composition of Alveolar Air and Its Relation to Atmospheric Air (p. 487)

The Concentrations of Gases in Alveolar Air Are Different from Those in Atmospheric Air. These differences are shown in Table 39–1 and can be explained as follows:

1. Alveolar air is only partially replaced by atmospheric air with each breath.
2. Oxygen is constantly being absorbed from the alveolar air.
3. Carbon dioxide is constantly diffusing from the pulmonary blood into the alveoli.
4. Dry atmospheric air is humidified before it reaches the alveoli.

Water Vapor Dilutes the Other Gases in the Inspired Air. Table 39–1 shows that atmospheric air is composed mostly of nitrogen and oxygen; it contains almost no carbon dioxide or water vapor. The atmospheric air becomes totally humidified as it passes through the respiratory passages. The water vapor at normal body temperature (47 mm Hg) dilutes the other gases in the inspired air. The oxygen partial pressure decreases from 159.0 mm Hg in atmospheric air to 149.3 mm Hg in humidified air, and the nitrogen partial pressure decreases from 597.0 mm Hg to 563.4 mm Hg (see Table 39–1).

Alveolar Air Is Renewed Slowly by Atmospheric Air. The amount of alveolar air replaced by new atmospheric air with each breath is only one seventh of the total; so many breaths are required to exchange the alveolar air completely. This slow replacement of

Table 39-1. Partial Pressures of Respiratory Gases as They Enter and Leave the Lungs (at Sea Level)

Gas	Partial Pressure (mm Hg)			
	Atmospheric Air*	Humidified Air	Alveolar Air	Expired Air
N_2	597.0 (78.62%)	563.4 (74.09%)	569.0 (74.9%)	566.0 (74.5%)
O_2	159.0 (20.84%)	149.3 (19.67%)	104.0 (13.6%)	120.0 (15.7%)
CO_2	0.3 (0.04%)	0.3 (0.04%)	40.0 (5.3%)	27.0 (3.6%)
H_2O	3.7 (0.50%)	47.0 (6.20%)	47.0 (6.20%)	47.0 (6.20%)
Total	760.0 (100%)	760.0 (100%)	760.0 (100%)	760.0 (100%)

*On an average cool, clear day.

alveolar air prevents sudden changes in gas concentrations in the blood.

The Alveolar Oxygen Concentration Is Controlled by the Rate of Oxygen Absorption into the Blood and the Rate of Entry of New Oxygen into the Lungs. The more rapidly oxygen is absorbed, the lower is its concentration in the alveoli. In comparison, the more rapidly new oxygen is breathed into the alveoli from the atmosphere, the higher is its concentration in the alveoli.

Expired Air Is a Combination of Dead Space Air and Alveolar Air. When air is expired from the lungs, the first portion of this air (dead space air) is typical humidified air (see Table 39–1). Then, more and more alveolar air becomes mixed with the dead space air until all the dead space air has been eliminated and only alveolar air is expired at the end of expiration. Normal expired air has approximate gas concentrations and partial pressures as shown (see Table 39–1).

Diffusion of Gases through the Respiratory Membrane (p. 489)

A Respiratory Unit Is Composed of a Respiratory Bronchiole, Alveolar Ducts, Atria, and Alveoli. There are about 300 million units in the two lungs. The alveolar walls are extremely thin, and within them is an almost solid network of interconnecting capillaries; the flow of blood in the alveolar wall has been described as a "sheet" of flowing blood. Gas exchange occurs through the membranes of all the terminal portions of the lungs, not merely in the alveoli themselves. These membranes are collectively known as the *respiratory membrane*, or the *pulmonary membrane*.

The Respiratory Membrane Is Composed of Several Layers. The exchange of oxygen and carbon dioxide between the blood and alveolar air requires diffusion through the following layers of the respiratory membrane:

- A layer of fluid lining the alveolus that contains surfactant
- The alveolar epithelium, which is composed of thin epithelial cells
- An epithelial basement membrane
- A thin interstitial space between the alveolar epithelium and the capillary membrane
- A capillary basement membrane that fuses in places with the epithelial basement membrane
- The capillary endothelial membrane

The Respiratory Membrane Is Optimized for Gas Exchange

- *Membrane thickness.* Despite the large number of layers, the overall thickness of the respiratory membrane averages about 0.6 μm.
- *Membrane surface area.* The total surface area of the respiratory membrane is about 70 square meters in the normal adult.
- *Capillary blood volume.* The capillary blood volume is 60 to 140 mL.
- *Capillary diameter.* The average diameter of the pulmonary capillaries is about 5 μm; the red blood cell membrane usually touches the capillary wall.

Multiple Factors Determine How Rapidly a Gas Passes through the Respiratory Membrane. The determining factors include the following:

- *Thickness of respiratory membrane.* The rate of diffusion through the membrane is inversely proportional to the membrane thickness. Edema fluid in the interstitial space and alveoli decreases diffusion because the respiratory gases must move not only through the membrane but also through this fluid. Fibrosis of the lungs can also increase the thickness of some portions of the respiratory membrane.
- *Surface area of respiratory membrane.* In the presence of emphysema, many of the alveoli coalesce, with dissolution of alveolar walls; this often causes the total surface area to decrease by as much as fivefold.
- *Diffusion coefficient.* The diffusion coefficient for the transfer of each gas through the respiratory membrane depends on its solubility in the membrane and, inversely, on the square root of its molecular weight.
- *Pressure difference across the respiratory membrane.* The difference between the partial pressure of gas in the alveoli and that of gas in the blood is directly proportional to the rate of gas transfer through the membrane in either direction.

Diffusing Capacity of the Respiratory Membrane (p. 491)

The Diffusing Capacity of the Lungs for Carbon Dioxide Is 20 Times Greater Than That for Oxygen. The ability of the respiratory membrane to exchange a gas between the alveoli and the pulmonary blood can be expressed in quantitative terms by its diffusing capacity; this is defined as the volume of a gas that diffuses through the membrane each minute for a 1 mm Hg difference in pressure. All the factors discussed that affect diffusion through the respiratory membrane can affect the diffusing capacity. The diffusing capacity of the lungs for oxygen when a person is at rest is about 21 mL/min/mm Hg. The diffusing capacity for carbon dioxide is about 20 times this value, or about 440 mL/min/mm Hg.

The Diffusion Capacity for Oxygen Increases During Exercise. During exercise, oxygenation of the blood is increased not only by greater alveolar ventilation but also by a greater capacity of the respiratory membrane for transmitting oxygen into the blood. During strenuous exercise, the diffusing capacity for oxygen can increase to about 65 mL/min/mm Hg, which is three times the diffusing capacity during resting conditions. This increase is caused by the following:

• *Increased surface area.* Opening up of closed pulmonary capillaries and dilation of open capillaries increases the surface area for diffusion of oxygen.
• *Improved ventilation-perfusion ratio* ($\dot{V}_A/\dot{Q}$).

Exercise improves the match between the ventilation of the alveoli and the perfusion of the alveolar capillaries with blood.

Effect of the Ventilation-Perfusion Ratio on Alveolar Gas Concentration *(p. 492)*

Even normally and especially with many lung diseases, some areas of the lungs are well ventilated but have almost no blood flow, whereas other areas have excellent blood flow but little or no ventilation. Under either of these conditions, gas exchange through the respiratory membrane is seriously impaired. A highly quantitative concept was developed to help understand respiratory exchange when there is imbalance between alveolar ventilation and alveolar blood flow; this concept is called the ventilation-perfusion ratio ($\dot{V}_A/\dot{Q}$).

The $\dot{V}_A/\dot{Q}$ is the Ratio of Alveolar Ventilation to Pulmonary Blood Flow. When $\dot{V}_A$ (alveolar ventilation) is normal for a given alveolus and $\dot{Q}$ (blood flow) is normal for the same alveolus, the $\dot{V}_A/\dot{Q}$ is also considered to be normal.

• *When the $\dot{V}_A/\dot{Q}$ equals zero* there is no alveolar ventilation, so the air in the alveolus comes to equilibrium with the oxygen and carbon dioxide in the blood. Because the blood that perfuses the capillaries is venous blood, it is the gases in this blood that come to equilibrium with the alveolar gases. Thus, the alveolar P_{O_2} is 40 mm Hg, and the P_{CO_2} is 45 mm Hg when $\dot{V}_A/\dot{Q}$ equals zero.

- *When $\dot{V}_A/\dot{Q}$ equals infinity,* there is no capillary blood flow to carry oxygen away or to bring carbon dioxide to the alveoli. The alveolar air now becomes equal to the humidified inspired air, which has a P_{O_2} of 149 mm Hg and a P_{CO_2} of 0 mm Hg.

- *When the $\dot{V}_A/\dot{Q}$ is normal,* there is both normal alveolar ventilation and normal alveolar capillary blood flow so that exchange of oxygen and carbon dioxide is nearly optimal. Alveolar P_{O_2} is normally at a level of 104 mm Hg, and alveolar P_{CO_2} is normally 40 mm Hg.

Concept of "Physiological Shunt" (When $\dot{V}_A/\dot{Q}$ Is Below Normal) *(p. 493)*

The Greater the Physiological Shunt, the Greater Is the Amount of Blood That Fails to Be Oxygenated as It Passes through the Lungs. Whenever $\dot{V}_A/\dot{Q}$ is below normal, a fraction of the venous blood passes through the pulmonary capillaries without becoming oxygenated. This fraction is called shunted blood. Some additional blood flows through the bronchial vessels rather than through the alveolar capillaries (normally about 2% of the cardiac output); this too is nonoxygenated, shunted blood. The total amount of shunted blood flow per minute is called the physiological shunt.

Concept of "Physiological Dead Space" (When $\dot{V}_A/\dot{Q}$ is Higher than Normal) *(p. 493)*

When the Physiological Dead Space Is Great, Much of the Work of Ventilation Is Wasted Because Some of the Ventilated Air Never Reaches the Blood. When alveolar ventilation is normal but the alveolar blood flow is low, there is far more available oxygen in the alveoli than can be transported away by the flowing blood; the ventilation of these nonperfused alveoli is said to be wasted. The ventilation of the anatomical dead space areas of the respiratory passageways is also wasted. The sum of these two types of wasted ventilation is called the *physiological dead space.*

Abnormalities of the Ventilation-Perfusion Ratio (p. 493)

The $\dot{V}_A/\dot{Q}$ Is High at the Top of the Lung and Low at the Bottom. Blood flow and ventilation both increase from the top to the bottom of the lung, but blood flow increases more progressively. The $\dot{V}_A/\dot{Q}$ is therefore higher at the top of the lung than at the bottom. In both extremes, inequalities of ventilation and perfusion decrease the effectiveness of the lung for exchange of oxygen and carbon dioxide. During exercise, however, the blood flow to the upper part of the lung increases markedly, so that far less physiological dead space occurs, and the effectiveness of gas exchange approaches optimum. The differences in ventilation and perfusion at the top and bottom of the upright lung and their effect on the regional P_{O_2} and P_{CO_2} are summarized in Table 39–2.

The $\dot{V}_A/\dot{Q}$ May Be Increased or Decreased in the Presence of Chronic Obstructive Lung Disease. Most chronic smokers develop bronchial obstruction, which can cause alveolar air to become trapped with resultant emphysema. The emphysema in turn causes many of the alveolar walls to be destroyed; thus two abnormalities occur in smokers to cause abnormal $\dot{V}_A/\dot{Q}$:

- *Low $\dot{V}_A/\dot{Q}$.* Because many of the small bronchioles are obstructed, the alveoli beyond the obstructions are unventilated.

- *High $\dot{V}_A/\dot{Q}$.* In areas where the alveolar walls have been destroyed but there is still alveolar ventilation, the ventilation is wasted because of inadequate blood flow.

Table 39-2. $\dot{V}_A/\dot{Q}$ Characteristics at the Top and Bottom of the Lung

Area of Lung	Ventilation	Perfusion (Blood Flow)	$\dot{V}_A/\dot{Q}$	Local Alveolar Po_2	Local Alveolar Po_2
Top	Low	Lower	Highest	Highest	Lowest
Bottom	High	Higher	Lowest	Lowest	Highest

CHAPTER 40

Transport of Oxygen and Carbon Dioxide in Blood and Tissue Fluids

Oxygen is transported principally in combination with hemoglobin to the peripheral tissue capillaries, where it is released for use by the cells. In the tissue cells, oxygen reacts with various foodstuffs to form large quantities of carbon dioxide. The carbon dioxide then enters the tissue capillaries and is transported back to the lungs. This chapter presents the physical and chemical principles of oxygen and carbon dioxide transport in the blood and body fluids.

Diffusion of Oxygen from the Alveoli to the Pulmonary Capillary Blood (p. 495)

The P_{O_2} of Pulmonary Blood Increases to Equal That of Alveolar Air within the First Third of the Capillary. The P_{O_2} averages 104 mm Hg in the alveolus, whereas in venous blood entering the capillary it averages only 40 mm Hg. The initial pressure difference that causes oxygen to diffuse into the pulmonary capillary is thus $104 - 40$ mm Hg, or 64 mm Hg. The P_{O_2} increases to equal that of alveolar air by the time the blood has moved one third of the distance through the capillary, becoming almost 104 mm Hg.

The Pulmonary Capillary Blood Becomes Almost Fully Saturated with Oxygen Even During Strenuous Exercise. Oxygen utilization can increase by 20-fold during strenuous exercise. An increase in cardiac output reduces the residence time of blood in the pulmonary capillaries to less than one half of normal. The blood, however, is still almost fully saturated with oxygen when it leaves the pulmonary capillaries for the following reasons:

- *Increased diffusing capacity.* As discussed in Chapter 39, the diffusing capacity for oxygen increases almost threefold during exercise because of increased capillary surface area and improved ventilation-perfusion ratio in the upper part of the lungs.
- *Transit time safety factor.* Again, blood becomes almost fully saturated with oxygen during its transit through the first one third of the pulmonary capillary bed, so that full saturation can still occur during large increases in cardiac output.

Bronchial Venous "Shunt" Flow Decreases the Arterial P_{O_2} from a Capillary Value of 104 mm Hg to an Arterial Value of about 95 mm Hg. About 2% of the blood that enters the left atrium has passed directly from the aorta through the bronchial circulation. This blood flow represents "shunt" flow because it is shunted past the gas exchange areas and its P_{O_2} value is typical of venous blood, about 40 mm Hg. This blood then mixes with oxygenated blood from the lungs; this mixing of the bloods is called *venous admixture of blood.*

Tissue P_{O_2} Is Determined by the Rate of Oxygen Transport to the Tissues and the Rate of Oxygen Utilization by the Tissues. The P_{O_2} in the initial portions of the peripheral capillaries is 95 mm Hg, and the P_{O_2} in the interstitial fluid surrounding the tissue cells averages 40 mm Hg. This pressure difference causes oxygen to diffuse rapidly from the blood into the tissues, and the P_{O_2} of the blood leaving the tissue capillaries is also about 40 mm Hg. Two main factors can affect the tissue P_{O_2}:

• *Rate of blood flow.* If the blood flow through a particular tissue becomes increased, greater quantities of oxygen are transported into the tissue during a given period, and the tissue P_{O_2} becomes correspondingly increased.

• *Rate of tissue metabolism.* If the cells use more oxygen for metabolism than normal, the interstitial fluid P_{O_2} tends to be reduced.

Carbon Dioxide Diffuses in a Direction Exactly Opposite to That of Oxygen. There is, however, one major difference between the diffusion of carbon dioxide and that of oxygen: carbon dioxide can diffuse about 20 times as rapidly as oxygen for a given difference in partial pressure.

Transport of Oxygen in Blood *(p. 496)*

About 97% of the Oxygen Is Carried to the Tissues in Chemical Combination with Hemoglobin. The remaining 3% is carried to the tissues in the dissolved state in the water of plasma and cells. Hemoglobin combines with large quantities of oxygen when the P_{O_2} is high and then releases the oxygen when the P_{O_2} level is low. When blood passes through the lungs, where the blood P_{O_2} rises to 95 mm Hg, hemoglobin picks up large quantities of oxygen. As it passes through the tissue capillaries, where the P_{O_2} falls to about 40 mm Hg, large quantities of oxygen are released from the hemoglobin. The free oxygen then diffuses to the tissue cells.

The Oxygen-Hemoglobin Dissociation Curve Shows the Percent Saturation of Hemoglobin Plotted as a Function of P_{O_2}. The oxygen-hemoglobin dissociation curve shown in Figure 40–1 demonstrates a progressive rise in the percentage of hemoglobin that is bound with oxygen as the blood P_{O_2} increases, which is called *percent saturation of the hemoglobin.* Note the following features in the curve:

- *When the P_{O_2} is 95 mm Hg (arterial blood),* the hemoglobin is about 97% saturated with oxygen and the oxygen content is about 19.4 mL/dL of blood; an average of nearly four molecules of oxygen are bound to each molecule of hemoglobin.
- *When the P_{O_2} is 40 mm Hg (mixed venous blood),* the hemoglobin is 75% saturated with oxygen and the oxygen content is about 14.4 mL/dL of blood; an average of three molecules of oxygen are bound to each molecule of hemoglobin.
- *When the P_{O_2} is 25 mm Hg (mixed venous blood during moderate exercise),* the hemoglobin is 50% saturated with oxygen, and the oxygen content is about 10 mL/dL of blood; an average of two molecules of oxygen are bound to each molecule of hemoglobin.

The Sigmoid Shape of the Oxygen-Hemoglobin Dissociation Curve Results from Stronger Binding of Oxygen to Hemoglobin as More Molecules of Oxygen Become Bound. Each molecule of hemoglobin can bind four molecules of oxygen. After one molecule of oxygen has bound, the affinity of hemoglobin for the second molecule is increased, and so forth. Note that the affinity for oxygen is high in the lungs where the P_{O_2} value

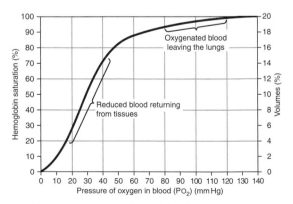

Figure 40–1. Oxygen-hemoglobin dissociation curve.

is about 95 mm Hg (flat portion of the curve) and low in the peripheral tissues where the P_{O_2} value is about 40 mm Hg (steep portion of the curve) (see Fig. 40–1).

The Maximum Amount of Oxygen Transported by Hemoglobin Is About 20 mL of Oxygen per 100 mL of Blood. In a normal person, each 100 mL of blood contains about 15 g of hemoglobin, and each gram of hemoglobin can bind with about 1.34 mL of oxygen when it is 100% saturated ($15 \times 1.34 = 20$ mL of oxygen per 100 mL of blood). However, the total quantity of oxygen bound with hemoglobin in normal arterial blood is about 97%, so about 19.4 mL of oxygen are carried in each 100 mL of blood. The hemoglobin in venous blood leaving the peripheral tissues is about 75% saturated with oxygen, so the amount of oxygen transported by hemoglobin in venous blood is about 14.4 mL of oxygen per 100 mL of blood. About 5 mL of oxygen is therefore normally transported to and used by the tissues in each 100 mL of blood.

Hemoglobin Functions to Maintain a Constant P_{O_2} in the Tissues. Although hemoglobin is necessary for the transport of oxygen to the tissues, it performs another major function essential to life as a *tissue oxygen buffer* system.

- *Under basal conditions,* the tissues require about 5 mL of oxygen from each 100 mL of blood. For the 5 mL of oxygen to be released, the P_{O_2} must fall to about 40 mm Hg. The tissue P_{O_2} level normally does not rise to 40 mm Hg because the oxygen needed by the tissues at that level is not released from the hemoglobin; therefore, the hemoglobin sets the tissue P_{O_2} level at an upper limit of about 40 mm Hg.

- *During heavy exercise,* oxygen utilization increases to as much as 20 times normal. This can be achieved with little further decrease in tissue P_{O_2}—down to a level of 15 to 25 mm Hg—because of the steep slope of the dissociation curve and the increase in tissue blood flow caused by the decreased P_{O_2} (i.e., a small fall in P_{O_2} causes large amounts of oxygen to be released).

The Oxygen-Hemoglobin Dissociation Curve Is Shifted to the Right in Metabolically Active Tissues in Which Temperature, P_{CO_2}, and Hydrogen Ion Concentration Are Increased. The oxygen-hemoglobin dissociation curve shown (see Figure 40–1) is for normal, average blood. A shift in the curve to the right occurs when the affinity for oxygen is low, facilitating the unloading of oxygen. Note that for any given value of P_{O_2} the percent saturation with oxygen is low when the curve is shifted to the right. The oxygen-hemoglobin dissociation curve is also shifted to the right as an adaptation to chronic hypoxemia associated with life at high altitude. Chronic hypoxemia increases the synthesis of 2,3-diphosphoglycerate, a factor that binds to hemoglobin decreasing its affinity for oxygen.

Carbon Monoxide Interferes with Oxygen Transport Because It Has About 250 Times the Affinity of Oxygen for Hemoglobin. Carbon monoxide combines with hemoglobin at the same point on the hemoglobin molecule as does oxygen and can therefore displace oxygen from the hemoglobin. Because it binds with about 250 times as much tenacity as oxygen, relatively small amounts of carbon monoxide can tie up a large portion of the hemoglobin, making it unavailable for oxygen transport. A patient with severe carbon monoxide poisoning can be helped by the administration of pure oxygen because oxygen at high alveolar pressures displaces carbon monoxide from its combination with hemoglobin more effectively than does oxygen at low alveolar pressures.

Transport of Carbon Dioxide in Blood (p. 502)

Under Resting Conditions, About 4 mL of Carbon Dioxide Are Transported from the Tissues to the Lungs in Each 100 mL of Blood. Approximately 70% of the carbon dioxide is transported in the form of bicarbonate ions, 23% in combination with hemoglobin and plasma proteins, and 7% in the dissolved state in the fluid of the blood.

- *Transport in the form of bicarbonate ions (70%).* Dissolved carbon dioxide reacts with water inside red blood cells to form carbonic acid. This reaction is catalyzed in the red blood cells by an enzyme called *carbonic anhydrase.* Most of the carbonic acid immediately dissociates into bicarbonate ions and hydrogen ions; the hydrogen ions in turn combine with hemoglobin. Many of the bicarbonate ions diffuse from the red blood cells into the plasma, and chloride ions diffuse into the red blood cells to maintain electrical neutrality, a phenomenon called the *chloride shift.*
- *Transport in combination with hemoglobin and plasma proteins (23%).* Carbon dioxide reacts directly

with amine radicals of the hemoglobin molecules and plasma proteins to form the compound carbamino-hemoglobin ($HbCO_2$). This combination of carbon dioxide with hemoglobin is a reversible reaction that occurs with a loose bond, so the carbon dioxide is easily released into the alveoli, where the P_{CO_2} is lower than that in the tissue capillaries.

- *Transport in the dissolved state (7%).* Only about 0.3 mL of carbon dioxide is transported in the form of dissolved carbon dioxide by each 100 mL of blood; this represents about 7% of all of the carbon dioxide transported.

CHAPTER 41

Regulation of Respiration

The nervous system adjusts the rate of alveolar ventilation to maintain the arterial blood oxygen pressure (PO_2) and carbon dioxide pressure (PCO_2) at relatively constant levels under a variety of conditions. This chapter describes the operation of this regulatory system.

Respiratory Center (p. 505)

The Respiratory Centers Are Composed of Three Main Groups of Neurons

- *The dorsal respiratory group* generates inspiratory action potentials in a steadily increasing ramplike fashion and is responsible for the basic rhythm of respiration. It is located in the distal portion of the medullae and receives input from peripheral chemoreceptors and other types of receptors via the vagus and glossopharyngeal nerves.

- *The pneumotaxic center,* located dorsally in the superior portion of the pons, helps control the rate and pattern of breathing. It transmits inhibitory signals to the dorsal respiratory group and thus controls the filling phase of the respiratory cycle. Because it limits inspiration, it has a secondary effect to increase respiratory rate.

- *The ventral respiratory group,* which is located in the ventrolateral part of the medulla, can cause either expiration or inspiration, depending on which neurons in the group are stimulated. It is inactive during normal quiet breathing but is important for stimulating the abdominal expiratory muscles when high levels of respiration are required.

The Hering-Breuer Reflex Prevents Overinflation of the Lungs. This reflex is initiated by nerve receptors located in the walls of the bronchi and bronchioles. When the lungs become overly inflated, the receptors send signals through the vagi into the dorsal respiratory group that "switches off" the inspiratory ramp and thus stops further inspiration. This is called the Hering-Breuer inflation reflex.

Chemical Control of Respiration (p. 507)

The Ultimate Goal of Respiration Is to Maintain Proper Concentrations of Oxygen, Carbon Dioxide, and Hydrogen Ions in the Tissues. Excess carbon dioxide or hydrogen ions mainly stimulate the respiratory center itself, causing increased strength of inspiratory and expiratory signals to the respiratory muscles. Oxygen, in contrast, acts on peripheral chemoreceptors located in the carotid and aortic bodies, and these in turn transmit appropriate nervous signals to the respiratory center for control of respiration.

Increased P_{CO_2} or Hydrogen Ion Concentration Stimulates a Chemosensitive Area of the Central Respiratory Center. The sensor neurons in the chemosensitive area are especially excited by hydrogen ions; however, hydrogen ions do not easily cross the blood-brain or blood-cerebrospinal fluid barrier. For this reason, changes in blood hydrogen ion concentration have little acute effect on stimulating the chemosensitive neurons compared with carbon dioxide, even though carbon dioxide is believed to stimulate these neurons secondarily by changing the hydrogen ion concentration. Carbon dioxide diffuses into the brain and reacts with the water of the tissues to form carbonic acid. This in turn dissociates into hydrogen ions and bicarbonate ions; the hydrogen ions then have a potent direct stimulatory effect.

Increased Blood Carbon Dioxide Concentration Has a Potent Acute Effect to Stimulate the Respiratory Drive but Only a Weak Chronic Effect. The excitation of the respiratory center by carbon dioxide is greatest during the first few hours of increased carbon dioxide concentration in the blood but then gradually declines over the next 1 to 2 days. This decline is caused by the following:

• The kidneys return the hydrogen ion concentration back toward normal after the carbon dioxide first increases the hydrogen ion concentration. The kidneys increase the blood bicarbonate, which binds with hydrogen ions in the blood and cerebrospinal fluid reducing their concentration.

• More importantly, the bicarbonate ions diffuse through the blood-brain and blood-cerebrospinal fluid barriers and combine directly with the hydrogen ions near the respiratory neurons.

Peripheral Chemoreceptor System for Control of Respiratory Activity—Role of Oxygen in Respiratory Control *(p. 508)*

Oxygen Is Unimportant for Direct Control of the Respiratory Center. Changes in oxygen concentration have virtually no direct effect on the respiratory center to alter the respiratory drive, but when the tissues do lack oxygen, the body has a special mechanism for respiratory control that is located in the peripheral chemoreceptors, outside the brain respiratory center. This mechanism responds when the arterial oxygen tension falls to 60 to 70 mm Hg.

Chemoreceptors Are Important for Detecting Changes in Arterial P_{O_2}. Peripheral chemoreceptors also respond to changes in P_{CO_2} and hydrogen ion concentration. The following two types of chemoreceptors transmit nervous signals to the respiratory center to help regulate respiratory activity:

- The *carotid bodies* are located in the bifurcations of the common carotid arteries; their afferent nerve fibers innervate the dorsal respiratory area of the medulla.
- The *aortic bodies* are located along the arch of the aorta; their afferent nerve fibers also innervate the dorsal respiratory area.

The Oxygen Lack Stimulus Is Often Counteracted by Decreases in Blood P_{CO_2} and Hydrogen Ion Concentration. When a person breathes air that has too little oxygen, the decrease in arterial P_{O_2} excites the carotid and aortic chemoreceptors, thereby increasing respiration. The increase in respiration leads to a decrease both arterial P_{CO_2} and hydrogen ion concentration. These two changes severely depress the respiratory center, so the final effect of increased respiration in response to low P_{O_2} is mostly counteracted. The effect of low arterial P_{O_2} on alveolar ventilation is far greater under some other conditions, including the following:

- *Pulmonary disease.* With pneumonia, emphysema, or other conditions that prevent adequate gas exchange through the pulmonary membrane, too little oxygen is absorbed into the arterial blood; and at the same time the arterial P_{CO_2} and hydrogen ion concentration remain near normal or are increased because of poor transport of carbon dioxide through the membrane.
- *Acclimatization to low oxygen.* When climbers ascend a mountain over a period of days rather than a period of hours, they can withstand far lower atmospheric oxygen concentrations. The reason is that the respiratory center loses about four fifths of its sensitivity to changes in arterial P_{CO_2} and hydrogen ions, and the low oxygen can drive the respiratory system to a much higher level of alveolar ventilation.

Regulation of Respiration During Exercise
_(p. 510)_

During Strenuous Exercise, the Arterial P_{O_2}, P_{CO_2}, and pH Values Remain Nearly Normal. Strenuous exercise can increase oxygen consumption and carbon dioxide formation by as much as 20-fold, but alveolar ventilation ordinarily increases almost exactly in step with the higher level of metabolism through two mechanisms:

- _Collateral impulses._ The brain, on transmitting impulses to the contracting muscles, is believed to transmit collateral impulses into the brain stem to excite the respiratory center.
- _Body movements._ During exercise, movements of the arms and legs are believed to increase pulmonary ventilation by exciting joint and muscle proprioceptors, which in turn transmit excitatory impulses to the respiratory center.

Chemical Factors Can Also Play a Role in the Control of Respiration During Exercise. When a person exercises, the nervous factors usually stimulate the respiratory center by the proper amount to supply the extra oxygen requirements for the exercise and to blow off the extra carbon dioxide. Occasionally, however, the nervous signals are either too strong or too weak in their stimulation of the respiratory center; then, the chemical factors play a significant role in bringing about the final adjustment in respiration required to keep blood gases as normal as possible.

CHAPTER 42

Respiratory Insufficiency—Pathophysiology, Diagnosis, Oxygen Therapy

The diagnosis and treatment of respiratory disorders require an understanding of the basic physiological principles of respiration and gas exchange. Pulmonary disease can result from inadequate ventilation, abnormalities of gas exchange in the lungs, or transport from the lungs to the peripheral tissues.

Methods for Studying Respiratory Abnormalities (p. 515)

The Most Fundamental Tests of Pulmonary Performance Are Determinations of the Blood P_{O_2}, P_{CO_2}, and pH. It is often important to make these measurements rapidly as an aid in determining the appropriate therapy for acute respiratory distress or acute abnormalities of acid-base balance.

Measurement of Maximum Expiratory Flow (p. 516)

A Forced Expiration Is the Simplest Test of Lung Function. Figure 42–1B shows the instantaneous relationship between pressure and flow when the patient expires with as much force as possible after having inspired as much air as possible. Thus expiration begins at total lung capacity (TLC) and ends at residual volume (RV) (see Fig. 42–1B). The middle curve shows the maximum expiratory flow at all lung volumes in a normal person. Note that the expiratory flow reaches a maximum value of more than 400 L/min at a lung volume of 5 L and then decreases progressively as the lung volume decreases. An important aspect of the curve is that the expiratory flow reaches a maximum value beyond which the flow cannot be increased further with additional effort. For this reason, the descending portion of the curve representing the maximum expiratory flow is said to be *effort-independent.*

The Maximum Expiratory Flow Is Limited by Dynamic Compression of the Airways. Figure 42–1A shows the effect of pressure applied to the outsides of the alveoli and respiratory passageways caused by compression of the chest cage. The arrows indicate that the same

Figure 42–1. *A,* Collapse of the respiratory passageway during a maximum expiratory effort, an effect that limits the expiratory flow rate. *B,* Effect of two respiratory abnormalities—constricted lungs and airway obstruction—on the maximum expiratory flow-volume curve.

amount of pressure is applied to the outsides of both the alveoli and bronchioles. Not only does this pressure force air from the alveoli into the bronchioles, it also tends to collapse the bronchioles at the same time, which opposes the movement of air to the exterior. Once the bronchioles have become almost completely collapsed, further expiratory force can still increase greatly the alveolar pressure, but it can also increase the degree of bronchiolar collapse and airway resistance by an equal amount, thus preventing a further rise in flow. Beyond a critical degree of expiratory force, a maximum expiratory flow has been reached.

The Maximum Expiratory Flow-Volume Curve Is Useful for Differentiating between Obstructive and Restrictive Lung Diseases. Figure 42–1*D* shows a normal maximum flow-volume curve along with curves generated from patients with obstructive lung disease or restrictive lung disease.

- *Restrictive lung disease.* The flow-volume curve in a restrictive lung disease (e.g., interstitial fibrosis) is characterized by low lung volumes and slightly higher than normal expiratory flow rates at each lung volume.
- *Obstructive lung diseases.* The flow-volume curve in obstructive lung diseases (e.g., chronic bronchitis, emphysema, asthma) is characterized by high lung volumes and lower than normal expiratory flow rates. The curve may also have a "scooped-out" appearance.

Physiologic Peculiarities of Specific Pulmonary Abnormalities *(p. 517)*

Obstructive Lung Disease Is Characterized by Increased Resistance to Airflow and High Lung Volumes. Patients with obstructive lung disease find it easier to breathe at high lung volumes because this increases the caliber of the airways (by increasing radial traction) and thus decreases the resistance to airflow. Mechanisms of airway obstruction include the following:

- *The airway lumen* may be partially obstructed by excessive secretions (chronic bronchitis), edema fluid, or aspiration of food or fluids.
- *The airway wall smooth muscle* may be contracted (asthma) or thickened because of inflammation and edema (asthma, bronchitis), or the mucous glands may be hypertrophied (chronic bronchitis).
- *Outside the airway*, the destruction of lung parenchyma may decrease radial traction, causing the airways to be narrowed (emphysema).

Restrictive Lung Disease Is Characterized by Low Lung Volumes. Patients with restrictive lung disease find it easier to breathe at low lung volumes because it is difficult to expand the lungs. Expansion of the lung may be restricted for the following reasons:

- Abnormal lung parenchyma in which excessive fibrosis increases lung elasticity (e.g., pulmonary fibrosis, silicosis, asbestosis, tuberculosis)
- Problems with the pleura (e.g., pneumothorax, pleural effusion)
- Neuromuscular problems (e.g., polio, myasthenia gravis)

Chronic Pulmonary Emphysema *(p. 517)*

The Term *Pulmonary Emphysema* Literally Means Excess Air in the Lungs. Chronic pulmonary emphysema, however, signifies a complex obstructive and destructive process of the lungs and is usually a consequence of long-term smoking. The following pathophysiological events contribute to its development:

- *Airway obstruction.* Chronic infection, excess mucus, and inflammatory edema of the bronchiolar epithelium combine to cause chronic obstruction of many of the smaller airways.
- *Destruction of alveolar walls.* The obstruction of the airways makes it especially difficult to expire, causing entrapment of air in the alveoli with subsequent overstretching of the alveoli. This, combined with lung infection, causes marked destruction of the epithelial cells lining the alveoli.

The Physiological Effects of Chronic Emphysema Are Extremely Varied. They depend on the severity of the disease and the relative degree of bronchiolar obstruction versus lung parenchymal destruction. Chronic emphysema usually progresses slowly over many years. Among the abnormalities are the following:

- *Increased airway resistance.* This is caused by bronchiolar obstruction. Expiration is especially difficult because the force on the outside of the lung compresses the bronchioles, which further increases their resistance.
- *Decreased diffusing capacity.* This is caused by the marked loss of alveolar walls and reduces the ability of the lungs to oxygenate the blood and remove carbon dioxide.
- *Abnormal ventilation-perfusion ratio* $(\dot{V}_A/\dot{Q})$. In the same lungs, areas of the lung with bronchiolar obstruction have a very low $\dot{V}_A/\dot{Q}$ (physiological shunt), resulting in poor aeration of blood, and other areas with loss of alveolar walls have a very high $\dot{V}_A/\dot{Q}$ (physiological dead space), resulting in wasted ventilation.
- *Increased pulmonary vascular resistance.* Loss of alveolar walls decreases the number of pulmonary capillaries. The loss of capillaries causes the pulmonary vascular resistance to increase, in turn causing pulmonary hypertension.

Pneumonia *(p. 518)*

The Term *Pneumonia* Includes Any Inflammatory Condition of the Lung in which Alveoli Are Filled with Fluid and Blood Cells. A common type of pneumonia is bacterial pneumonia, caused most often by pneumococci.

The infected alveoli become progressively filled with fluid and cells. Eventually, large areas of the lungs, sometimes whole lobes or even a whole lung, become "consolidated," which means they are filled with fluid and cellular debris.

Atelectasis *(p. 519)*

Atelectasis Is a Collapse of Lung Tissue Affecting All or Part of One Lung. The following are two common causes:

- *Airway obstruction.* Air trapped beyond a bronchial obstruction is absorbed, causing alveolar collapse. If the lung cannot collapse, negative pressure develops in the alveoli, causing edema fluid to collect.
- *Lack of surfactant.* With hyaline membrane disease (also called respiratory distress syndrome), the quantity of surfactant secreted by the alveoli is greatly depressed. As a result, the surface tension of the alveolar fluid is increased, causing the lungs to collapse or become filled with fluid.

Asthma *(p. 520)*

Asthma Is an Obstructive Lung Disease. The usual cause is hypersensitivity of the bronchioles to foreign substances in the air. The allergic reaction produces (1) localized edema in the walls of the small bronchioles as well as secretion of thick mucus into the bronchiolar lumens and (2) spasm of the bronchiolar smooth muscle. In both instances the airway resistance increases greatly.

The Asthmatic Person Can Usually Inspire Adequately but Has Great Difficulty Expiring. Clinical measurements show a greatly reduced maximum expiratory rate, resulting in dyspnea, or "air hunger." The functional residual capacity and residual volume of the lung are increased during the asthmatic attack because of the difficulty expiring air.

Tuberculosis *(p. 520)*

With tuberculosis, the tubercle bacilli cause (1) invasion of the infected region by macrophages and (2) walling off of the lesion by fibrous tissue to form the so-called tubercle. Tuberculosis in its late stages causes many areas of fibrosis and reduces the total amount of functional lung tissue.

Hypoxia and Oxygen Therapy (p. 520)

Hypoxia Can Result from Multiple Causes. The following is a descriptive classification of the causes of hypoxia:

- Inadequate oxygenation of the lungs because of extrinsic reasons
  1. Deficiency of oxygen in the atmosphere
  2. Hypoventilation (neuromuscular disorders, narcotic abuse)
- Pulmonary disease
  1. Hypoventilation due to increased airway resistance or decreased pulmonary compliance
  2. Uneven alveolar ventilation-perfusion ratio
  3. Diminished respiratory membrane diffusion
- Venous-to-arterial shunts ("right-to-left" cardiac shunts)
- Inadequate oxygen transport by the blood to the tissues
  1. Anemia or abnormal hemoglobin
  2. General circulatory deficiency
  3. Localized circulatory deficiency (peripheral, cerebral coronary vessels)
  4. Tissue edema
- Inadequate tissue capability of using oxygen
  1. Poisoning of cellular enzymes (cyanide)
  2. Diminished cellular metabolic capacity because of toxicity, vitamin deficiency, or other factors

Oxygen Therapy for the Various Types of Hypoxia (p. 521)

Oxygen Therapy Is of Great Value in Certain Types of Hypoxia but of Almost No Value in Others. Recalling the basic physiological principles of the various types of hypoxia, one can readily decide when oxygen therapy may be of value and, if so, how valuable.

- *Atmospheric hypoxia.* Oxygen therapy can correct the depressed oxygen level in the inspired gases and therefore provide 100% effective therapy.
- *Hypoventilation hypoxia.* A person breathing 100% oxygen can move five times as much oxygen into the alveoli with each breath as when breathing normal air. Again, here oxygen therapy can be extremely beneficial.
- *Hypoxia caused by impaired alveolar membrane diffusion.* Essentially the same result occurs as with hypoventilation hypoxia because oxygen therapy can

increase the P_{O_2} in the lungs from a normal value of about 100 mm Hg to as high as 600 mm Hg, thus raising the oxygen diffusion gradient.

- *Hypoxia caused by oxygen transport deficiencies.* For hypoxia caused by anemia, abnormal hemoglobin transport of oxygen, circulatory deficiency, or physiological shunt, oxygen therapy is of less value because oxygen is already available in the alveoli. Instead, the problem is deficient transport of oxygen to the tissues. Extra oxygen can be transported in the dissolved state in the blood when alveolar oxygen is increased to the maximum level; this extra oxygen may be the difference between life and death.

- *Hypoxia caused by inadequate tissue use of oxygen.* With this type of hypoxia, the tissue metabolic enzyme system is simply incapable of utilizing the oxygen that is delivered. It is therefore doubtful that oxygen therapy can be of any measurable benefit.

Hypercapnia *(p. 522)*

Hypercapnia Means Excess Carbon Dioxide in the Body Fluids. When the alveolar P_{CO_2} rises higher than about 60 to 75 mm Hg, the person is breathing about as rapidly and deeply as possible, and air hunger, or *dyspnea*, becomes severe. As the P_{CO_2} rises to 80 to 100 mm Hg, the person becomes lethargic and sometimes even semicomatose.

Cyanosis Means Bluish Skin. It is caused by deoxygenated hemoglobin in the skin blood vessels, especially capillaries. This deoxygenated hemoglobin is dark blue-purple. In general, definite cyanosis appears whenever the arterial blood contains more than 5 g of deoxygenated hemoglobin in each 100 mL of blood. A person with anemia almost never becomes cyanotic because there is not enough hemoglobin for 5 g of it to be deoxygenated in the arterial blood. By comparison, in a person with excess red blood cells (polycythemia), the great excess of available hemoglobin leads often to cyanosis, even under otherwise normal conditions.

Aviation, Space, and Deep-Sea Diving Physiology

CHAPTER 43

Aviation, High-Altitude, and Space Physiology

Technological advancements have made it increasingly more important to understand the effects of altitude and low gas pressures as well as other factors—acceleratory forces, weightlessness—on the human body. This chapter discusses each of these problems.

Effects of Low Oxygen Pressure on the Body (p. 527)

A Decrease in Barometric Pressure Is the Basic Cause of High-Altitude Hypoxia. Note in Table 43–1 that as altitude increases the barometric pressure decreases and P_{O_2} decreases proportionately. The alveolar P_{O_2} is also reduced by carbon dioxide and water vapor.

- *Carbon dioxide.* The alveolar P_{CO_2} falls from a sea level value of 40 mm Hg to lower values as the altitude increases. In the acclimatized person with a fivefold increase in ventilation, the P_{CO_2} can be as low as 7 mm Hg because of increases in ventilation.
- *Water vapor pressure.* In the alveoli, it remains at 47 mm Hg so long as the body temperature is normal, regardless of altitude.

Carbon Dioxide and Water Vapor Pressure Reduce the Alveolar Oxygen. The barometric pressure is 253 mm Hg at the top of 29,028-foot Mount Everest; 47 mm Hg of this must be water vapor, leaving 206 mm Hg for other gases. In the acclimatized person, 7 mm of the 206 mm Hg must be carbon dioxide, leaving 199 mm Hg. If there were no use of oxygen by the body, one fifth of this 199 mm Hg would be oxygen and four fifths would be nitrogen, or the P_{O_2} in the alveoli would be 40 mm Hg. However, some of this alveolar oxygen is normally absorbed by the blood, leaving an alveolar P_{O_2} of about 35 mm Hg.

Breathing Pure Oxygen Increases Arterial Oxygen Saturation at High Altitudes. Table 43–1 shows arterial oxygen saturation while breathing air and while breathing pure oxygen.

- *Breathing air.* Up to an altitude of about 10,000 feet, the arterial oxygen saturation remains at least as high as 90%; it falls progressively until it is only about 70% at 20,000 feet and much less at still higher altitudes.

Table 43–1. Effects of Acute Exposure to Low Atmospheric Pressures on Alveolar Gas Concentrations and Arterial Oxygen Saturation

Altitude (feet)	Barometric Pressure (mm Hg)	Po2 in Air (mm Hg)	Breathing Air*			Breathing Pure Oxygen		
			P_{CO_2} in Alveoli (mm Hg)	P_{O_2} in Alveoli (mm Hg)	Arterial Oxygen Saturation (%)	P_{CO_2} in Alveoli (mm Hg)	P_{O_2} in Alveoli (mm Hg)	Arterial Oxygen Saturation (%)
0	760	159	40 (40)	104 (104)	97 (97)	40	673	100
10,000	523	110	36 (23)	67 (77)	90 (92)	40	436	100
20,000	349	73	24 (10)	40 (53)	73 (85)	40	262	100
30,000	226	47	24 (7)	18 (30)	24 (38)	40	139	99
40,000	141	29				36	58	84
50,000	87	18				24	16	15

*Numbers in parentheses are acclimatized values.

- *Breathing pure oxygen.* When pure oxygen is breathed, the space in the alveoli formerly occupied by nitrogen becomes occupied by oxygen. At 30,000 feet, aviators could have an alveolar P_{O_2} as high as 139 mm Hg instead of the 18 mm Hg they would have when breathing air.

A Person Remaining at High Altitudes For Days, Weeks, or Years Becomes More and More Acclimatized to the Low P_{O_2}. Acclimatization makes it possible for a person to work harder without hypoxic effects or to ascend to still higher altitudes. The principal means by which acclimatization comes about are the following:

- Increased pulmonary ventilation
- Increased concentration of red blood cells
- Increased diffusing capacity of the lungs
- Increased vascularity of the tissues
- Increased ability of the cells to use oxygen despite the low P_{O_2}

Pulmonary Ventilation Can Increase Fivefold in the Acclimatized Person but Only 65% in the Unacclimatized Person. Acute exposure to a hypoxic environment increases alveolar ventilation to a maximum of about 65% above normal. If the person remains at a very high altitude for several days, the ventilation gradually increases to an average of about five times normal (400% above normal).

- *Acute increase in pulmonary ventilation.* The immediate 65% increase in pulmonary ventilation on rising to a high altitude blows off large quantities of carbon dioxide, reducing the P_{CO_2} and increasing the pH of body fluids. Both these changes inhibit the respiratory center and thereby oppose the effect of low P_{O_2} to stimulate the peripheral respiratory chemoreceptors in the carotid and aortic bodies.
- *Chronic increase in pulmonary ventilation.* The acute inhibition fades away within 2 to 5 days, allowing the respiratory center to respond with full force, increasing the ventilation by about fivefold. The decreased inhibition results mainly from a reduction in bicarbonate ion concentration in the cerebrospinal fluid and the brain tissues. This in turn decreases the pH in the fluids surrounding the chemosensitive neurons of the respiratory center, thereby increasing the activity of the center.

Hematocrit and Blood Volume Increase During Acclimatization. Hypoxia is the principal stimulus for an increase in red blood cell production. With full acclimatization to low oxygen, the hematocrit rises from a normal value of 40 to 45 to an average of about 60, with a proportionate increase in hemoglobin concentration. In addition, the blood volume increases, often by 20% to 30%, resulting in a total rise in circulating hemoglobin of 50% or more. This increase in hemoglobin and blood volume begins after 2 weeks, reaching half development within a month or so and full development only after many months.

The Pulmonary Diffusing Capacity Can Increase as Much as Threefold After Acclimatization. The normal diffusing capacity for oxygen through the pulmonary membrane is about 21 mL/mm Hg/min. The following factors contribute to the threefold increase after acclimatization:

- *Increased pulmonary capillary blood volume* expands the capillaries and increases the surface area through which oxygen can diffuse into the blood.
- *Increased lung volume* expands the surface area of the alveolar membrane.
- *Increased pulmonary arterial pressure* forces blood into greater numbers of alveolar capillaries—especially in the upper parts of the lungs, which are poorly perfused under usual conditions.

Chronic Hypoxia Increases the Number of Capillaries in the Tissues. The cardiac output often increases as much as 30% immediately after a person ascends to high altitude but then decreases back toward normal as the blood hematocrit increases, so the amount of oxygen transported to the tissues remains about normal. The number of capillaries in the tissues increases, especially in animals born and bred at high altitudes. The greater capillarity is especially marked in tissues with high metabolic rates.

A Person Who Remains at a High Altitude Too Long Can Develop *Chronic Mountain Sickness*. The following effects contribute to the development of mountain sickness: (1) the red blood cell mass and hematocrit become exceptionally high, (2) the pulmonary arterial pressure increases even more than normal, (3) the right side of the heart becomes greatly enlarged, (4) the peripheral arterial pressure begins to fall, (5) congestive heart failure ensues, and (6) death often follows unless the person is removed to a lower altitude.

Weightlessness in Space (p. 533)

Physiological Problems Exist with Weightlessness. Most of the problems that occur appear to be related to three effects of weightlessness: (1) motion sickness during the first few days of travel, (2) translocation of fluids in the body because of the failure of gravity to cause normal hydrostatic pressure gradients, and (3) diminished physical activity because no strength of muscle contraction is required to oppose the force of gravity. The physiological consequences of prolonged periods in space are the following:

- Decreased blood volume
- Decreased red blood cell mass
- Decreased muscle strength and work capacity
- Decreased maximum cardiac output
- Loss of calcium and phosphate from bones and loss of bone mass

The physiological consequences of prolonged weightlessness are similar to those experienced by people who lie in bed for an extended time. For this reason, extensive exercise programs are carried out during prolonged space missions, and most of the effects mentioned are greatly reduced, except for some bone loss. In previous space expeditions in which the exercise program had been less vigorous, astronauts had severely decreased work capacities for the first few days after returning to earth. They also had a tendency to faint when they stood up during the first day or so after return to gravity because of their diminished blood volume and perhaps diminished responses of the acute arterial pressure control mechanisms. Even with an exercise program, fainting continues to be a problem after prolonged weightlessness.

CHAPTER 44

Physiology of Deep-Sea Diving and Other Hyperbaric Conditions

The pressure around a diver increases progressively during descent to deeper levels. Air must be supplied also under high pressure, exposing the blood in the lungs to extremely high alveolar gas pressure, a condition called *hyperbarism*. These high pressures can cause tremendous alterations in the body physiology.

As One Descends into the Sea, the Pressure Increases and the Gases Are Compressed to Smaller Volumes

- *Increase in pressure.* A column of sea water 33 feet deep exerts the same pressure at its bottom as the entire atmosphere above the earth. A person 33 feet underneath the ocean surface is therefore exposed to a pressure of 2 atmospheres: the first atmosphere of pressure caused by the air above the water and the second atmosphere by the weight of the water itself (Table 44–1).
- *Decrease in volume.* If a bell jar at sea level contains 1 L of air, the volume has been compressed to ½ L at 33 feet underneath the sea surface where the pressure is 2 atmospheres; at 8 atmospheres (233 feet) the volume is ⅛ L. The volume to which a given quantity of gas is compressed is inversely proportional to the pressure, as shown in Table 44–1. This is the physical principle called *Boyle's law.*

Effect of High Partial Pressures of Individual Gases on the Body (p. 535)

Nitrogen Narcosis Can Occur When Nitrogen Pressure Is High. When a diver remains deep in the sea for an hour or more and is breathing compressed air, the depth at which the first symptoms of mild narcosis appear is about 120 feet. At this level, divers begin to exhibit joviality and seem to lose many of their cares. At 150 to 200 feet, they become drowsy. At 200 to 250 feet, strength wanes considerably. Beyond 250 feet, the divers usually become almost useless as a result of nitrogen narcosis.

The Amount of Oxygen Transported in the Blood Markedly Increases at Extremely High P_{O_2}. As the pressure rises progressively into the thousands of millimeters of mercury, a large portion of the total oxygen is then dissolved, rather than being bound with hemoglobin.

Table 44–1. Effect of Sea Depth on Pressure and on Gas Volumes

Depth (feet)	Atmospheres (s)	Volume (liters)
Sea level	1	1.0000
33	2	0.5000
66	3	0.3333
100	4	0.2500
133	5	0.2000
166	6	0.1667
200	7	0.1429
300	10	0.1000
400	13	0.0769
500	16	0.0625

If the P_{O_2} in the lungs is about 3000 mm Hg (4 atmospheres pressure), the total amount of oxygen dissolved in the blood's water is 9 mL/dL of blood.

The Brain Is Especially Susceptible to Acute Oxygen Poisoning. Exposure to 4 atmospheres of oxygen (P_{O_2} 3040 mm Hg) causes seizures followed by coma in most people after 30 minutes.

Nervous System Oxygen Toxicity Is Caused by "Oxidizing Free Radicals". Molecular oxygen (O_2) must first be converted to an "active" form before it can oxidize other chemical compounds. There are several forms of active oxygen; they are called oxygen free radicals. One of the most important of these is the superoxide free radical O_2^-, and another is the peroxide radical in the form of hydrogen peroxide.

- *Normal tissue P_{O_2}.* Even when the tissue P_{O_2} is normal (40 mm Hg), small amounts of free radicals are continually being formed from the dissolved molecular oxygen. The tissues also contain enzymes that remove these free radicals, especially peroxidases, catalases, and superoxide dismutases.

- *High tissue P_{O_2}.* Above about 2 atmospheres, the tissue P_{O_2} markedly increases and large amounts of oxidizing free radicals overwhelm the enzyme systems for removing them. One of the principal effects of the oxidizing free radicals is to oxidize the polyunsaturated fatty acids of the membranous structures of the cells, and another effect is to oxidize some of the cellular enzymes, thus damaging severely the cellular metabolic systems.

Chronic Oxygen Poisoning Causes Pulmonary Disability. A person can be exposed to 1 atmosphere pressure of oxygen almost indefinitely without developing acute oxygen toxicity of the nervous system. However, lung passageway congestion, pulmonary edema, and atelectasis begin to develop after only 12 hours or so of 1 atmosphere oxygen exposure. This increase in susceptibility of the lungs to high oxygen results from direct exposure to the high oxygen pressure.

When a Person Breathes Air under High Pressure for a Long Time, the Amount of Nitrogen Dissolved in the Body Fluids Becomes Excessive. The blood flowing through the pulmonary capillaries becomes saturated with nitrogen to the same high pressure as that in the breathing mixture. Over several hours, enough nitrogen is carried to all the tissues of the body to saturate them also with high levels of dissolved nitrogen.

Decompression Sickness Results from Formation of Nitrogen Bubbles in Tissues. If large amounts of nitrogen have become dissolved in a diver's body and the diver suddenly returns to the surface of the sea, significant quantities of nitrogen bubbles can cavitate in body fluids either intracellularly or extracellularly causing minor or serious damage, depending on the number and size of bubbles formed; this phenomenon is called *decompression sickness.*

Many of the Symptoms of Decompression Sickness Are Caused by Gas Bubbles Blocking Blood Vessels. At first, only the smallest vessels are blocked by minute bubbles, but as the bubbles coalesce, progressively larger vessels are affected. Tissue ischemia and sometimes tissue death are the result.

- *Joint pain.* In about 89% of people with decompression sickness, the symptoms are pain in the joints and muscles of the legs or arms. The joint pain accounts for the term "the bends" that is often applied to this condition.
- *Nervous system symptoms.* In 5% to 10% of those with decompression sickness, nervous system symptoms range from dizziness in about 5% to paralysis or collapse and unconsciousness in 3%.

- *The "chokes."* About 2% of those with decompression sickness develop "the chokes," caused by massive numbers of microbubbles that obstruct the capillaries of the lungs; this is characterized by serious shortness of breath often followed by severe pulmonary edema and occasionally death.

Tank Decompression Is Used to Treat Decompression Sickness. The diver is placed in a pressurized tank, and the pressure is then lowered gradually back to normal atmospheric pressure allowing sufficient time for accumulated nitrogen to be expelled from the lungs.

Hyperbaric Oxygen Therapy *(p. 540)*

Hyperbaric Oxygen Can Be Therapeutic in Several Important Clinical Conditions. The oxygen is usually administered at a P_{O_2} of 2 to 3 atmospheres of pressure. It is believed that the same oxidizing free radicals responsible for oxygen toxicity are also responsible for the therapeutic benefits. Some of the conditions for which hyperbaric oxygen therapy has been especially beneficial are the following:

- *Gas gangrene.* The bacteria that cause this condition, clostridial organisms, grow best under anaerobic conditions and stop growing at oxygen pressures higher than about 70 mm Hg. Hyperbaric oxygenation of the tissues can often stop the infectious process entirely and thus convert a condition that formerly was almost 100% fatal to one that is cured in most instances when treated early.
- *Leprosy.* Hyperbaric oxygenation might have almost as dramatic an effect in curing leprosy as in curing gas gangrene—also because of the susceptibility of the leprosy bacillus to destruction by high oxygen pressures.
- *Other conditions.* Hyperbaric oxygen therapy has also been valuable in the treatment of decompression sickness, arterial gas embolism, carbon monoxide poisoning, osteomyelitis, and myocardial infarction.

IX

The Nervous System: A. General Principles and Sensory Physiology

Organization of the Nervous System, Basic Functions of Synapses, and Neurotransmitters

General Design of the Nervous System (p. 543)

The Nervous System Includes Both Sensory (Input) and Motor (Output) Systems Interconnected by Complex Integrative Mechanisms. The fundamental unit of operation is the *neuron,* which typically consists of a cell body *(soma),* several *dendrites,* and a single *axon.* Although most neurons exhibit the same three components, there is enormous variability in the morphology of individual neurons throughout the brain. It is estimated that the nervous system is composed of more than 100 billion neurons.

Much of the activity in the nervous system arises from mechanisms that stimulate *sensory receptors* located at the distal termination of a *sensory neuron.* Signals travel over peripheral nerves to reach the spinal cord and are then transmitted throughout the brain. Incoming sensory messages are processed and integrated with information stored in various pools of neurons such that the resulting signals can be used to generate an appropriate *motor response.*

The motor division of the nervous system is responsible for controlling a variety of bodily activities such as contraction of striated and smooth muscles and secretion by exocrine and endocrine glands. Actually, only a relatively small proportion of the sensory input received by the brain is used to generate an immediate motor response. Much of it is discarded as irrelevant to the function at hand. Sensory input can be stored in the form of *memory.*

Information stored as memory can become part of the processing mechanism used to manage subsequent sensory input. The brain compares new sensory experiences with those stored in memory and in this way develops successful strategies to form a motor output.

Central Nervous System Synapses (p. 546)

Nervous System Function Is Based on Interactions That Occur between Neurons at Specialized Junctions Called Synapses. At a termination site, an axon typically forms a number of branches that exhibit small dilated regions called *synaptic terminals* or *synaptic boutons.* The synaptic bouton is apposed to, but separated from, an adjacent postsynaptic structure (dendrite or soma) by a narrow space (200 to 300 angstroms) called the *synaptic cleft.* Synaptic boutons contain a variety of organelles, including numerous mitochondria, and they exhibit an aggregation of relatively small spheroidal *synaptic vesicles*, which contain molecules of a chemical *neurotransmitter* agent. When released from the axon terminal, this transmitter agent binds to receptors on the postsynaptic neuron and alters its membrane permeability to certain ions.

Chemical Synapses and Electrical Synapses Are the Two Major Types of Synapse in the Brain. The overwhelming majority are *chemical synapses.* One neuron, the *presynaptic element,* releases a transmitter agent that binds to the *postsynaptic neuron,* which is then excited or inhibited. The transmission of signals at chemical synapses is typically "one way"—from the presynaptic axon terminal to the postsynaptic dendrite or soma.

The least common type of synapse (in mammals) is the *electrical synapse.* These synapses consist of gap junctions that form low resistance channels between the presynaptic and postsynaptic elements. At these synapses, various ions can freely move between the two related neurons, thereby mediating rapid transfer of signals that can spread through large pools of neurons.

When a synaptic bouton is invaded by an action potential, the transmitter agent is released into the synaptic cleft, where it can bind with specific receptors located in the membrane of the postsynaptic dendrite or soma. The excitatory or inhibitory action of the transmitter agent is determined by the response of the postsynaptic receptors.

Neurotransmitter Release Is Calcium-Dependent (p. 548)

- When invaded by an action potential, voltage-gated *calcium channels* in the surface membrane of the synaptic bouton are opened, and calcium moves *into* the terminal.
- Inward calcium flux allows synaptic vesicles to move to release sites at the presynaptic membrane. The vesicles fuse with the presynaptic membrane and exocytose their transmitter agent into the synaptic cleft. The quantity of transmitter released is directly related to the amount of calcium entering the terminal.

Action of the Transmitter Substance on the Postsynaptic Neuron (p. 548)

Receptors are complex proteins with (1) a *binding domain* extending into the synaptic cleft and (2) an *ionophore* that extends through the membrane into the interior of the postsynaptic structure. The ionophore can be either an ion channel specific for a certain ion, or it can form a "second messenger" activator. In both cases, the receptors are linked to *ligand-gated* ion channels.

- *Ligand-gated ion channels* can be *cationic*—passing sodium, potassium, or calcium ions—or *anionic*—passing mainly chloride ions.
- In general, ligand-gated channels that allow sodium to enter the postsynaptic neuron are *excitatory*, whereas channels that allow chloride to enter (or potassium to exit) are *inhibitory*. Channels open and close within fractions of a millisecond, and therefore these mechanisms provide for rapid interaction between neurons.
- *Second messenger activators* are commonly *G-proteins* attached to a portion of the receptor that protrudes into the postsynaptic element. When the receptor is activated, a portion of the G-protein is released and moves within the cytoplasm of the postsynaptic neuron (as a "second messenger"), where it performs one of four possible activities: (1) opens a membrane channel specific for an ion species such as sodium or potassium and keeps it open for a longer period of time than is generally seen with a typical ligand-gated channel; (2) activates cyclic adenosine monophosphate (cAMP) or cyclic guanosine monophosphate (cGMP), which stimulates specific metabolic machinery in the neuron; (3) activates enzymes, which then initiate biochemical reactions in the postsynaptic neuron; or (4) activates gene transcription and protein synthesis that may alter the metabolism or morphology of the cell. Each of these activities is especially well suited to the induction of long-term changes in the excitability, biochemistry, or functional activity of the postsynaptic neuron.

Chemical Substances That Function as Neurotransmitters (p. 550)

At present more than 50 substances have been reported to fulfill the criteria as neurotransmitters. Generally, these substances can be divided into two groups: *small-molecule transmitters* and *neuroactive peptides.*

Small-Molecule, Rapidly Acting Transmitters Can Be Synthesized and Packaged into Synaptic Vesicles in the Axon Terminal. The effect of these agents on the postsynaptic membrane is brief in duration (1 millisecond or less) and typically opens or closes an ion channel. In some instances, the small-molecule agents can stimulate receptor-activated enzymes and alter the metabolism of the postsynaptic neuron. The synaptic vesicles used by these neurotransmitters are *recycled* at the axon terminal. That is, they fuse with the presynaptic membrane near the synaptic active site, and newly formed vesicles are released from the axon terminal membrane more peripherally and are subsequently replenished with the transmitter agent. *Acetylcholine* is one of the typical small-molecule transmitters. It is synthesized from acetyl coenzyme A and choline in the presence of the enzyme *choline acetyltransferase.* The latter substance is synthesized in the soma and delivered to synaptic boutons via axonal transport mechanisms. When acetylcholine is released from vesicles into the synaptic cleft, it binds to receptors on the postsynaptic membrane. Within milliseconds it is broken down into acetate and choline by the enzyme *acetylcholinesterase,* which is also present in the synaptic cleft. As a general rule, the small-molecule transmitters are rapidly inactivated shortly after they bind to their receptor. In this example, choline is actively transported back into the synaptic bouton for subsequent reuse in the synthesis of acetylcholine.

Neuropeptides Form the Second Group of Transmitter Agents and Are Typically Synthesized in the Soma as Integral Components of Large Proteins. These large molecules are cleaved in the cell body and packaged into vesicles in the Golgi apparatus either as the active peptidergic agent or as a precursor of the neuroactive substance. The vesicles are delivered to axon terminals, and the transmitter is released into the synaptic cleft as described later. Commonly, however, smaller amounts of the neuroactive peptide are released compared with the small-molecule transmitters, and their vesicles do not appear to be recycled. An important feature of the neuropeptides is a more prolonged duration of activity than that of the small-molecule agents. The peptides can alter ion channel function and modify cell metabolism or gene expression, and these actions can be sustained for minutes, hours, days, or presumably even longer.

In most instances, neurons utilize only one neurotransmitter agent. However, examples are being reported in which a small-molecule substance and a neuropeptide are *co-localized* in a single synaptic bouton. How the neuron might coordinate the use of the two substances remains to be established.

Electrical Events During Neuronal Excitation *(p. 552)*

- The neuronal membrane exhibits a *resting membrane potential* of about −65 millivolts. Moving this potential to a more positive value (depolarization) makes the cell more excitable, whereas lowering it to a more negative value (hyperpolarization) makes the cell less excitable.

- At rest, the concentrations of ions external and internal to the cell membrane are different. Extracellular sodium concentration is much higher than its intracellular concentration, whereas just the opposite is true for potassium. The distribution of chloride ions is similar to sodium, although their concentration gradient is less than that for sodium.

- Recall that the Nernst potential for an ion is *the* electrical potential that opposes movement of that ion down its concentration gradient:

Nernst Potential (millivolts)

$$EMF = \pm 61 \times \log \frac{(\text{Ion Concentration Inside})}{(\text{Ion Concentration Outside})}$$

- For sodium, the Nernst potential is +61 millivolts. Because the resting membrane potential in neurons is approximately −65 millivolts, one might expect sodium to move into the cell at rest. It cannot move inward, however, because the voltage-gated sodium channels are closed. A small amount does "leak" in, and potassium "leaks" out; but a sodium/potassium pump exchanges sodium ions for potassium ions and moves sodium out and potassium back into the cell, thereby maintaining the resting potential.

- The neuronal membrane at rest is maintained at about −65 millivolts because it is much more permeable to *potassium* ions than to sodium ions. As a result, positively charged potassium ions move out of the cell, leaving behind negatively charged ion species, and the interior becomes negatively charged with respect to the extracellular environment. The interior of the soma (and dendrites) consists of a highly conductive fluid environment with essentially no electrical resistance. Therefore, changes in electrical potential that occur in one part of the cell can easily spread throughout the neuron.

- When a transmitter-receptor interaction results in the opening of *ligand-gated sodium channels* in the postsynaptic membrane, sodium enters the postsynaptic neuron, and the membrane potential depolarizes toward the Nernst potential for sodium (+61 millivolts). This new, more positive local potential is called an *excitatory postsynaptic potential* (EPSP). If the membrane potential of the postsynaptic neuron moves above *threshold* at the axon initial segment, an action potential is generated. The action potential is thought to be initiated at the axon initial segment because this region contains approximately seven times the number of voltage-gated membrane channels found in other parts of the neuron. In most instances, the simultaneous discharge of *many* axon terminals is required to bring the postsynaptic neuron to threshold. This is called *summation,* a concept discussed later.

Electrical Events During Neuronal Inhibition *(p. 554)*

- Neurotransmitters that selectively open *ligand-gated chloride channels* are the basis for production of an *inhibitory postsynaptic potential* (IPSP).
- The Nernst potential for chloride is −70 millivolts. Generally, this is more negative than the postsynaptic neuron resting membrane potential; as a result, chloride ions move into the cell, the membrane potential becomes more negative (hyperpolarized), and the cell is less excitable (inhibited). Similarly, if a transmitter selectively opens potassium channels, positively charged potassium ions would exit the cell, making the interior more negative.

EPSPs and IPSPs Are Summated Over Time and Space *(p. 554)*

- *Temporal summation* occurs when a second postsynaptic potential (excitatory or inhibitory) arrives before the membrane has returned to its resting level. Because a typical postsynaptic potential may last about 15 milliseconds and ion channels are open for

about 1 millisecond (or less), there is usually sufficient time for several channel openings to occur over
the course of a single postsynaptic potential. The
effects of these two potentials are additive (summed
over time).

• *Spatial summation* occurs when a number of axon
terminals over the surface of a neuron are active
simultaneously. Their aggregate effects are summed,
and the combined postsynaptic potential is greater
than any one individual potential. Commonly, the
magnitude of a single EPSP might be only 0.5 to 1.0
millivolt—far less than the 10 to 20 millivolts that
are often required to reach threshold. Spatial summation enables the combined EPSP to exceed threshold.

• At any given point in time, a neuron is combining the
effects of *all* the EPSPs and IPSPs that are occurring
over its surface. Consequently, the postsynaptic neuron might become (1) more excitable and increase its
firing rate or (2) may become less excitable and
decrease its level of firing.

Special Functions of Dendrites for Exciting Neurons *(p. 555)*

Because the dendritic surface forms such a large
proportion of the total surface of the neuron, it is
estimated that 80% to 95% of all synaptic boutons terminate on dendritic elements. Dendrites contain a relatively small number of voltage-gated ion channels in
their surface membrane and therefore are not able to
propagate action potentials. However, they can support
the spread of electrical current by *electrotonic conduction,* although this mode of transmission is subject to
decay (decrement) over time and space. Excitatory (or
inhibitory) postsynaptic potentials that arise at distal
points on the dendritic tree may decrease to such a
low level by the time they reach the soma and axon initial segment there is insufficient current to bring the
neuron to threshold. Conversely, synapses on proximal
dendrites or soma have more influence over the initiation of action potentials because they are simply closer
to the axon initial segment, and the synaptic potentials
do not decrement to a subthreshold level.

Firing Rate of a Neuron: Related to Its State of Excitation *(p. 556)*

Many factors contribute to determination of the firing
threshold, and this functional characteristic varies widely

among neurons. Some neurons are inherently more excitable than others (i.e., it takes less current to reach threshold), whereas others fire at a more rapid rate once threshold is exceeded. The firing rate of a neuron is directly related to the degree to which the threshold is exceeded; the farther it is above threshold, the greater is firing rate, although there is an upper limit.

Synaptic Transmission Exhibits Special Characteristics *(p. 557)*

- When synapses are repetitively stimulated at a rapid rate, the response of the postsynaptic neuron diminishes over time, and the synapse is said to be *fatigued*. This decreased responsiveness is mainly the result of increased build-up of calcium in the synaptic bouton and an inability to replenish the supply of neurotransmitter agent rapidly.
- When repetitive (tetanic) stimulation is applied to an excitatory synapse followed by a brief rest period, subsequent activation of that synapse may require less current and produce an enhanced response. This is called *post-tetanic facilitation.*
- The pH of the extracellular synaptic environment influences the excitability of neuronal function. More acidic values *decrease* excitability, whereas more alkaline levels *increase* neuronal activity.
- A *decrease* in the supply of oxygen diminishes synaptic activity.
- The effects of drugs and chemical agents on neuronal excitability are diverse, complex, and variable. For example, caffeine increases the excitability of many neurons, whereas strychnine indirectly increases the activity of neurons by inhibiting certain populations of inhibitory interneurons.
- Passage of current across a synapse requires a certain amount of time that varies from one neuronal pool to another. This is called *synaptic delay,* and it is influenced by the time (1) required to release transmitter, (2) needed for the transmitter to diffuse across the synaptic cleft, (3) required for transmitter-receptor binding, (4) needed by receptors to carry out their action, and (5) required for ions to diffuse into the postsynaptic cell and alter the membrane potential.

CHAPTER 46

Sensory Receptors, Neuronal Circuits for Processing Information

Sensory Receptors (p. 559)

Five Basic Types of Sensory Receptor

- *Mechanoreceptors* detect physical deformation of the receptor membrane or the tissue immediately surrounding the receptor.
- *Thermoreceptors* detect changes (warm or cold) in the temperature of the receptor.
- *Nociceptors* detect the presence of physical or chemical damage to the receptor or the tissue immediately surrounding it.
- *Photoreceptors* (electromagnetic) detect light (photons) striking the retina.
- *Chemoreceptors* are responsible for taste and smell, O_2 and CO_2 levels in the blood, and osmolality of tissue fluids.

Sensory Receptors Are Highly Sensitive to One Particular Type of Stimulus (Modality)—"The Labeled Line" Principle. Once activated, a receptor initiates action potentials in its associated sensory fiber, which then conveys these impulses to the spinal cord in the form of a "labeled line" via a peripheral nerve. These impulses or action potentials are similar in all sensory fibers. They may exhibit qualitative differences in amplitude or frequency, but an action potential initiated by a painful stimulus is not perceived as uniquely distinguishable from an action potential initiated by any other receptor or *sensory modality.*

What does allow us to differentiate one type of sensation from another is the location in the nervous system where the fiber leads or terminates. Each fiber or collection of neurons linked by related sensory fibers is referred to as a "labeled line." For example, action potentials traveling along the fibers and neurons that comprise the *anterolateral system* (spinothalamic tract) are perceived as pain, whereas action potentials carried over the dorsal column–medial lemniscal system are distinguished as touch or pressure.

Sensory Receptors (p. 560)

Receptors Transduce a Physicochemical Stimulus into a Nerve Impulse. When activated by the appropriate stimulus, a local current is generated at the receptor—referred to as a receptor potential. No matter whether the stimulus is mechanical, chemical, or physical (heat, cold, light), the transduction process results in a change in the ionic permeability of the receptor membrane and consequently a change in the potential difference across this membrane. The maximum receptor potential amplitude of about 100 millivolts is achieved when the membrane sodium permeability is at its maximum level.

The Sensory Fiber Linked to Each Receptor Exhibits "Threshold Phenomena". Only when the receptor potential exceeds a set value (threshold) is a self-propagating action potential initiated in the fiber. The receptor potential is a graded potential, meaning that it decrements (diminishes) over time and space.

The Receptor Potential Is Proportional to the Stimulus Intensity. As the stimulus intensity increases, subsequent action potentials usually increase in *frequency.* The receptor potential amplitude may change substantially with a relatively small intensity change but then increase only minimally with greater stimulus intensity.

Sensory Receptors Adapt to Their Stimuli Either Partially or Completely Over Time. This adaptation occurs by one of two mechanisms. First, the physicochemical properties of the receptor may be altered by the stimulus; for example, when a pacinian corpuscle is initially deformed (and its membrane permeability increased), the fluid in its concentric lamellae redistributes the applied pressure. This redistribution is reflected as a decrease in membrane permeability, and the receptor potential diminishes or adapts. Second, a process of *accommodation* may occur in the sensory fiber itself. Although poorly understood, this may involve a gradual "inactivation" of sodium channels over time.

Receptors Are Classified as Slowly Adapting or Rapidly Adapting. *Slowly adapting receptors* continue to transmit signals with little change in frequency so long as the stimulus is present. For this reason, they are called "tonic receptors" and are able to signal stimulus strength for extended periods of time. Some examples are muscle spindles, Golgi tendon organs, pain receptors, baroreceptors, and chemoreceptors. *Rapidly adapting receptors* are activated only when the stimulus intensity changes. Therefore these receptors are referred to as "rate receptors" or "movement detectors." The Pacinian corpuscle is the best example of the latter receptor category, along with the receptors of the semicircular ducts and joint receptors (proprioceptors).

Physiological Classification of Nerve Fibers (p. 563)

Two Schemes Have Been Devised to Classify the Entire Range of Peripheral Nerve Fibers

- In the more general scheme, all peripheral fibers are divided into types A and C, with type A fibers subdivided into four categories (Fig. 46–1). This scheme is based on the diameter and conduction velocity of

Figure 46–1. Physiological classifications and functions of nerve fibers.

each fiber, with type Aα being the largest and most rapidly conducting variety.
- A second scheme, devised mainly by sensory physiologists, distinguishes five main categories that are again based on fiber diameter and conduction velocity.

Intensity of a Stimulus (p. 564)

Intensity Is Represented in Sensory Fibers Using the Features of Spatial and Temporal Summation. Commonly, a single sensory nerve trunk in a peripheral nerve contains several fibers each related to a variable number of receptors (more than 100 in the case of free nerve endings in the skin) at its distal termination. The aggregate of all the receptors and fibers related to a single nerve defines the *receptive field* of that nerve. An intense stimulus that extends to the entire receptive field activates all the fibers in the sensory nerve trunk, and a less intense stimulus activates proportionally fewer fibers.

Gradations of stimulus intensity are signaled by involving a variable number of "parallel" fibers in the same nerve (spatial summation) or by changing the frequency of impulses traveling in a single fiber (temporal summation).

Transmission and Processing of Signals in Neuronal Pools (p. 564)

Any aggregate of neurons, such as the cerebral cortex, thalamus, or an individual nucleus in the thalamus, can be referred to as a *neuronal pool.* Typically, each neuronal pool has a set of several inputs (afferents), its *receptive field,* and one or several "targets" to which it projects via a set of organized efferent axons.

Afferent Systems Can Provide Either *Threshold or Subthreshold Stimulation* to the Neuronal Pool. Threshold stimulation obviously increases the membrane potential above firing levels in several cells, and they generate action potentials. In others, the membrane potential may be slightly depolarized but not quite enough to reach threshold (subthreshold). These cells are said to be *facilitated;* that is, they are more excitable because smaller excitatory postsynaptic potentials (EPSPs) than normal bring the cell to threshold and fire action potentials.

In Some Neuronal Pools, *Divergence* of Incoming Signals Is a Common Feature. This divergence may take one of two forms. With an *amplification* mechanism, an input fiber may branch to contact many neurons in the pool, and these postsynaptic cells then project in a unified manner to one or a restricted number of targets. With the other form of divergence, the activated neurons in the pool project to multiple, unrelated targets.

The Processing in Neuronal Pools Might Utilize the Mechanism of *Convergence*. Multiple inputs from a single afferent system may terminate on a single neuron in the pool. Alternatively, convergence can result when input signals from multiple afferent sources reach a single neuron in the pool.

On the Afferent Side, a Single Neuron or Pool of Neurons Can Give Rise to Both Excitatory and Inhibitory Output Signals. A single efferent axon may provide excitatory output to one neuron in the next (postsynaptic) pool that is itself an excitatory (relay) neuron, or it may synapse with an inhibitory interneuron in the next pool, which might then inhibit relay neurons in the postsynaptic pool. This is called *feedforward inhibition.*

Signal Processing in Neuronal Pools Can Involve a *Reverberating Circuit* or *Oscillating Circuits*. In these circuits, the output axons of the pool give rise to collateral branches that synapse with *excitatory* interneurons located *within* the pool. These excitatory interneurons then provide feedback to the same output neurons of the pool, leading to a self-propagating sequence of signals. The EPSPs produced by the excitatory interneurons can be facilitatory or may actually stimulate firing by the pool output neurons. The latter situation is the substrate for a neuronal cell group that emits a *continuous train* of efferent signals. Some neuronal pools generate a *rhythmical output signal*—such as the respiratory centers in the medullary reticular formation. This function utilizes a reverberating circuit.

Instability and Stability of Neuronal Circuits *(p. 569)*

Extensive and Diverse Connectivity in the Nervous System Can Produce *Functional Instability* in the Brain when Operations Go Awry. One of the most obvious examples of this instability is an *epileptic seizure.* Two mechanisms are used by the nervous system to combat functional instability:

- The most prominent of these mechanisms is *feedback inhibition.* In this circuit, the output of a neuronal pool activates *inhibitory interneurons* located in the pool, and these cells then provide inhibitory feedback to the main output neurons of the pool. Such a circuit forms an internally regulated "brake" on the output of the pool. When the brake fails, as during a seizure, the pool output fires in an uncontrolled manner.

- The second method used to limit instability is called *synaptic fatigue*. The substrate for this feature is not well understood. It may have a molecular basis, such as a decrease in the uptake or utilization of calcium. Alternatively, it may be related to a more long-term change in receptor sensitivity involving the process of receptor number (sensitivity) up-regulation or down-regulation, which is known to occur in the brain.

CHAPTER 47

Somatic Sensations:
I. General Organization, the Tactile
and Position Senses

Classification of Somatic Senses *(p. 571)*

1. *Mechanoreception* includes both tactile and position (proprioceptive) sensations.
2. *Thermoreception* detects increases or decreases in temperature.
3. *Nociception* detects tissue damage or the release of specific pain-mediating molecules.

The sensory modalities conveyed over the somatic sensory systems include discriminative (precisely localized) touch, crude (poorly localized) touch, pressure, vibration, and the senses of static body position and body movement, which are collectively referred to as *proprioception. Exteroceptive* sensations are those that originate from stimulation of body surface structures, such as the skin and subcutaneous tissues, as well as deeper structures including muscle, fascia, and tendons. In contrast, sensory signals that arise from internal organs (endodermally derived structures) are called *visceral* sensations.

Detection and Transmission of Tactile Sensations *(p. 571)*

Even Though Touch, Pressure, and Vibration Are Often Classified as Separate and Distinct Sensations, They Are Each Detected by the Same General Class of Tactile Receptors: The *Mechanoreceptors*. At least six types of mechanoreceptor are classified as *tactile* receptors:

- *Free nerve endings* are found in varying density in all areas of the skin as well as the cornea of the eye.
- *Meissner's corpuscle* is an encapsulated, rapidly adapting receptor found in the nonhairy (glabrous) areas of skin such as the fingertips and lips, areas that are particularly sensitive to even the lightest touch stimulation.
- *Merkel's discs* (known as expanded tip receptors) are found in glabrous skin but are also present in moderate numbers in hairy skin surfaces. These receptors are relatively slowly adapting and are thought to signal continuous touch of objects against the skin.

- *Hair end-organs* (peritrichal endings) are entwined about the base of each hair on the body surface. They are rapidly adapting and detect movement of objects over the skin surface that displaces the hairs.

- *Ruffini's end-organs* are encapsulated endings located in the skin and deeper tissues, as well as joint capsules. They exhibit little adaptation and thus signal continuous touch and pressure applied to the skin or movement around the joint where they are located.

- *Pacinian corpuscles* are present in the skin and deeper tissues such as fascia. They adapt rapidly and are thought to be especially important for detecting vibration or other rapid change in the mechanical state of the tissues.

Most of these categories of tactile receptors transmit signals over relatively large myelinated fibers that exhibit rapid conduction velocities. In contrast, free nerve endings are linked to small myelinated fibers and unmyelinated type C fibers that conduct at relatively slow velocities.

Each of the tactile receptors is also involved in the detection of vibration. Pacinian corpuscles detect the most rapid vibratory stimuli (30 to 800 cycles per second) and are linked to the large, rapidly conducting myelinated fibers. Low-frequency vibration (up to about 80 cycles per second) stimulates Meissner's corpuscles and the other tactile receptors, which generally transmit at relatively slow conduction velocities and are less rapidly adapting than the Pacinian corpuscles.

The sense of tickle or itch is related to highly sensitive, rapidly adapting free nerve endings in the superficial layers of the skin that mainly transmit over type C fibers. The function of this sensory modality is presumably to call attention to light skin irritations that can be relieved by movement or scratching, a stimulus that appears to override the itch signals.

Sensory Pathways for Transmitting Somatic Signals into the Central Nervous System
(p. 573)

The Main Pathways for Transmission of Somatosensory Signals Are the *Dorsal Column–Medial Lemniscal System* and the *Anterolateral System*. With a few exceptions, sensory information carried by nerve fibers from the

body surface (exclusive of the face) enters the spinal
cord through dorsal roots. Once in the central nervous
system, the signals are segregated into one of two pathways. Signals that originate at thermoreceptors and
nociceptors are processed along the anterolateral system (they are described in Chapter 48). Signals
that arise from mechanoreceptors travel in the dorsal
column–medial lemniscal (DC-ML) system. These
modalities include discriminative touch, vibration, and
proprioception. In a similar manner, somatosensory
information from the face is carried mainly in branches
of the trigeminal nerve; when such fibers enter the
brain stem, they also segregate into two pathways: one
is specialized for processing pain, temperature, and
crude touch; the other is responsible for discriminative
touch, vibration, and proprioception.

Transmission in the DC–ML System *(p. 573)*

The *Anatomy* of the DC-ML System Is Characterized by a High Degree of Somatotopic (Spatial) Organization as Follows

- **Primary sensory neurons.** The central processes of
  dorsal root ganglion primary sensory neurons that
  enter the spinal cord through the medial division of
  the dorsal root entry zone are the larger, myelinated
  fibers carrying signals related to discriminative touch,
  vibration, and proprioception. On entering the cord,
  some of these fibers form local synapses in the gray
  matter, whereas many simply pass into the dorsal
  column area and ascend without synapsing until they
  reach the *dorsal column nuclei* in the caudal medulla.
  Here, fibers carrying information from the lower
  extremities synapse in the nucleus gracilis, whereas
  those from the upper extremity terminate in the
  nucleus cuneatus.
- **Dorsal column nuclei.** Axons of cells in the cuneate
  and gracile nuclei form the *medial lemniscus,* which
  crosses the midline in the caudal medulla as the sensory decussation. This fiber bundle continues rostrally to the thalamus, where the axons terminate in
  the ventrobasal complex, mainly the ventrolateral
  posterior nucleus (VPL). Axons of VPL neurons then
  enter the posterior limb of the internal capsule and
  project to the *primary somatosensory cortex* (SI) in
  the postcentral gyrus.

- **Medial lemniscal pathway.** The fibers of the DC-ML system exhibit a high degree of somatotopic organization *(spatial orientation).* Fibers carrying signals from the lower extremity pass upward through the medial portion of the dorsal column, terminate in the gracile nucleus, and form the ventral and lateral portion of the medial lemniscus. They eventually terminate laterally in the VPL; neurons here project to the most medial part of the SI, on the medial wall of the hemisphere. Information from the upper extremity travels in the lateral part of the dorsal column, terminates in the cuneate nucleus, and enters the dorsal and medial portion of the medial lemniscus. These fibers synapse in the medial part of the VPL and finally reach the arm territory of SI in the hemisphere contralateral to the body surface, where the signals originated. Throughout the system, there is a point-to-point relationship between the origin in the periphery and the termination in the SI.

- **Somatosensory signals from the face.** Tactile somatosensory signals from the face travel in the trigeminal nerve and enter the brain stem at midpontine levels, where the primary sensory fibers terminate in the principal trigeminal sensory nucleus. From here, axons cross the midline and course rostrally, adjacent to the medial lemniscus, and eventually terminate medially in a portion of the ventrobasal complex, the ventral posteromedial nucleus (VPN). This system of fibers is comparable to the DC-ML system and conveys similar types of somatosensory information from the face.

- **Somatosensory areas of the cerebral cortex.** The postcentral gyrus comprises the primary somatosensory cortex, which corresponds to Brodmann's areas 3, 1, and 2. A second somatosensory area (SII) is much smaller than SI and is located just posterior to the face region of SI bordering on the lateral fissure. Within SI, segregation of body parts is maintained such that the face region is ventrally located nearest the lateral fissure, the upper extremity continues medially and dorsally from the face region and extends toward the convexity of the hemisphere, and the lower extremity projects onto the medial surface of the hemisphere. In fact, there is a complete but separate body representation in areas 3, 1, and 2. Within each of these body representations, there is an *unequal* volume of cortex devoted to each body part. Those body surfaces with a high density of sensory receptors are represented by larger areas in the cortex than those with a relatively low density of receptors.

Functional Anatomy of the Primary Somatosensory Cortex (p. 576)

- Contains six horizontally arranged cellular layers numbered I to VI beginning with layer I at the cortical surface. The most characteristic is layer IV because it receives the important projections from VPL and VPM of the ventrobasal thalamus. From here, information is spread dorsally into layers I to III and ventrally to layers V and VI.

- Contains an army of vertically organized columns of neurons that extend through all six layers. These are *functionally* determined columns that vary in width from 0.3 to 0.5 mm and are estimated to contain about 10,000 neurons each. In the most anterior part of area 3 in SI, the vertical columnar arrays are concerned with muscle afferents, whereas in the posterior part of area 3, they process cutaneous input. In area 1 the vertical columns process additional cutaneous input whereas in area 2 they are concerned with pressure and proprioception.

The Functions of the *Primary* and *Association* Somatosensory Areas Can Be Inferred from Studies of Patients with Lesions in These Areas as Follows

- Lesions that involve *primary somatosensory cortex* result in (1) the inability to localize precisely the cutaneous stimuli on the body surface, although some crude localizing ability may be retained; (2) the inability to judge degrees of pressure or the weight of objects touching the skin; and (3) the inability to identify objects by touch or texture *(astereognosis)*.

- Lesions that involve Brodmann's areas 5 and 7 damage the *association cortex for somatic sensation.* Common signs and symptoms include (1) the inability to recognize objects that have a relatively complex shape or texture when palpated with the contralateral hand; (2) the loss of the awareness of the contralateral side of the body *(hemineglect)* (this symptom is most acute with lesions in the nondominant parietal lobe); and (3) when feeling an object, patients explore only the side that is ipsilateral to their lesion and ignore the contralateral side *(amorphosynthesis)*.

Overall Characteristics of Signal Transmission and Analysis in the DC-ML System *(p. 577)*

The *receptive field* of an SI cortical neuron is determined by the combination of primary sensory neurons, dorsal column nuclear neurons, and thalamic neurons that provide afferent projections to that SI neuron.

Two-Point Discrimination Is Used to Test the DC-ML System. This method is often used to determine the individual's ability to distinguish two simultaneously applied cutaneous stimuli as two separate "points" *(two-point discrimination)*. This capability varies substantially over the body surface. On the fingertips and lips two points of stimulation as close together as 1 to 2 mm can be distinguished as separate points, whereas on the back the two points must be separated by at least 30 to 70 mm. This function depends on the central processing elements in the DC-ML pathway to recognize that the two excitatory signals generated peripherally are separate and nonoverlapping.

Lateral Inhibition Is a Mechanism Used throughout the Nervous System to "Sharpen" Signal Transmission. This process uses inhibition of the input from the peripheral portion of a receptive field to define better the boundaries of the excited zone. In the DC-ML system, lateral inhibition occurs at the level of the dorsal column nuclei and in thalamic nuclei.

The DC-ML System Is Particularly Effective in Sensing *Rapidly Changing* and *Repetitive* Stimuli, Which Is the Basis for *Vibratory Sensation*. This capability resides in the rapidly adapting pacinian corpuscles, which are able to detect vibrations up to 700 cycles per second, and in Meissner's corpuscles, which detect somewhat lower frequencies, such as 200 cycles per second and below.

The Awareness of Body Position or Body Movement Is Called *Proprioceptive Sensation*. The sense of body movement is also called the kinesthetic sense or dynamic proprioception. A combination of tactile, muscle, and joint capsule receptors are used by the nervous system to produce the sense of proprioception. For movements of small body parts such as the fingers, tactile receptors in the skin and in joint capsules are thought to be most important when determining the proprioceptive signal. For complex movements of the upper or lower limbs where some joint angles are increasing and others decreasing, muscle spindles are an important determinant of proprioceptive sensation. At the extremes of joint angulation, the stretch imposed on ligaments and deep tissues around the joint can activate Pacinian corpuscles and Ruffini endings. The latter, being rapidly adapting receptors, are probably responsible for detecting the rate of change in movement.

Transmission of Less Critical Sensory Signals in the Anterolateral Pathway *(p. 580)*

Signals traveling on small myelinated fibers and unmyelinated C fibers can arise from tactile receptors (typically free nerve endings) in the skin. This information is transmitted along with pain and temperature signals in the anterolateral portion of the spinal cord white matter. As discussed in Chapter 48, the anterolateral system extends to the ventrobasal thalamus as well as to the intralaminar and posterior thalamic nuclei. Although some painful stimuli are fairly well localized, the precise point-to-point organization in the DC-ML system and the relative diffuseness of the anterolateral system probably account for the less effective localizing ability of the latter system.

The characteristics of transmission in the anterolateral pathway are similar to that of the DC-ML except for the following differences: (1) the velocity of transmission are one half to one third those of the DC-ML, (2) the degree of special localization is poor, (3) the gradations of intensity are far less pronounced, and (4) the ability to transmit rapid repetitive signals is poor. In addition to pain and temperature this system transmits the sensations of tickle and itch, crude touch, and sexual sensations.

CHAPTER 48

Somatic Sensations: II. Pain, Headache, and Thermal Sensations

Pain is mainly a protective mechanism for the body because it is not a pure sensation but, rather, a response to tissue injury that is created, as it were, within the nervous system.

Pain Sensation: Fast and Slow Pain Classification (p. 583)

Fast pain is felt within about 0.1 second after the stimulation, whereas *slow pain* begins 1 second or more following the painful stimulus. Slow pain is usually associated with tissue damage and can be referred to as burning pain, aching pain, or chronic pain.

All pain receptors are free nerve endings. They are found in largest number and density in the skin, periosteum, arterial walls, joint surfaces, the dura, and its reflections inside the cranial vault.

Three Types of Stimuli (p. 583)

Pain Receptors Are Activated by Mechanical, Thermal, and Chemical Stimuli

- *Mechanical* and *thermal* stimuli tend to elicit *fast pain.*
- *Chemical* stimuli tend to produce *slow pain,* although this is not always the case. Some of the more common chemical agents that elicit pain sensations are bradykinin, serotonin, histamine, potassium ions, acids, acetylcholine, and proteolytic enzymes. The tissue concentration of these substances appears to be directly related to the degree of tissue damage and, in turn, the perceived degree of painful sensation. In addition, prostaglandins and substance P enhance the sensitivity of pain receptors but do not directly excite them.
- Pain receptors adapt very slowly or essentially not at all. In some instances, the activation of these receptors becomes progressively *greater* as the pain stimulus continues; this is called *hyperalgesia.*

Dual Pathways for Transmission of Pain Signals into the Central Nervous System (p. 584)

Fast pain signals elicited by mechanical or thermal stimuli are transmitted over Aδ fibers in peripheral nerves at velocities between 6 and 30 m/sec. In contrast, the slow, chronic type of pain signals are transmitted over type C fibers at velocities ranging from 0.5 to 2.0 m/sec. As these two types of fiber enter the spinal cord through dorsal roots, they are segregated such that Aδ fibers primarily excite neurons in lamina I of the dorsal horn, whereas C fibers synapse with neurons in the substantia gelatinosa. The latter cells then project deeper into the gray matter and activate neurons mainly in lamina V but also in laminae VI and VII. The neurons that receive Aδ fiber input (fast pain) give rise to the *neospinothalamic* tract, whereas those that receive C fiber input form the *paleospinothalamic* tract.

The Neospinothalamic Tract Is Used During Pain Localization. Axons from neurons in lamina I that form the neospinothalamic tract cross the midline close to their origin and ascend the white matter of the spinal cord as part of the anterolateral system. Some of these fibers terminate in the brain stem reticular formation, but most project all the way to the ventral posterolateral nucleus (VPL) of the thalamus (ventrobasal thalamus). From here, thalamic neurons project to the primary somatosensory (SI) cortex. This system is primarily used during the localization of pain stimuli.

Activity in the Paleospinothalamic System May Impart the Unpleasant Perception of Pain. The *paleospinothalamic pathway* is the phylogenetically older of the two pain pathways. The axons of cells in lamina V, like those from lamina I, cross the midline near their level of origin and ascend in the anterolateral system. The axons of lamina V cells terminate almost exclusively in the brain stem, rather than in the thalamus. In the brain stem, these fibers reach the reticular formation, the superior colliculus, and the periaqueductal gray. A system of ascending fibers, mainly from the reticular formation, proceed rostrally to the intralaminar nuclei and posterior nuclei of the thalamus, as well as to portions of the hypothalamus. Pain signals transmitted over this pathway are typically localized only to a major part of the body. For example, if the stimulus originates in the hand, it may be localized to "somewhere" in the upper extremity.

- The role of SI cortex in pain perception is not entirely clear. Complete removal of the SI cortex does not eliminate the perception of pain. Such lesions do, however, interfere with the ability to interpret the quality of pain and to determine its precise location.

- The fact that the brain stem reticular areas and the intralaminar thalamic nuclei that receive input from the paleospinothalamic pathway are part of the brain stem activating or alerting system may explain why individuals with chronic pain syndromes have difficulty sleeping.

Pain Suppression ("Analgesia") System in the Brain and Spinal Cord (p. 586)

There is marked variability in the degree to which individuals react to painful stimuli; this is in large part because of the existence of a mechanism for pain suppression (analgesia) that resides in the central nervous system. This pain suppression system consists of three major components.

- The *periaqueductal gray* of the mesencephalon and rostral pons receives input from the ascending pain pathways in addition to descending projections from the hypothalamus and other forebrain regions.
- The *nucleus raphe magnus* (serotonin) and *nucleus paragigantocellularis* (norepinephrine) in the medulla receive input from the periaqueductal gray and project to neurons in the spinal cord dorsal horn.
- In the dorsal horn, *enkephalin interneurons* receive input from descending serotonergic raphe magnus axons, and the latter form direct synaptic contact with incoming pain fibers causing both presynaptic and postsynaptic inhibition of the incoming signal. This effect is thought to be mediated by calcium channel blockade in the membrane of the sensory fiber terminal.

Brain's Opiate System—Endorphins and Enkephalins

Neurons in the periaqueductal gray and nucleus raphe magnus (but not the noradrenergic medullary reticular neurons) have *opiate receptors* on their surface membranes. When stimulated by exogenously administered opioid compounds (analgesics) or by endogenous opioid neurotransmitter agents (endorphins and enkephalins) found in the brain, the pain suppression circuitry is activated, which leads to reduced pain perception.

Pain Sensation: Inhibited by Certain Types of Tactile Stimulation

Activation of the large, rapidly conducting tactile sensory fibers of the dorsal roots appears to suppress the transmission of pain signals in the dorsal horn, probably through lateral inhibitory circuits. Although poorly understood, such circuitry probably explains the relief of pain achieved by the simple maneuver of rubbing the skin in the vicinity of a painful stimulus.

Electrical Stimulation: Relief of Pain

Stimulating electrodes implanted over the spinal cord dorsal columns or stereotactically positioned in the thalamus or periaqueductal gray has been used to reduce chronic pain. The level of stimulation can be regulated upward or downward by the patient to manage pain suppression more effectively.

Referred Pain *(p. 588)*

Most often, referred pain involves signals originating in an internal (visceral) organ or tissue. The mechanism is not well understood but is thought to be due to the fact that visceral pain fibers may synapse with neurons in the spinal cord that also receive pain input from cutaneous areas seemingly unrelated to the visceral stimulation site. A common example is pain from the heart wall being *referred* to the surface of the left side of the jaw and neck or the left arm. Rather than associating the pain with the heart, the patient perceives the pain sensation as coming from the face or arm. This implies that visceral afferent signals from the heart converge on the same spinal cord neurons that receive cutaneous input from the periphery (or the convergence may occur in the thalamus).

In other instances, leakage of gastric secretions from a perforated or ulcerated gastrointestinal tract may directly stimulate pain endings in the peritoneum and lead to severe painful sensations in the body wall. The pain may localize to the dermatomal surface related to the embryonic location of the visceral structure. Spasms in the muscular wall of the gut or distention of a muscular wall of an organ such as the urinary bladder may also lead to painful sensations.

Pain from an internal organ such as an inflamed appendix may be experienced in two locations. If the involved appendix touches the parietal peritoneum, pain may be felt in the wall of the right lower abdominal quadrant or it can be referred to the region around the umbilicus, or both, because of the termination of visceral pain fibers in the T-10 or T-11 segments of the spinal cord, which receive cutaneous input from those dermatomes.

Clinical Abnormalities of Pain and Other Somatic Sensations (p. 590)

- *Hyperalgesia* involves a heightened sensitivity to painful stimuli. Local tissue damage or the local release of certain chemicals can lower the threshold for activation of pain receptors and the subsequent generation of pain signals.

- Interruption of the blood supply or damage to the ventrobasal thalamus (somatosensory region) may cause the *thalamic pain syndrome.* This is initially characterized by a loss of all sensation over the contralateral body surface. Sensations may return after a few weeks to months, but they are poorly localized and nearly always painful. Eventually, a state is reached in which even minor skin stimulation can lead to excruciatingly painful sensations; this is known as *hyperpathia.*

- Viral infection of a dorsal root ganglion or cranial nerve sensory ganglion may lead to segmental pain and a severe skin rash in the area subserved by the affected ganglion. This is known as *herpes zoster (shingles).*

- Severe lancinating pain may occur in the cutaneous distribution of one of the three main branches of the trigeminal nerve (or glossopharyngeal nerve); this is called *tic douloureux or trigeminal neuralgia* (or glossopharyngeal neuralgia). In some instances, it is caused by the pressure of a blood vessel compressing the surface of the trigeminal nerve in the cranial cavity; often it can be surgically corrected.

- The *Brown-Séquard syndrome* is caused by extensive damage to either the right or left half of the spinal cord such as occurs with hemisection. A characteristic set of somatosensory deficits ensues. Transection of the anterolateral system results in loss of pain and temperature sensation *contralaterally* that typically begins one or two segments caudal to the level of the lesion. On the side *ipsilateral* to the lesion, there is a loss of dorsal column sensations beginning at about the level of the lesion and extending through all levels caudal to the lesion. If the lesion involves several segments of the cord, there may be an ipsilateral loss of *all* sensation in those dermatomes that correspond to the location of the cord lesion. These patients, of course, exhibit motor deficits as well.

Headache (p. 590)

Headache Can Result When Pain from Deeper Structures Is Referred to the Surface of the Head. The source of the pain stimuli may be intra- or extracranial; in this chapter we focus on intracranial sources. The brain itself is insensitive to pain, but the dura mater and cranial nerve sheaths contain pain receptors that transmit signals traveling with cranial nerves X and XII that enter spinal cord levels C-2 and C-3. When somatosensory structures are damaged, the patient experiences the sensation of tingling, or *pins and needles*. The exceptions, as described previously, are tic douloureux and the thalamic pain syndrome.

Headache of Intracranial Origin. *Pressure on the venous sinuses and stretching of the dura or blood vessels and cranial nerves passing through the dura lead to the sensation of headache.* When structures above the tentorium cerebelli are affected, pain is referred to the frontal portion of the head, whereas involvement of structures below the tentorium results in occipital headaches.

Meningeal inflammation typically produces pain involving the entire head. Likewise, if a small volume of cerebrospinal fluid is removed (as little as 20 mL) and the patient is not recumbent, gravity causes the brain to "sink"; this leads to stretching of meninges, vessels, and cranial nerves, resulting in a diffuse headache. The headache that follows an alcoholic binge is thought to be due to the direct toxic irritation of alcohol on the meninges. Constipation may also cause headache as a result of direct toxic effects of circulating metabolic substances or from circulatory changes related to the loss of fluid into the gut.

Although the mechanism is still not completely understood, *migraine headaches* are thought to be the result of vascular phenomena. Prolonged unpleasant emotions or anxiety produces spasm in brain arteries and leads to local ischemia in the brain. This may result in prodromal visual or olfactory symptoms. As a result of the prolonged spasm and ischemia, the muscular wall of the vessel loses its ability to maintain normal tone. The pulsation of circulating blood alternately stretches (dilates) and relaxes the vessel wall, which stimulates pain receptors in the vascular wall or in the meninges surrounding the entry points of vessels into the brain or cranium. The result is an intense headache. Other causative theories are being investigated, and a number of new and effective treatments for this condition should soon be available.

Headache of Extracranial Origin *(p. 591)*

Emotional tension can cause the muscles of the head especially those attached to the scalp and neck to become spastic and irritate the attachment areas. Irritation of the nasal and accessory nasal structures that are highly sensitive can lead to the phenomenon of sinus headache. Difficulty in focusing the eyes can lead to excessive contraction of the ciliary muscle as well as the muscles of the face in an effort to squint to sharpen the focus on the object at hand. This can lead to eye and facial pain commonly known as an eyestrain type of headache.

Thermal Sensations

Thermal Receptors and Their Excitation *(p. 592)*

- *Pain receptors* are stimulated only by extreme degrees of cold or warmth. In this case, the perceived sensation is one of pain, not temperature.
- Specific *warmth receptors* have not yet been identified, although their existence is suggested by psychophysical experiments; at present, they are simply regarded as free nerve endings. Warmth signals are transmitted over type C sensory fibers.
- The *cold receptor* has been identified as a small nerve ending, the tips of which protrude into the basal aspect of basal epidermal cells. Signals from these receptors are transmitted over $A\delta$ type sensory fibers. There are 3 to 10 times as many cold receptors as warmth receptors, and their density varies from 15 to 25 per square centimeter on the lips to 3 to 5 receptors per square centimeter on the fingers.

Cold and Warmth Receptors: Temperatures in the Range of 7°C to 50°C *(p. 592)*

Temperatures below 7°C and above 50°C activate pain receptors, and both of these extremes are perceived similarly as very painful, not as cold or warm. The peak temperature for activation of cold receptors is about 24°C, and the warmth receptors are maximally active at about 45°C. Both cold and warm receptors can be stimulated with temperatures in the range of 31°C to 43°C.

When the cold receptor is subjected to an abrupt temperature decrease, it is strongly stimulated initially; but then, after the first few seconds, the generation of action potentials falls off dramatically. However, the decrease in firing progresses more slowly over the next 30 minutes or so. This means that the cold and warm receptors respond to *steady state temperature* as well as *changes in temperature.* This explains why a cold outdoor temperature "feels" so much colder at first as one emerges from a warm environment.

The stimulatory mechanism in thermal receptors is believed to be related to the change in metabolic rate in the nerve fiber induced by the temperature change. It has been shown that for every 10°C temperature change there is a twofold change in the rate of intracellular chemical reactions.

The density of thermal receptors on the skin surface is relatively small. Therefore, temperature changes that affect only a small surface area are not as effectively detected as temperature changes that affect a large skin surface area. If the entire body is stimulated, a temperature change as small as 0.01°C can be detected. Thermal signals are transmitted through the central nervous system in parallel with pain signals.

X

The Nervous System:
B. The Special Senses

CHAPTER 49

The Eye: I. Optics of Vision

Physical Principles of Optics (p. 597)

- Light travels through transparent objects at a *slower velocity* than it does through air. The *refractive index* of a transparent substance is the ratio of its velocity in air to its velocity in the transparent object.
- The direction that light travels is always *perpendicular* to the plane of the wave front. When a light wave passes through an angulated surface, it is bent (refracted) at some angle if the refractive indices of the two media are different. The angle depends on the refractive index of the barrier material and the angle between the two surfaces.

Application of Refractive Principles to Lenses

- A *convex* lens focuses light rays. Light rays that pass through the lens perimeter are bent (refracted) toward those (to make themselves perpendicular to the wave front) that pass through the central region. The light rays are said to *converge.*
- A *concave* lens diverges light rays. At the lens perimeter, light waves are refracted so they travel perpendicular to the wave front, or interface, and are bent away from those passing through the central region. This is called *divergence.*
- The *focal length* of a lens is the distance beyond a convex lens at which parallel light rays converge to a single point.
- Each point source of light in front of a convex lens is focused on the opposite side of the lens in line with the lens center. That is, the object appears to be upside down and reversed from left to right.
- The more a lens bends light rays, the greater is its refractive power. The unit of measure for refractive power is the *diopter.* A spherical (or convex) lens that converges parallel light rays to a point 1 meter beyond the lens has a refractive power of +1 diopter; if the light rays are bent twice as much, the diopter is +2.

Optics of the Eye (p. 600)

The eye is optically equivalent to a photographic camera. It has a lens, a variable aperture (pupil), and the retina, which corresponds to the film. The lens system of the eye focuses an inverted, upside down image on the retina. However, we perceive the image as right side up because the brain has "learned" that this is the correct or normal orientation.

Accommodation Depends on a Change in the Shape of the Lens and Allows the Eye to Focus on a Near Object. When shifting the gaze from a far to a near object, the process of *accommodation* involves (1) making the lens more convex, (2) narrowing the pupillary diameter, and (3) adduction (vergence) of both eyes. When the lens is in a "relaxed" state with no tension exerted on the edges of its capsule, it assumes a nearly spherical shape owing to its own intrinsic elastic properties. When the inelastic zonule fibers attached to the lens perimeter become taut and are pulled radially by their attachment to the *inactive* ciliary muscle (and ciliary body), the lens is relatively flat or less convex. When the ciliary muscle is *activated* by postganglionic parasympathetic fibers in the oculomotor nerve, the circular fibers of the ciliary muscle contract, producing a sphincter-like action that relaxes the tension on the zonule fibers and allows the lens to become more convex owing to its own inherent elasticity. This increases its refractive capability and allows the eye to focus on near objects. At the same time, the sphincter pupillae muscle is activated, the pupil constricts, and the two eyes are medially deviated.

Presbyopia Is the Loss of Accommodation by the Lens. As an individual ages, the lens begins to lose its intrinsic elastic properties and becomes less responsive and unable to focus on near objects. This condition (*presbyopia*) is corrected with reading glasses designed to magnify near objects or with bifocals in which one lens (the upper portion) is designed to enhance distance vision and the second lens (lower portion) has greater refractive capability to improve near vision.

The Diameter of the Pupil (Iris) Is Also a Factor in Accommodation. The greater the diameter, the more light there is that enters the eye. Squinting (narrowing the pupil opening) improves the sharpness of the image by increasing the focal plane.

Errors of Refraction (p. 602)

- *Emmetropia* refers to the normal eye. When the ciliary muscle is completely relaxed, all distant objects are in sharp focus on the retina.
- *Hyperopia*, also known as "farsightedness," is due to an eyeball that is too short from top to bottom,

causing light rays to focus behind the retina; this condition is corrected with a convex lens.

- *Myopia*, also known as "nearsightedness," is due to an eye that is elongated from front to back causing light rays to focus in front of the retina; this condition is corrected with a concave lens that decreases refraction by producing divergence of the entering light rays.

- *Astigmatism* is caused by substantial differences in the curvature over different planes through the eye. For example, the curvature in a vertical plane through the eye may be much less than the curvature through a horizontal plane. As a result, light rays entering the eye from different directions are focused at different points. This condition requires a cylindrical lens for correction.

- *Cataracts* are caused by an opacity that forms in a portion of the lens. The treatment of choice is to remove the lens and substitute an artificial lens implant.

- *Keratoconus* is a condition that results from the formation of an oddly shaped cornea with a prominent bulge on one side causing a severe refractive problem that cannot be corrected by a single lens. The best solution is a contact lens that adheres to the surface of the cornea and is held in place by a film of tear fluid. This lens is ground to compensate for the bulge in the cornea such that the anterior surface of the contact lens becomes a far more uniform and effective refractive surface.

Visual Acuity: Sharpest within the Foveal Region of the Retina *(p. 604)*

The *fovea* is made up entirely of cone photoreceptors, each having a diameter of about 1.5 μm. Normal visual acuity in humans allows discrimination of two points of light as being distinct when they are separated by at least 25 seconds of arc on the retina.

The fovea is normally about 0.5 mm in diameter. Maximal acuity occurs in less than 2 degrees of the visual field. The reduction in acuity outside the foveal region is due in part to the presence of rod photoreceptors intermixed with cones and to the linkage of some rod and cone receptors to the same ganglion cells.

The test chart for visual acuity is usually placed 20 feet from the individual being tested. If letters of a particular size can be recognized at a distance of 20 feet, the individual is said to have 20/20 vision. If the individual can only see letters at 20 feet that should be visible all the way out to 200 feet, that individual has 20/200 vision.

Determination of Distance of an Object from the Eye—Depth Perception (p. 605)

Knowing the size of an object allows the brain to calculate its distance from the eye. If an individual looks at a distant object without moving the eyes, no *moving parallax* is apparent. However, if the head is moved from side to side, close objects move rapidly across the retina, whereas distant objects move very little or not at all.

Binocular vision also aids in determining the distance of an object. Because the eyes are typically about 2 inches apart, an object placed 1 inch in front of the bridge of the nose is seen by a small part of the peripheral retina in the left and right eyes. In contrast, the image of an object at 20 feet falls on closely corresponding points in the middle of each retina. This type of binocular parallax (stereopsis) provides the ability to judge distances from the eyes accurately.

Ophthalmoscope (p. 605)

The ophthalmoscope allows the retina of the observed eye to be illuminated by means of an angled mirror or prism and a small bulb. The observer positions the instrument to view the subject's retina through the subject's pupil. If either the subject's eyes or the examiner's eyes are not emmetropic, refraction can be adjusted using a series of movable lenses in the instrument.

Fluid System of the Eye—Intraocular Fluid (p. 606)

- *Vitreous humor* lies between the lens and retina and is more of a gelatinous body than a liquid. Substances can diffuse through the vitreous, but there is little movement or flow in this liquid.
- *Aqueous humor* is a watery fluid secreted by the epithelial lining of ciliary processes on the ciliary body at a rate of 2 to 3 µL/min. This fluid migrates between the ligaments supporting the lens and through the pupil into the anterior chamber of the eye (between the lens and cornea). From here, the fluid flows into the angle between the cornea and iris and then through a trabecular meshwork to enter the canal of Schlemm, which empties directly into extraocular veins.

The *intraocular pressure* is normally about 15 mm Hg, with a range of 12 to 20 mm Hg. A tonometer is usually used to measure intraocular pressure. This device consists of a small footplate that is placed on the anesthetized cornea. A small force is applied to the footplate, which displaces the cornea inward, and the distance of inward displacement is calibrated in terms of intraocular pressure.

Glaucoma is a condition in which intraocular pressure can reach dangerously high levels (in the range of 60 to 70 mm Hg). As the pressure rises above 20 to 30 mm of Hg, axons of retinal ganglion cells that form the optic nerve are compressed to the extent that axonal flow is interrupted, causing permanent injury to the parent neuron. Compression of the central retinal artery may also lead to neuronal death in the retina. Glaucoma can be treated with eyedrops that reduce the secretion of aqueous humor or increase its absorption. If drug therapy fails, surgical procedures are performed to open the trabecular spaces or to drain the trabecular meshwork directly into subconjunctival spaces outside the eyeball.

CHAPTER 50

The Eye: II. Receptor and Neural Function of the Retina

Anatomy and Function of the Structural Elements of the Retina (p. 609)

The Retina Is Composed of 10 Cellular Layers or Boundaries. These are listed below in sequence, beginning with the most external layer (most distant from the center of the eyeball):

1. Pigment layer
2. Layer of rods and cones
3. Outer limiting membrane
4. Outer nuclear layer
5. Outer plexiform layer
6. Inner nuclear layer
7. Inner plexiform layer
8. Ganglionic layer
9. Layer of optic nerve fibers
10. Inner limiting membrane

When light passes through the lens system of the eye, it first encounters the inner limiting membrane, the optic nerve fibers, and the ganglion cell layer; it then continues through the remaining layers to reach the receptors, the rods and cones. The *fovea* is a specialized region of approximately 1 square millimeter in the central region of the retina. In the center of the fovea is an area 0.3 mm in diameter called the *central fovea*. This is the region of maximal visual acuity, and it is here that the photoreceptor layer contains only cones. In addition, the subjacent retinal layers—all the way to the optic nerve fibers and blood vessels—are displaced laterally to enable more direct access to the receptor elements.

Each photoreceptor consists of (1) an outer segment, (2) an inner segment, (3) a nuclear region, and (4) the synaptic body or terminal. The receptors are referred to as *rods* or *cones,* depending primarily on the shape of their outer segment (Fig. 50–1).

The light sensitive photopigment *rhodopsin* is found in the rod outer segment, whereas a similar material called a color-sensitive pigment, *photopsin,* or cone pigment, is found in the cone outer segment. These photopigments are proteins incorporated into a stacked array of membranous discs in the receptor outer segment, which represent infolding of the photoreceptor outer

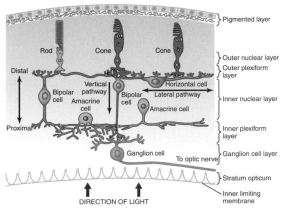

Figure 50–1. Layers of the retina.

cell membrane. This is not readily apparent in the distal portion of the rod outer segment, however, where the membranous discs become secondarily detached from, and entirely contained within, the limiting membrane of the outer segment.

The inner segments of the rods and cones are essentially indistinguishable and contain the cytoplasmic components and organelles common to other neuronal cell bodies. Individual photoreceptor nuclei are continuous with their own inner segment, but the outer limiting membrane of the retina forms an incomplete separation or boundary between the layer of inner segments and the layer of photoreceptor nuclei (outer nuclear layer).

The *synaptic body* contains those elements such as mitochondria and synaptic vesicles that are typically found in axon terminals in the brain. The black pigment *melanin* in the pigment layer reduces light reflection throughout the globe of the eye and thus performs a function similar to the black coloring inside the bellows of a camera. The importance of this pigment is best illustrated by its absence in albino individuals. Because of the large amount of reflection inside the globe of the eye, albinos rarely exhibit better than 20/100 visual acuity. The pigment layer also stores large quantities of vitamin A used in the synthesis of visual pigments.

The *central retinal artery* provides the blood supply only to the innermost layers of the retina (ganglion cell axons to the inner nuclear layer). The outermost layers of the retina receive their blood supply by diffusion from the highly vascularized choroid, which is situated between the sclera and retina.

When an individual suffers traumatic retinal detachment, the line of separation occurs between the neural retina and pigment epithelium. Because of the independent blood supply to the inner layers of the retina via the central retinal artery, the retina can survive for several days and may resist functional degeneration if the retina is surgically returned to its normal apposition to the pigment epithelium.

Photochemistry of Vision *(p. 611)*

Rhodopsin-Retinal Cycle, and Excitation of the Rods

Rhodopsin Is Decomposed by Light Energy. The rod photopigment rhodopsin is concentrated in that portion of the outer segment that protrudes into the pigment layer. This substance is a combination of the protein *scotopsin* and the carotenoid pigment *retinal* or, more specifically, 11-*cis* retinal. When light energy is absorbed by rhodopsin, the retinal portion is transformed into the all-*trans* configuration, and the retinal and scotopsin components begin to separate. In a series of reactions that occur extremely rapidly, the retinal component is converted to lumirhodopsin, metarhodopsin I, metarodopsin II, and finally scotopsin; and all-*trans* retinal is cleaved. During this process, metarhodopsin II is believed to elicit the electrical changes in the rod membrane that lead to subsequent impulse transmission through the retina.

Rhodopsin Reformation Occurs. During the first stage of the reformation of rhodopsin, all-*trans* retinal is converted to the 11-*cis* configuration, which then immediately combines with scotopsin to form rhodopsin. There is also a second pathway leading to the formation of rhodopsin that involves conversion of all-*trans* retinal into all-*trans* retinol, which is a form of vitamin A. The retinol is converted enzymatically to 11-*cis* retinol and then to 11-*cis* retinal, which is able to combine with scotopsin to form rhodopsin. If excess retinal is present in the retina, it is converted to vitamin A, thereby reducing the total amount of rhodopsin in the retina. Night blindness occurs in vitamin A–deficient individuals because rods are the photoreceptors maximally used under

relatively dim lighting conditions, and the formation
of rhodopsin is dramatically decreased owing to the
absence of vitamin A. This condition can be reversed
in about 1 hour or less with an intravenous injection of
vitamin A.

Excitation of the Rod When Rhodopsin Is Activated by Light *(p. 612)*

Rod photoreceptors behave quite differently from other
neural receptor elements. In the dark (in the absence of
photic stimulation), rod outer segment membranes are
"leaky" to sodium; that is, sodium ions *enter* the outer
segment and alter its membrane potential from the typical level of −70 to −80 millivolts observed in sensory
receptors to a more positive value of −40 millivolts.
This is known as a sodium current or the "dark current," and it causes a small amount of transmitter
release in the dark. When light strikes the rod outer
segment, rhodopsin molecules undergo the series of
reactions described previously, and this *decreases* the
conductance of sodium into the outer segment and
diminishes the dark current. Some sodium ions continue
to be pumped out through the cell membrane, and
this loss of positive ions causes the interior to become
more negative; the membrane potential becomes more
negative and is said to *hyperpolarize.* The flow of transmitter is halted.

When light strikes a photoreceptor, the transient
hyperpolarization in rods reaches a peak in about 0.3
second and lasts for more than 1 second. In addition,
the magnitude of the receptor potential is proportional
to the *logarithm* of the light intensity. This has great
functional significance because it allows the eye to discriminate light intensity through a range many thousand times as great as would otherwise be possible. It
is the result of an extremely sensitive chemical cascade
that amplifies the stimulatory effects about a million-
fold as follows. Activated rhodopsin (metarhodopsin II)
acts as an enzyme to activate many molecules of *transducin,* a protein also found in the outer segment disc
membrane. The activated transducin in turn activates
phosphodiesterase, an enzyme that immediately hydrolyzes many molecules of *cyclic guanosine monophosphate*
(cGMP). The loss of cGMP results in closure of many
sodium channels, which is then accompanied by an
increasingly more negative (hyperpolarized) membrane
potential. Within about 1 second, metarhodopsin II is

inactivated, and the entire cascade reverses: the membrane potential becomes more depolarized as sodium channels are reopened, and sodium once again enters the outer segment as the dark current is reestablished. Cone photoreceptors behave similarly, but the amplification factor is 30 to 300 times less than in the rods.

Photochemistry of Color Vision by the Cones (p. 614)

As in the rods described previously, the photochemical transduction process in cones involves an opsin and a retinal. In cones, the opsin is called *photopsin*, which has a chemical composition different from that of rhodopsin, whereas the retinal component is exactly the same as in rods. There are three types of cone, each characterized by a different photopsin that is maximally sensitive to a particular wavelength of light in either the blue, green, or red portion of the light spectrum.

Light and Dark Adaptation (p. 614)

If exposed to bright light for long periods of time, large proportions of the photochemicals in both rods and cones are depleted, and much of the retinal is converted to vitamin A. As a result, the overall sensitivity to light is reduced; this effect is called *light adaptation.* Conversely, when an individual remains in the dark for a long period of time, the opsins and retinal are converted back to light-sensitive pigments. In addition, vitamin A is converted to retinal, providing even more photosensitive pigment; this is the process of *dark adaptation.* The latter process occurs about four times as rapidly in cones as in rods, but cones exhibit less sensitivity change in the dark. Cones cease adapting after only a few minutes, whereas the more slowly adapting rods continue to adapt for minutes to hours, and their sensitivity increases over a broad range.

Adaptation can also occur through changes in pupillary size. This change can be on the order of 30-fold within a fraction of a second. Neural adaptation can also take place in the circuits that exist within the retina and brain. If light intensity increases, transmission from bipolar cell to horizontal cell to amacrine and ganglion cell may also increase. Although the latter form of adaptation is less substantial than pupillary changes, neural adaptation, like pupillary adaptation, occurs rapidly.

The value of light and dark adaptive processes is that they provide the eye with the ability to change its sensitivity by as much as 500,000-fold to 1 million-fold. This can be appreciated when entering a dark room from a brightly lit environment. The sensitivity of the retina is low because it is light-adapted, and little can be seen in the dark room. As dark adaptation occurs, vision in the dark improves. The intensity of sunlight is estimated to be 10 billion times greater than light intensity on a starlit night. Yet the eye can function to some degree under both conditions because of its enormous adaptive range.

Color Vision *(p. 615)*

Tricolor Mechanism of Color Detection

Spectral sensitivity of the three types of cone is based on the light absorption curves for the three cone pigments. All visible color (other than blue, green, or red) is the result of combined stimulation of two or more types of cone. The nervous system then interprets the ratio of activity of the three types as a color. About equal stimulation of blue, green, and red cones is interpreted as white light.

Changing the color of the light that illuminates a scene does not substantially alter the hues of color in the scene. This is called *color constancy*, and it is believed that the mechanism for this phenomenon resides in the primary visual cortex.

When a particular type of cone is missing from the retina, some colors cannot be distinguished from others. An individual who lacks red cones is called a *protanope*. The overall spectrum is shortened at the long-wavelength end by the absence of red cones. Red-green color blindness is a genetic defect in males but is transmitted by the female. Genes on the female X chromosome code for the respective cones. This defect rarely occurs in females because by having two X chromosomes they almost always have one normal copy of the gene.

Neural Functions of the Retina *(p. 616)*

Neural Circuitry of the Retina

- *Photoreceptors* consist of rod and cone outer segments and inner segments in the photoreceptor layer, a cell body in the outer nuclear layer, and a synaptic terminal in the outer plexiform layer.

- *Horizontal cells, bipolar cells, and amacrine cells* receive synaptic input in the outer plexiform layer, have their somas in the inner nuclear layer, and form presynaptic contacts in the inner plexiform layer.
- *Ganglion cells* receive synaptic input in the inner plexiform layer, have a soma in the ganglion cell layer, and give rise to axons that course within the optic nerve fiber layer.
- *Interplexiform cells* transmit signals in the opposite direction—from the inner plexiform to the outer plexiform layer.

In the fovea, the pathway from a cone to a ganglion cell is relatively direct and can involve a receptor, a bipolar cell, and a ganglion cell. Horizontal cells can be involved in the outer plexiform layer, whereas amacrine cells are active in the inner plexiform layer. More peripherally in the retina, where rod photoreceptors are most abundant, the input from several photoreceptors can converge on a single bipolar neuron, which may have output only to an amacrine cell that then projects to a ganglion cell. This represents the pure rod vision pathway. Horizontal and amacrine cells can provide lateral connectivity.

Neurotransmitters present in the retina include glutamate (used by rods and cones) and γ-aminobutyric acid (GABA), glycine, dopamine, acetylcholine, and indoleamines (used by amacrine cells). The transmitter used by horizontal, bipolar, or interplexiform cells is unclear.

Beginning with the photoreceptors, transmission of signals up to the ganglion cell layer occurs only by *electrotonic conduction* (graded potentials) and not action potentials. The ganglion cell is the only retinal neuron capable of generating an action potential; this ensures that signals in the retina accurately reflect illumination intensity, and it gives retinal neurons more flexibility in their response characteristics.

Lateral Inhibition to Enhance Visual Contrast— Function of the Horizontal Cells

Horizontal cell processes connect laterally with photoreceptor synaptic terminals and bipolar cell dendrites. The photoreceptors that lie in the center of a light beam are maximally stimulated, whereas those at the periphery are inactivated by horizontal cells, which are themselves activated by the light beam. It is said that the *surround* is inhibited, whereas the central region is *excited* (although these terms may not be precisely correct). This is the basis for the enhancement of visual contrast. Amacrine cells may also contribute to contrast enhancement through their lateral projections in the inner plexiform layer. Interestingly, whereas horizontal cells may have axons, amacrine cells do not and therefore their physiological properties are highly complex.

Some Bipolar Cells Are Excited by Light

Some bipolar cells depolarize when their related photoreceptor or receptors are stimulated by light, whereas others hyperpolarize. There are two possible explanations for this observation. One is that the two bipolar cells simply respond differently to glutamate release by the photoreceptor; one bipolar cell is excited by glutamate, and the other type of bipolar cell is inhibited. Another explanation is that one type of bipolar cell may receive direct (excitatory) input from the photoreceptor, and the other may receive indirect inhibitory input from a horizontal cell. Having some bipolar cells excited and others inhibited may also contribute to the lateral inhibition scheme.

Amacrine Cells and Their Functions

Nearly 30 types of amacrine cell have been identified by morphological or histochemical means. Some amacrine cells respond vigorously at the onset of a visual stimulus, others at the offset, and still others at both onset and offset. Another type responds only to a moving stimulus. Because of the variety of neurotransmitters used by this class of cell, there can be no generalization regarding its effect on its target neuron.

Ganglion Cells and Optic Nerve Fibers *(p. 619)*

There are about 1.6 million ganglion cells in the retina; yet it is estimated that 100 million rods are present with 3 million cones. This means that an average of 60 rods and 2 cones converge on each retinal ganglion cell. The population of ganglion cells is divided into W-, X-, and Y-type cells.

- *W-type ganglion cells* constitute nearly 40% of the entire pool, are small, and have a somal diameter of 10 μm; they transmit action potentials at the relatively slow velocity of 8 m/sec. They receive most of their input from rod photoreceptors (via bipolar and amacrine cells) and exhibit a relatively broad dendritic field. These cells appear to be especially sensitive to movement in the visual field, and because of their dominant input from rods, they are probably responsible for dark-adapted vision.

- *X-type ganglion cells* are somewhat more numerous than W-cells and represent about 55% of all ganglion cells. They have a somal diameter of 10 to 15 μm and conduct at about 14 m/sec. These cells exhibit relatively small dendritic fields and therefore represent discrete locations in the visual field. Each X cell receives input from at least one cone photoreceptor, so this class of cell is probably responsible for color vision.

- *Y-type ganglion cells* are the largest; they exhibit somal diameters up to 35 μm and conduct at velocities of about 50 m/sec. As might be predicted, their dendritic spread is broad. They are the fewest in number, however, constituting only about 5% of the total pool. These cells respond rapidly to changes anywhere in the visual field (either intensity or movement) but are not capable of specifying with accuracy where the change occurred.

Excitation of the Ganglion Cells *(p. 619)*

It is the ganglion cell axons that form the optic nerve fibers. Even when unstimulated, they transmit action potentials at rates varying between 5 and 40 per second. Visual signals are thus superimposed on this background or spontaneous level of firing.

Many ganglion cells are particularly sensitive to changes in light intensity. Some cells respond with increased firing when light intensity increases, whereas others increase their firing when light intensity decreases. These effects are due to the presence of depolarizing and hyperpolarizing bipolar cells. The responsiveness to light intensity fluctuation is equally well developed in the peripheral and foveal regions of the retina.

Contrast Levels and Lateral Inhibition *(p. 620)*

Ganglion cells are said to be responsive to contrast borders, rather than absolute levels of illumination. When photoreceptors are activated by flat, diffuse light, depolarizing bipolar cells provide excitatory output, but at the same time hyperpolarizing bipolar cells and horizontal cells can produce inhibitory output. When a light stimulus has sharp contrast, at the light-dark border one photoreceptor in the light is hyperpolarized, and a depolarizing signal is transmitted through its bipolar cell to a ganglion cell, which then increases its firing. A neighboring photoreceptor in the dark region is depolarized and its bipolar-ganglion cell line is inactivated. At the same time, a horizontal cell linked to the hyperpolarized (illuminated) photoreceptor is inactivated because the photoreceptor stops releasing a transmitter substance that depolarizes that horizontal cell. Therefore, the hyperpolarizing influence exerted by this horizontal cell on the neighboring (depolarized) photoreceptor in the dark is lost, and that photoreceptor depolarizes even further. The dark is made "darker," and the light is made "lighter" (i.e., contrast is enhanced).

Transmission of Color Signals by the Ganglion Cells
(p. 620)

Some ganglion cells are stimulated by all three types of cone photoreceptor. Such a ganglion cell is thought to signal "white" light. Most ganglion cells, however, are stimulated by light of one wavelength and inhibited by another. For example, red light may excite and green inhibit a particular ganglion cell; this is called a *color-opponent mechanism* and is thought to be the process used to differentiate color. Because the substrate for such a process is present in the retina, recognition and perception of color may actually begin in the retina at the level of the primary sensory receptive element.

CHAPTER 51

The Eye: III. Central Neurophysiology of Vision

Visual Pathways *(p. 623)*

Axons of retinal ganglion cells form the *optic nerve.* Axons that originate from the nasal retina cross at the *optic chiasm,* and those from the temporal retina pass through the lateral aspect of the chiasm without crossing each other (Fig. 51–1). Retinal axons continue posterior to the chiasm as the *optic tract,* and most terminate in the *dorsal lateral geniculate nucleus.* From here, the axons of geniculate neurons proceed further posteriorly as the *geniculocalcarine (optic) radiations* and terminate in the *primary visual (striate) cortex.* In addition, retinal axons extend to other regions of the brain including the (1) suprachiasmatic nucleus (control of circadian rhythms), (2) pretectal nuclei (for pupillary light reflexes), (3) superior colliculus (control of rapid eye movements), and (4) ventral lateral geniculate nucleus.

Functions of the Dorsal Lateral Geniculate Nucleus (DLGN) of the Thalamus

The DLGN is a laminated structure that consists of six concentrically arranged layers. The most internal layer is layer 1, and the most superficial is layer 6. Retinal axons that terminate in the DLGN arise from the contralateral nasal retina and the ipsilateral temporal retina and thus carry point-to-point information from the contralateral visual field. The contralateral nasal fibers terminate in layers 1, 4, and 6, and the ipsilateral temporal fibers terminate in layers 2, 3, and 5. Information from the two eyes remains segregated in the DLGN as does input from X and Y retinal ganglion cells. The Y cell input terminates in layers 1 and 2, which are termed the *magnocellular* layers because they contain relatively large neurons. This is a rapidly conducting pathway that is color-blind but carries effective localizing information. Layers 3 to 6 are termed the *parvocellular* layers because they contain relatively small neurons that receive input from X cells that transmit color and form information. Thus, information from the retina is processed along at least two parallel pathways: (1) a dorsal stream carrying information from rod photoreceptors and large (Y) ganglion cells that specify location and movement information and (2) a ventral stream carrying color and

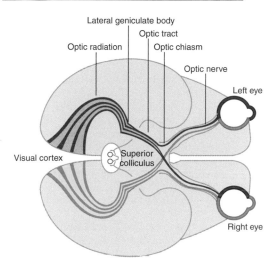

Figure 51–1. Principal visual pathways from the eyes to the visual cortex. (Modified from Polyak SL: The Retina. Chicago: University of Chicago, 1941.)

form (shape) information from cone photoreceptors and small (X) ganglion cells.

Organization and Functions of the Visual Cortex *(p. 624)*

The *primary visual cortex,* or area 17 of Brodmann, is also referred to as V-1. It is located on the medial surface of the hemisphere lining both walls of the calcarine sulcus near the occipital pole. It receives visual input from each eye and contains the representation of the entire contralateral visual field, with the lower visual field contained in the upper bank of the calcarine sulcus and the upper visual field located in the lower bank. The macular portion of the retina is represented posteriorly near the occipital pole, and more peripheral retinal input reaches more anterior territories.

Secondary visual cortex (called V-2 to V-5) surrounds the primary area and corresponds to areas 18 and 19 of Brodmann as well as the middle temporal (MT) gyrus and areas 7a and 37 of Brodmann.

The Primary Visual Cortex Has a Layered Structure. Like all other areas of the neocortex, the primary visual cortex is organized into six horizontally arranged layers. The Y-type incoming geniculate fibers terminate most heavily in a subdivision of layer IV called IVcα, whereas the X-type fibers terminate primarily in layers IVa and IVcβ.

There Is Also a Vertical, Columnar Organization in V-1. A vertical array of neurons is approximately 50 μm in width and extends through the entire thickness of the cortex from the pial surface to the underlying subcortical white matter. As thalamic input terminates in layer IV, signals are spread by local circuits upward and downward in the column.

Interspersed Among These Columns Are the So-Called *Color Blobs*. These aggregates of neurons respond specifically to color signals mediated by surrounding cortical columns.

Visual Signals from the Two Eyes Remain Segregated through Projections from the DLGN to V-1. The cells in one vertical column in layer IV are primarily responsive to input from one eye, and neurons in the next adjacent column are preferentially responsive to the other eye. These are called *ocular dominance columns.*

Two Major Pathways for Analysis of Visual Information *(p. 626)*

Neuronal linkages in the Y cell pathway follow a more *dorsal* stream from V-1 into the rostrally adjacent area 18 (V-2) and then on to the parietal cortex. This path signals the "where" of the stimulus by conveying information concerning precise localization of the visual image in space, the gross form of the image, and whether it is moving.

Conversely, a more *ventral* pathway, from V-1 into adjacent V-2, and temporal association cortex carry the X cell information necessary for analysis of visual details. These signals are used to recognize textures, letters, and words along with the color of objects; they therefore determine "what" the object is and its meaning.

Neuronal Patterns of Stimulation During Analysis of the Visual Image *(p. 626)*

The visual cortex detects the orientation of lines and borders. We discussed earlier (see Chapter 50) that a major function of the visual system involves detection of contrast, particularly the edges formed by lines and borders. Neurons in layer IV of V-1, called *simple cells,* are maximally responsive to lines or edges that are aligned in a preferred orientation.

Other cells in V-1, called *complex cells,* are responsive to lines or edges with a preferred orientation, but the line can be displaced laterally or vertically for some defined distance.

A third class of cell, called the *hypercomplex cell,* is primarily located in visual association areas. These cells detect lines or edges that have a specific length, a specific angulated shape, or some other relatively complex feature.

Neurons of various types in the visual cortex participate in some circuits that are *serially* organized as well as pathways in which information is transmitted in a *parallel* manner. Both of these categories of functional organization are important to normal vision.

Detection of Color

Color is detected by means of color contrast. Often, color is contrasted with a white portion of the scene, which is the basis for the *color constancy* concept discussed in Chapter 50. Color contrast is detected by an opponent process in which certain colors excite certain neurons and inhibit others.

Removal of V-1 Causes Loss of Conscious Vision. Individuals may still be able to react "reflexively" to changes in light intensity, movement in the visual scene, and gross patterns of light stimuli. This activity is mainly due to activity in subcortical visual centers such as the superior colliculus.

Fields of Vision; Perimetry *(p. 627)*

The visual field—the area seen by an eye—is divided into a nasal (medial) portion and a temporal (lateral) portion. The process of testing the visual field of each eye independently is called *perimetry.* The subject fixates on a single point in the center of the visual field while a second small spot is moved in and out of the visual field. The subject then identifies its location.

A *blind spot* exists in that portion of the visual field occupied by the *optic disc.* A blind spot in any other portion of the visual field is called a *scotoma.* With *retinitis pigmentosa,* portions of the retina degenerate, and excessive melanin pigment is deposited in these areas. The process usually begins in the peripheral retina and then spreads centrally.

Effects of Lesions in the Optic Pathways on Fields of Vision. Interruption of the crossing fibers in the optic chiasm causes a visual field loss in the temporal portion of the visual field of each eye; this is called *bitemporal heteronymous hemianopsia.* Section of one optic tract leads to loss of the nasal visual field in the ipsilateral eye and the temporal field contralaterally; this condition is called *contralateral homonymous hemianopsia.* A lesion involving the optic radiations in one hemisphere produces a similar defect. These two lesions can be differentiated by the presence or absence of the pupillary light reflexes. If the reflexes are preserved, the lesion is in the optic radiations; if they are lost, the lesion must involve the optic tracts that carry retinal signals to the pretectal region.

Eye Movements and Their Control *(p. 627)*

For a visual scene to be interpreted correctly, the brain must be able to move the eyes into position to view the scene properly. Eye movement is accomplished by three pairs of muscles: the medial and lateral recti, the superior and inferior recti, and the superior and inferior oblique muscles. These muscles are innervated by motoneurons in the nuclei of the third, fourth, and sixth cranial nerves. The activity of these motoneurons is influenced by a variety of areas in the brain, including cells in the frontal, parietal, and occipital lobes; the brain stem reticular formation; the superior colliculus; the cerebellum; and the vestibular nuclei. Three general eye movement categories are considered: fixation, saccadic, pursuit.

Fixation **Involves Moving the Eyes to Bring a Discrete Portion of the Visual Field into Focus on the Fovea.** Voluntary fixation is controlled by the frontal eye fields, Brodmann's area 8, and an area in the occipital lobe that represents a portion of the secondary visual cortex (area 19).

Saccadic **Movement of the Eyes Is a Mechanism of Successive Fixation Points.** When the eyes rapidly jump from one object to another, each jump is called a *saccade.* These movements are rapid, and the brain suppresses the visual image during the movement so one typically is not conscious of the point-to-point movement.

Pursuit **Movements Occur When the Eyes Fixate on a Moving Target.** The control system for such movements involves the transmission of visual information to the cerebellum by various routes. The brain then computes the trajectory of the target and activates the appropriate motoneurons to move the eyes so the target is kept in focus on the fovea.

The superior colliculi are mainly responsible for orienting the eyes and head toward a visual (or auditory) stimulus. The visual field is mapped in the superior colliculus independent of a similar map in the visual cortex. This activity is thought to be mediated by input via Y-type retinal ganglion cells (and perhaps also W-type cells). The superior colliculus also directs turning of the head and body toward a visual stimulus through its descending projections in the tectospinal tract. Interestingly, other sensory inputs, such as audition and somatosensation, are funneled through the superior colliculus and its descending connections such that the superior colliculus performs a global integrating function with respect to orientation of the eyes and body toward various stimulus points.

Autonomic Control of Accommodation and Pupillary Aperture (p. 631)

Parasympathetic fibers to the eye originate in the Edinger-Westphal nucleus and course via the oculomotor nerve to the ciliary ganglion, where postganglionic fibers originate and extend to the eye with ciliary nerves. *Sympathetic fibers* originate in the intermediolateral cell column of the spinal cord and pass to the superior cervical ganglion. Postganglionic sympathetic fibers course on the *internal* carotid and ophthalmic arteries eventually reaching the eye.

When the fixation point of the eyes changes, the focusing power of the lens is adjusted in the proper direction by appropriate activation of the autonomic innervation of the ciliary and sphincter pupillae muscles in each eye.

When the eyes focus from far to near (or vice versa), they must also converge. This involves bilateral activation of the medial rectus muscles in each eye. The areas of the brain that control pupillary changes and convergence are sufficiently separated, as lesions may disrupt one function but not the other. For example, an Argyll-Robertson pupil is one that does not exhibit normal light reflexes but accommodates. Such a pupil is commonly seen in individuals afflicted with syphilis.

CHAPTER 52

The Sense of Hearing

Tympanic Membrane and the Ossicular System (p. 633)

Conduction of Sound from the Tympanic Membrane to the Cochlea

The tympanic membrane is cone-shaped. Attached to its center is the handle of the *malleus*, which is the first in the series of bony elements that comprise the ossicular chain. The *incus* is attached to the malleus by ligaments, so the two bones move together when the tympanic membrane moves the malleus. At its other end, the incus articulates with the *stapes*, which in turn is attached to the oval window of the membranous labyrinth. The malleus is also attached to the *tensor tympani* muscle, which keeps the tympanic membrane taut.

Impedance Matching between Sound Waves in Air and Sound Waves in the Cochlear Fluid Is Mediated by the Ossicular Chain. The amplitude of stapes movement at the oval window is only three fourths as large as the movement of the handle of the malleus. The ossicular chain does not amplify sound waves by increasing the *movement* of the stapes as is commonly believed; instead, the system increases the *force* of the movement about 1.3-fold. Because the area of the tympanic membrane is so great relative to the surface area of the oval window (55 square millimeters vs. 3.2 square millimeters), the lever system multiplies the pressure of the sound wave exerted against the tympanic membrane by a factor of 22. The fluid in the membranous labyrinth has far greater inertia than air; the pressure amplification added by the ossicular chain is necessary to cause vibration in the fluid. The tympanic membrane and ossicles together provide *impedance matching* between sound waves in air and sound vibrations in the fluid of the membranous labyrinth. In the absence of a functioning ossicular chain, normal sounds are barely perceptible.

Contraction of the Stapedius and Tensor Tympani Muscles Attenuates Sound Conduction. When extremely loud sounds are transmitted through the ossicular chain, there is reflex damping of the malleus by the *stapedius* muscle, which acts as an antagonist to the tensor tympani. In this way, the rigidity of the ossicular chain is increased, and the conduction of sound, particularly at lower frequencies, is greatly reduced. Interestingly, this same mechanism is used to diminish the sensitivity to one's own speech.

Transmission of Sound through Bone (p. 634)

Because the cochlea is entirely embedded in bone, vibration of the skull can stimulate the cochlea itself. When a tuning fork is vibrated and applied to the skull on the forehead or mastoid region, a humming sound can be heard. Generally, however, even relatively loud sounds in the air do not have sufficient energy to enable effective hearing via bone conduction.

Cochlea (p. 634)

Functional Anatomy of the Cochlea

The cochlea consists of three tubes coiled side by side. The *scala vestibuli* and *scala media* are separated by the vestibular membrane (Reissner's membrane), and the scala media and the scala tympani are separated by the basilar membrane. The *organ of Corti* lies on the surface of the basilar membrane and within the scala media. The roof of the organ of Corti is formed by the tectorial membrane. At the end of the cochlea opposite the round and oval windows, the scala vestibuli is continuous with the scala tympani at the helicotrema. The overall stiffness of the basilar membrane is 100 times less at the helicotrema than it is near the oval window. This means that the stiffest portion near the oval window is most sensitive to high-frequency vibrations, whereas the more compliant end near the helicotrema is responsive to low-frequency vibration.

Transmission of Sound Waves in the Cochlea— "Traveling Wave" (p. 635)

When a sound wave strikes the tympanic membrane, the ossicles are set into motion, and the footplate of the stapes is pushed into the membranous labyrinth at the oval window. This initiates a wave that travels along the basilar membrane toward the helicotrema.

Vibration Patterns Are Induced by Different Sound Frequencies. The pattern of vibration initiated in the basilar membrane is different for different sound frequencies. Each wave is relatively weak at its outset but becomes strongest at that portion of the basilar membrane that has a resonant frequency equal to that of the sound wave. The wave essentially dies out at this point and does not affect the remainder of the basilar membrane. In addition, the velocity of the traveling wave is greatest near the oval window and then gradually decreases as it proceeds toward the helicotrema.

Vibration Patterns Are Induced by Different Sound Amplitudes. The maximal amplitude of vibration for sound frequency is spread in an organized way over the surface of the basilar membrane. For example, maximal vibration for an 8000 cycle per second (Hertz or Hz) sound occurs near the oval window, whereas that for a 200 Hz sound is located near the helicotrema. The principal method for sound discrimination is the "place" of maximal vibration on the basilar membrane for that sound.

Function of the Organ of Corti *(p. 636)*

The receptor cells of the organ of Corti are of two types: the *inner* and the *outer hair cells.* There is a single row of inner hair cells that number about 3500 and three to four rows of outer hair cells that total about 12,000. Nearly 95% of the eighth cranial nerve sensory fibers that innervate the cochlea form synaptic contact with inner hair cells. The cell bodies of the sensory fibers are found in the spiral ganglion, which is located in the bony modiolus (the center) that serves as support for the basilar membrane at one end. The central processes of these ganglion cells enter the brain stem in the rostral medulla to synapse in the cochlear nuclei.

Vibration of the Basilar Membrane Excites the Hair Cells. The apical surface of the hair cells gives rise to many stereocilia and a single kinocilium that project upward into the overlying tectorial membrane. When the basilar membrane vibrates, the hair cell cilia embedded in the tectorial membrane are bent in one direction and then in the other; and it is this movement that mechanically opens ion channels and leads to depolarization of the hair cell.

Hair Cell Receptor Potentials Activate Auditory Nerve Fibers. The approximately 100 cilia protruding from the apical surface of the hair cells progressively increase in length from the region of the attachment of the basilar membrane to the modiolus. The longest of these cilia is referred to as a kinocilium. When the stereocilia are bent toward the kinocilium, potassium channels in the cilial membrane are opened, potassium enters, and the hair cell is depolarized. Exactly the reverse occurs when the cilia move away from the kinocilium;

that is, the hair cell is hyperpolarized. The fluid bathing the cilia and apical surface of the hair cells is *endolymph*. This watery fluid is different from the *perilymph* in the scala vestibuli and scala tympani, which, like extracellular fluid, is high in sodium and low in potassium. The endolymph is secreted by the stria vascularis (specialized epithelium in the wall of the scala media), and it is *high* in potassium and *low* in sodium. The electrical potential across the endolymph, called the endocochlear potential, is about +80 millivolts. However, the interior of the hair cell is about −70 millivolts. Therefore the potential difference across the membrane of the cilia and apical surface of the hair cells is about 150 millivolts; this greatly increases their sensitivity.

Determination of Sound Frequency—The "Place" Principle *(p. 638)*

The nervous system determines sound frequency by the point of maximal stimulation along the basilar membrane. Sounds at the high-frequency end of the spectrum maximally stimulate the basal end near the oval window. Low-frequency stimulation maximally stimulates the apical end near the helicotrema. Sound frequencies below 200 Hz, however, are discriminated differently. These frequencies cause synchronized *volleys* of impulses at the same frequency in the eighth cranial nerve, and cells in the cochlear nuclei that receive input from these fibers can distinguish the frequencies.

Determination of Loudness *(p. 638)*

1. As the sound becomes louder, the amplitude of vibration in the basilar membrane increases, and hair cells are activated more rapidly.
2. With increased amplitude of vibration, more hair cells are activated, and spatial summation enhances the signal.
3. Outer hair cells are activated by large-amplitude vibrations; somehow this signals the nervous system that the sound has surpassed a certain level that delimits high intensity.

The auditory system can discriminate between a soft whisper and a loud noise that might represent as much as a 1 trillion times increase in sound energy. Thus, the intensity scale is compressed by the brain to provide a wide range of sound discrimination.

Because of the wide range in sound sensitivity, intensity is expressed as the logarithm of the actual intensity.

The unit of sound intensity is the *bel,* and sound levels are most often expressed in 0.1 bel units or as 1 *decibel.*

The threshold for hearing in humans is different at different intensities. For example, a 3000 Hz tone can be heard at an intensity level of 70 decibels, whereas a 100 Hz tone can be heard only if the intensity is increased to a level 10,000 times as great.

The range of hearing is typically listed as 20 to 20,000 Hz. Again, however, the intensity level is significant because at a level of 60 decibels the frequency range is only 500 to 5000 Hz. To hear the full range of sound, the intensity level must be very high.

Central Auditory Mechanisms *(p. 639)*

Auditory Nervous Pathways

Primary sensory fibers from the spiral ganglion enter the brain stem and terminate in the *dorsal* and *ventral cochlear nuclei.* From here, signals are sent to the contralateral (and ipsilateral) *superior olivary nucleus,* where cells give rise to fibers that enter the lateral lemniscus, which terminates in the *inferior colliculus.* Cells in the inferior colliculus project to the *medial geniculate nucleus* of the thalamus, and from here signals are transmitted to the primary auditory cortex, the *transverse temporal gyrus of Heschel.* It is important to understand that (1) beginning with the output from the cochlear nuclei, signals are transmitted bilaterally through central pathways with a contralateral predominance; (2) collaterals from central pathways synapse in the brain stem reticular formation; and (3) spatial representations of sound frequency (tonotopic organization) are found at many levels in the various cell groups of the central auditory pathways.

Function of the Cortex in Hearing *(p. 640)*

The primary auditory cortex corresponds to Brodmann's areas 41 and 42. Surrounding these areas is area 22, a portion of which is considered the secondary auditory cortex.

At least six tonotopic representations (maps) of sound frequency have been described in the primary auditory cortex. The question of why these various maps exist is unanswered at the moment, but it is presumed that each region selects some particular feature of sound or sound perception and performs an analysis of that feature.

Bilateral destruction of the primary auditory cortex does not eliminate the ability to detect sound; it does, however, cause difficulty when *localizing* sounds in the environment. Lesions in the secondary auditory cortex interfere with the ability to interpret the *meaning* of particular sounds. This is particularly true for spoken words and is referred to as a *receptive aphasia.*

Determination of the Direction from Which Sound Comes *(p. 641)*

The superior olivary nucleus is divided into *medial* and *lateral* subdivisions. The lateral subnucleus determines sound direction by detecting the difference in sound intensity transmitted from the two ears. The medial subnucleus localizes sound by detecting the difference in the time of arrival of sound in the two ears. The input to individual cells in the latter nucleus is segregated such that signals from the right ear reach one dendritic system and input from the left ear synapses with a separate dendritic system on the same neuron.

Centrifugal Signals from the Central Nervous System to Lower Auditory Centers *(p. 641)*

Each processing level in the central auditory pathway gives rise to descending or retrograde fibers that project back toward the cochlear nuclei as well as to the cochlea itself. These centrifugal connections are more pronounced in the auditory system than in any other sensory pathway. It is speculated that these connections allow one to attend to particular sound features selectively.

Hearing Abnormalities *(p. 642)*

Hearing difficulties can be assessed with an audiometer, which allows specific sound frequencies to be individually delivered to each ear. When a patient suffers *nerve deafness,* both air and bone conduction of sound are affected, and the damage usually involves one or more of the neural components of the auditory system. When only air conduction is affected, damage to the ossicular chain is usually the cause. This is often due to chronic middle ear infections.

CHAPTER 53

The Chemical Senses—Taste and Smell

The senses of taste and smell allows an individual to separate undesirable or even lethal foods from those that are pleasant to eat and nutritious. The sense of taste is mainly a function of the *taste buds*, but the sense of smell contributes substantially to taste perception. The texture of food as sensed by tactile receptors in the mouth also contributes to the taste experience.

The Primary Sensations of Taste *(p. 645)*

At present, receptors for at least 13 chemical substances are identified. They include the following:

Sodium receptors (2)
Potassium receptors (2)
Chloride receptor (1)
Adenosine receptor (1)
Hydrogen ion receptor (1)
Inosine receptor (1)
Sweet receptors (2)
Bitter receptors (2)
Glutamate receptor (1)

For practical purposes, the activity of these receptors has been grouped into five categories called the *primary sensations of taste*, which are *sour, salty, sweet, bitter and umami.*

- *Sour* taste is caused by acidic substances, and the taste intensity is proportional to the logarithm of the hydrogen ion concentration.
- *Salty* taste is attributed mainly to the cations of ionized salts, but some salts also activate additional receptors, which explains the slight difference among salty-tasting items.
- *Sweet* taste is the result of activation of several receptor types, including sugars, glycols, alcohols, aldehydes, and other organic chemicals.
- *Bitter* taste is also caused by the activation of several receptors associated with organic chemicals. Two of the more common substances are long-chain, nitrogen-containing items and alkaloids. This group includes medicinal compounds such as quinine, caffeine, strychnine, and nicotine. A strong bitter taste often causes a substance to be rejected, which is related to the fact that dangerous toxins found in some plants are alkaloids.

- *Umami,* a Japanese word meaning delicious, is a fifth category and is the dominant taste of foods containing L-glutamate, such as meat extract and aging cheese.

Threshold for Taste

To be recognized as salty a substance's concentration need be only 0.01M, whereas for quinine to be perceived as bitter its concentration need only be 0.000008M. This correlates with the notion that bitter serves a protective function against dangerous alkaloids; thus, its sensitivity is high. Some individuals are "taste blind" for certain substances. This is probably due to the normal variation one sees in the presence of, or the number of certain classes of, receptors.

Taste Bud and Its Function *(p. 646)*

A taste bud is composed of about 50 modified epithelial cells, some of which, the *sustentacular cells,* serve a supporting function and others are the actual *receptor cells.* The latter are continuously replaced by the surrounding epithelial cells via mitotic division. The life span of a taste cell in lower mammals is about 10 days but is unknown for humans. The apical surfaces of the taste cells are arranged around a *taste pore.* Microvilli or taste hairs protrude from the pore and provide the receptor surface for taste molecules. Intertwined among the cell bodies are sensory nerve fibers, which form postsynaptic elements and respond to activity in taste cells.

The 3000 to 10,000 Taste Buds in the Adult Are Found in Relation to Three Types of *Papillae* on the Tongue. *Fungiform* papillae are found on the anterior two thirds of the tongue, *circumvallate* papillae form a V-shaped configuration on the posterior one third of the tongue, and *foliate* papillae are found along the lateral margins of the tongue. A small number of taste buds are also found on the palate, tonsils, and epiglottis and in the proximal esophagus. Each taste bud typically responds to only one of the five primary taste substances; the exception is when an item is present in very high concentration—then it may stimulate more than one receptor type.

Like Other Receptors, Taste Cells Produce a *Receptor* Potential. Application of the substance to which it is sensitive causes the taste cell to be depolarized, and the degree of depolarization correlates with the concentration of the taste substance. The binding of a taste substance to its receptor opens ion-specific channels that allow sodium to enter the cell. The taste substance elicits a rapid response in the associated sensory fibers that adapts to a lower level within a few seconds. The taste substance is washed away from the receptor by saliva.

Transmission of Taste Signals into the Central Nervous System (p. 647)

Taste fibers from the anterior two thirds of the tongue first travel in branches of the trigeminal nerve and then join the chorda tympani, a branch of the facial nerve. Taste sensation from the posterior one third of the tongue is carried by fibers in the glossopharyngeal nerve, whereas any taste fibers from the epiglottis or other areas course within branches of the vagus nerve. From their entry into the brain stem, all taste fibers are funneled into the *solitary tract* and eventually synapse in the rostral portion of the *nucleus of the solitary tract.* From here, axons pass rostrally in rather ill-defined pathways to the *ventromedial nucleus* of the thalamus and then onto the cerebral cortex in the ventral region of the postcentral gyrus, which curls into the lateral fissure.

In addition to the cortical pathway for taste perception, *taste reflexes* involve fibers that course from the solitary tract directly to the superior and inferior salivatory nuclei, which contain preganglionic parasympathetic neurons for the eventual activation of saliva secretion by the submandibular, sublingual, and parotid glands. Although some of the adaptive qualities of taste are the result of activity at the receptor level, most taste adaptation apparently occurs through central mechanisms, which are not well defined at present.

Sense of Smell (p. 648)

In humans, the sense of smell is probably the least understood sense, perhaps because it is largely a subjective phenomenon. Compared with some animals, it is poorly developed in humans.

Olfactory Membrane (p. 648)

The receptor surface for smell is located in the upper part of the nasal cavity and typically exhibits a surface area of only about 2.4 square centimeters. Olfactory receptor cells are bipolar neurons derived from the central nervous system. There are usually about 100 million of these cells in each individual, interspersed with a much smaller number of *sustentacular cells.*

The apical surface of the receptor cell exhibits a knob that emits 4 to 25 olfactory hairs or cilia, which contain the receptors and project into the mucus present on the epithelial surface. Spaced among the receptor cells are the glands of Bowman, which secrete mucus onto the epithelial surface.

Stimulation of the Olfactory Cells *(p. 649)*

Odorant molecules diffuse into the mucus and bind to receptor proteins that are linked to a cytoplasmic G-protein. On activation, the *α-subunit* of the G-protein separates away and activates adenyl cyclase, which in turn leads to the formation of cyclic adenosine monophosphate (cAMP). Sodium channels are then activated by cAMP, and sodium ions enter the cell and depolarize it, leading to the production of action potentials in the olfactory sensory fibers. This depolarization process multiplies the excitatory effect of a weak odorant molecule and greatly enhances the sensitivity of the system.

Like the taste system, the intensity of olfactory stimulation is proportional to the logarithm of the stimulus strength. The receptors adapt about 50% during the first, second, and thereafter adapt very little and very slowly. Although most odors appear to adapt to extinction within a minute or two, this is not a physiological process at the level of the receptor but, rather, a function of central mechanisms that alter perception. This may be correlated with the large number of centrifugal fibers that course from the olfactory regions of the brain back into the olfactory bulb.

Search for the Primary Sensations of Smell *(p. 650)*

As many as 100 smell sensations have been reported, but they have been narrowed to seven primary odor sensations: *camphoraceous, musky, floral, peppermint, ethereal, pungent, and putrid.*

Smell, even more than taste, is associated with pleasant or unpleasant affective qualities. The threshold for some odorant molecules is extremely low, on the order of 1/25 billionth of a milligram. The range of sensitivity, however, is only 10 to 50 times that of the threshold level, which is relatively low compared with other sensory systems.

Transmission of Smell Signals into the Central Nervous System *(p. 651)*

The olfactory bulb lies over the cribriform plate of the ethmoid bone that separates the cranial and nasal cavities. The olfactory nerves pass through perforations in the cribriform plate and enter the olfactory bulb, where they terminate in relation to glomeruli. This is a tangled knot of mitral and tufted cell dendrites and olfactory nerve fibers. Mitral and tufted cell axons leave the olfactory bulb via the olfactory tract and enter specialized regions of the cortex without first passing through the thalamus.

The *medial olfactory area* is represented by the septal nuclei, which project to the hypothalamus and other regions that control behavior. This system is thought to be involved in primitive functions such as licking, salivation, and other feeding behavior.

The *lateral olfactory area* is composed of the prepiriform, piriform, and cortical amygdaloid regions. From here, signals are directed to less primitive limbic structures, such as the hippocampus. This apparently is the system that associates certain odors with specific behavioral responses.

Another, phylogenetically newer pathway projects to the dorsomedial thalamic nucleus and then onto the orbitofrontal cortex.

Fibers that originate in the brain course centrifugally to reach granule cells in the olfactory bulb. The latter cells inhibit mitral and tufted neurons of the bulb, and in this way one's ability to distinguish different odors is sharpened.

XI

The Nervous System: C. Motor and Integrative Neurophysiology

CHAPTER 54

Motor Functions of the Spinal Cord; the Cord Reflexes

The spinal cord is often relegated to a role secondary to that of the brain when nervous system functions are analyzed. Circuits exist in the spinal cord, however, that process sensory information and are capable of generating complex motor activity. In addition, it is clear that even the most advanced and complicated functions involving the control of movement performed by the brain cannot be implemented if the spinal cord and its direct connections with skeletal muscles are not intact.

Organization of the Spinal Cord for Motor Functions *(p. 655)*

Anterior horn motor neurons are present at all levels of the cord and give rise to axons that exit the cord via its ventral roots and then pass distally in peripheral nerves to innervate skeletal striated muscles. A motor neuron and all the muscle fibers it innervates are referred to collectively as a *motor unit.*

Spinal cord ventral horn motor neurons are of two varieties: alpha and gamma motor neurons. The largest are the *alpha motor neurons,* which give rise to myelinated axons that average about 14 micrometers in diameter and conduct action potentials very rapidly. The *gamma motor neurons* are much smaller and give rise to smaller axons that average about 5 µm in diameter and conduct action potentials at a slower velocity than the alpha motor neurons.

A third cell type that contributes to motor and sensory functions in the spinal cord is the *interneuron.* There are several varieties of these cells; they are about 30 times more numerous than motor neurons, are highly excitable, and may have spontaneous firing rates as high as 1500 per second. The interneurons actually receive the bulk of synaptic input that reaches the spinal cord, as either incoming sensory information or as signals descending from higher centers in the brain.

The *Renshaw cell* is one variety of interneuron that receives input from collateral branches of motor neuron axons and then, via its own axonal system, provides inhibitory connections with the same or neighboring motor neurons. This suggests that the motor system, like the sensory systems, uses the mechanism of lateral inhibition to focus or sharpen its signals. Other inter-neurons are responsible for interconnecting one or several adjacent segments of the cord in an ascending or descending direction; the latter cells are called *propriospinal neurons*.

Muscle Sensory Receptors—Muscle Spindles and Golgi Tendon Organs—and Their Roles in Muscle Control *(p. 657)*

Receptor Function of the Muscle Spindle

The sensory feedback from skeletal muscles includes (1) the current length of the muscle and (2) the current tension in the muscle. The length value is derived from a *muscle spindle*, whereas tension is signaled by a *Golgi tendon organ*.

A *muscle spindle* is 3 to 10 mm in length and consists of 3 to 12 thin intrafusal muscle fibers that are actually striated muscle fibers. Each is attached at its distal ends to the associated extrafusal skeletal muscle. The central region of each intrafusal fiber is devoid of actin-myosin contractile elements and, instead, forms a capsule containing several nuclei. When the nuclei are arranged more or less linearly, the fiber is called a *nuclear chain fiber*; when nuclei are simply aggregated or clumped in the central region, the fiber is called a *nuclear bag fiber*. Typically, a muscle spindle contains one to three nuclear bag fibers and three to nine nuclear chain fibers. The distally located contractile elements of each intrafusal fiber are innervated by relatively small *gamma motor neuron axons*.

Two types of sensory fiber are associated with muscle spindle intrafusal fibers. One is called the *primary* ending, or the annulospiral ending. The primary ending is a type Ia myelinated primary sensory fiber with an average diameter of 17 μm and a rapid conduction velocity of 70 to 120 m/sec. Typically, a spindle also has at least one type II, secondary or flower-spray, ending that exhibits an average diameter of 8 μm, is lightly myelinated, and conducts at a slower velocity than the type Ia fibers. The primary ending wraps itself around the central (nuclear) region of both a nuclear bag and a nuclear chain intrafusal fiber, whereas the secondary ending forms numerous small terminal branches that cluster around the nuclear region of only the nuclear chain intrafusal fibers.

Dynamic and Static Responses of the Muscle Spindle *(p. 657)*

When the central region of a spindle is *slowly* stretched, the number of impulses in both the primary and secondary endings increases in proportion to the degree of stretch; this is called the *static response*. Because the nuclear chain fibers are innervated by both the primary and secondary sensory fibers, the static response is thought to be mediated by these intrafusal fibers.

When the length of a spindle is *suddenly* increased, the primary sensory fiber exhibits a vigorous response. This is called the *dynamic response*, and it appears to signal the rate of change in length. Because most nuclear bag fibers are mainly associated with primary endings, it is assumed that they are responsible for the dynamic response.

Control of Intensity of the Static and Dynamic Responses by the Gamma Motor Nerves

Gamma motor neurons are divided into two categories based on the type of intrafusal fiber they innervate. Gamma motor neurons distributing to nuclear bag fibers are called *dynamic*, whereas those distributing to nuclear chain fibers are *static*. Stimulation of a dynamic gamma motor neuron enhances only the dynamic response, and static gamma motor neuron stimulation enhances the static response.

Muscle spindles exhibit a continuous or background level of activity that can be modulated upward (increased firing) or downward (decreased firing) as necessary for the ongoing muscle activity.

Muscle Stretch Reflex *(p. 658)*

Type Ia sensory fibers enter the spinal cord through the dorsal roots and give rise to branches that either terminate in the cord near their level of entry or ascend to the brain. Those that terminate in the cord synapse directly (monosynaptic) with alpha motor neurons in the ventral horn, which innervate extrafusal fibers in the *same* muscle where the primary sensory fibers originated. This circuitry is the substrate for the *stretch reflex*. This reflex has two components: a dynamic phase while the spindle is being stretched and a static phase when the muscle has stopped increasing in length and has reached a new static length. An important function of the stretch reflex is its *damping effect* on oscillatory or jerky movements. In the absence of normally functioning spindle sensory mechanisms, an unusual repetitive contraction of muscles called *clonus* appears.

Role of the Muscle Spindle in Voluntary Motor Activity *(p. 659)*

Approximately 31% of the axons distributing to any given muscle are from gamma motor neurons. However, when signals are transmitted from the motor cortex or other control centers, both alpha and gamma motor neurons are *co-activated*. The stimulation of gamma motor neurons during contraction of a muscle maintains the sensitivity of the spindle and prevents it from going "slack" and stopping its output. The gamma motor neuron system is most strongly influenced by descending projections from the facilitatory regions of the brain stem reticular formation, which are in turn influenced by output from the cerebellum, basal ganglia, and cerebral cortex as well as ascending spinoreticular pain fibers.

Clinical Applications of the Stretch Reflex *(p. 660)*

The physician can assess the general state of reflex activity by testing the stretch reflex at a number of key joint locations. For example, tapping on the patellar tendon at the knee stretches spindles in the quadriceps and normally elicits a reflex contraction of that muscle group (stretch reflex), which produces a knee jerk. A reflex that is too strong or too brisk can indicate one type of problem, whereas a reflex that is weak or absent suggests other problems.

Clonus—alternating contraction of the agonist and antagonistic muscles crossing a joint—is a sign of abnormal stretch reflex function. This sign is often prominent at the ankle, where rapid, maintained dorsiflexion induced by the examiner might elicit sustained jerking movements (alternate flexion and extension) of the foot at the ankle joint. This is a sign that the spinal cord circuits that mediate the stretch reflex are not being properly influenced by the descending projections from the brain.

Golgi Tendon Reflex *(p. 661)*

The Golgi tendon organ is an encapsulated receptor through which a small bundle of muscle tendon fibers pass just prior to their bony insertion. Sensory fibers intermingle with and entwine the tendon fibers and are stimulated when the *tension* imposed by muscle contraction is increased. Like the muscle spindle, the tendon organ responds vigorously when the tendon is undergoing stretch (dynamic response) and then settles down to a steady-state level that is proportional to the degree of tension (static response).

Signals from the Tendon Organ Are Conducted through Large Myelinated Type Ib Fibers, Which Conduct Nearly as Rapidly as the Type Ia Fibers from the Muscle Spindles. On entering the cord, these fibers form branches, with some terminating locally on the pool of interneurons and others entering a long ascending pathway. Local inhibitory interneurons link the tendon organ input to the alpha motor neurons that innervate those muscles with which the tendon organ is associated. In contrast to muscle spindle input, which excites its related motor neurons, the tendon organ produces *inhibition* of the motor neurons innervating the muscle with which the tendon organ is associated. This negative feedback prevents injury to the muscle when it exceeds its upper limit of tension. In addition, via their ascending projections the tendon organs provide input to the cerebellum and motor areas of the cerebral cortex that are used by these centers for controlling movement.

Flexor Reflex and the Withdrawal Reflexes (p. 661)

The *withdrawal (flexor) reflex* is elicited by pain receptors, usually those located in the skin. The muscles activated are the ones required to remove the body part away from the painful stimulus. Typically, they are flexor muscles in the limbs, but the reflex is not limited to these muscles. The sensory fibers that carry these signals terminate on the pool of spinal cord interneurons, most of which provide excitatory input to the appropriate ventral horn motor neurons, whereas others inhibit motor neurons that innervate antagonistic muscles. The latter mechanism is called *reciprocal inhibition.*

Crossed Extensor Reflex (p. 663)

The *crossed extensor reflex* often occurs in conjunction with the flexor reflex. Removing a limb from a painful stimulus may require support from one or more body parts. For example, withdrawing the foot might require that the other foot support the entire body. In this situation, interneurons that receive the incoming pain signal from one foot can project across the midline to excite the appropriate contralateral motor neurons to support the body; often they are extensor motor neurons. It also is possible, if the lower extremity is initially affected by the pain stimulus, for impulses to spread to more rostral cord levels through propriospinal neurons that synapse with motor neurons, innervating upper extremity musculature that might be needed to stabilize the body.

Reflexes of Posture and Locomotion (p. 663)

Postural and Locomotor Reflexes of the Cord

In experimental animals in which the spinal cord has been isolated from the remainder of the brain by a cervical level transection, certain reflex motor patterns are released from the normal descending control mechanisms from the brain.

- Pressure on a footpad causes the limb to be extended against the applied pressure. In some animals, when held in place on all four limbs, this reflex can generate sufficient muscle force to support the entire body. This reflex is called the *positive supportive reaction.*
- Similarly, when an animal with a cervical cord transection is placed on its side, it tries to raise itself to a standing position, although this maneuver is rarely successful. This reflex is called the *cord righting reflex.*
- If a cord-transected animal is suspended on a treadmill so each of the limbs can touch the surface of the treadmill, all four limbs move in a synchronous and coordinated manner as if the animal was trying to walk on the treadmill.

These observations indicate that circuits intrinsic to the spinal cord are capable of generating movements in a single extremity, a pair of extremities, or all four extremities. This circuitry involves connections between flexor and extensor motor neurons in a single cord segment, across the midline, and rostrally and caudally through the propriospinal system.

Spinal Cord Transection and Spinal Shock (p. 665)

When the spinal cord is transected, all cord functions below the transection become substantially depressed; this is referred to as *spinal shock.* The condition may persist for a few hours, days, or weeks. It is thought to represent a period during which the excitability of spinal neurons is dramatically reduced owing to the loss of all descending projections. As is the case in other areas of the nervous system, the affected neurons gradually regain their excitability as they reorganize and adapt to the new levels of reduced synaptic input.

Some of the more common symptoms that appear during spinal shock include the following:

- *Arterial blood pressure may fall significantly,* indicating that the output of the *sympathetic* nervous system is completely interrupted.
- *All skeletal muscle reflexes are nonfunctional.* In humans, 2 weeks to several months may be required for reflex activity to return to normal. If the transection is incomplete and some descending pathways remain intact, some reflexes become hyperactive.
- *Sacral autonomic reflexes that regulate bladder and bowel function may be suppressed for several weeks.*

CHAPTER 55

Cortical and Brain Stem Control of Motor Function

Essentially, each purposeful or voluntary movement that an individual consciously decides to make has at least some component controlled by the cerebral cortex. However, not all movement is "voluntary," and much of the control over muscles and their coordinated activity involves a variety of brain centers—including the basal ganglia, cerebellum, brain stem, and spinal cord—that work in concert with areas of the cerebral cortex.

Motor Cortex and Corticospinal Tract (p. 667)

Primary Motor Cortex

The primary motor cortex is located in the frontal lobe within the gyrus immediately anterior to the central sulcus, called the *precentral gyrus* or *Brodmann's area 4*. Many years ago, during neurosurgical procedures in humans, Penfield and Rasmussen discovered that stimulation of points in the precentral gyrus led to movement or activation of muscles in various parts of the body. They observed that muscle activation was *somatotopically* organized in this gyrus such that stimulation of the lateral-most portion caused activation of head and neck muscles; activation of the middle portion led to movement in the hand, arm, or shoulder; and stimulation in the medial portion of the gyrus caused activation of trunk and lower extremity muscles. At some stimulation points individual muscles were activated, whereas at others a group of muscles was activated.

Premotor Area (p. 668)

Immediately anterior to the lateral portion of the primary motor cortex is the *premotor cortex*. This cortex forms a portion of *Brodmann's area 6* and contains a somatotopically organized map of the body musculature. Stimulation in this cortex, however, typically produces movements that involve groups of muscles. For example, the arm and shoulder may be activated to place the hand in position to perform a certain task.

Supplementary Motor Area (p. 668)

The *supplementary motor area* is located in the medial portion of area 6 on the dorsal convexity and medial wall of the hemisphere just anterior to the lower extremity portion of the precentral gyrus. Stimulation here requires greater intensity and typically causes bilateral muscle activation, usually involving the upper extremities.

Some Specialized Areas of Motor Control Found in the Human Motor Cortex (p. 668)

- *Broca's area (motor speech area)* lies just anterior to the face portion of the primary motor cortex near the sylvian fissure. Activity in this area engages the musculature needed to convert simple vocal utterances into whole words and complete sentences.

- *The frontal eye field (Brodmann's area 8)* also lies just anterior to the precentral gyrus but somewhat more dorsal than Broca's area. This cortical region controls the conjugate eye movements required to shift gaze from one object to another.

- A *head rotation area* associated with the frontal eye field is functionally linked to area 8 and serves to enable movements of the head correlated with eye movement.

- An area related to the control of *fine movements of the hand* is located in the premotor cortex just anterior to the hand region of area 4. When this area is damaged, the muscles of the hand are not paralyzed, but certain hand movements are lost; this is called *motor apraxia.*

Transmission of Signals from the Motor Cortex to the Muscles (p. 669)

Corticospinal (Pyramidal) Tract

Primary Output Pathway from the Motor Cortex. The corticospinal tract mainly originates from the primary motor cortex (30%), and the premotor cortex (30%); the remainder is divided among several other areas, including the primary somatosensory cortex (postcentral gyrus), supplementary cortex, parietal lobe areas, and portions of the cingulate gyrus. After leaving the cortex, axons of this tract enter the posterior limb of the internal capsule and pass caudally through the brain stem to the ventral surface of the medulla, where they are contained in the medullary pyramids. At the junction of the medulla and spinal cord, most of the fibers cross the midline to enter the lateral funiculus of the spinal cord and form the *lateral corticospinal tract,* which extends throughout the length of the cord.

The fibers that do not cross continue as far as the thoracic spinal cord in the *ventral corticospinal tract.*

The largest fibers in the pyramidal tract are about 16 μm in diameter and are believed to originate from the giant cells of Betz found in the precentral gyrus. There are approximately 34,000 Betz cells, and the total number of fibers in the corticospinal tract is about 1 million, so the large fibers represent only about 3% of the entire tract.

Other Fiber Pathways from the Motor Cortex

In addition to projections to the spinal cord, branches of pyramidal tract fibers reach many other areas, including the caudate and putamen, red nucleus, reticular formation, basilar pontine nuclei, and inferior olive. The projections to the red nucleus may provide an alternate pathway for the motor cortex to influence the spinal cord via the rubrospinal tract if corticospinal axons are damaged at a level caudal to the red nucleus.

Incoming Pathways to the Motor Cortex *(p. 670)*

It is also important to consider the areas of the brain that provide *input* to the motor areas that give rise to the corticospinal system; they are surrounding areas of cortex in the same and contralateral hemispheres, including the somatosensory cortex as well as fibers from a variety of thalamic nuclei that carry information from the ascending somatosensory pathways, cerebellum, basal ganglia, and reticular activating system.

Excitation of the Spinal Cord Motor Control Areas by the Primary Motor Cortex and Red Nucleus *(p. 670)*

Like neurons in the visual cortex, those in the motor cortex are organized into vertical modules. Each vertical unit may control the activity of a synergistic group of muscles or an individual muscle. It is estimated that 50 to 100 pyramidal neurons must be activated simultaneously or in rapid succession to cause muscle contraction. Often, if a strong signal is needed to cause initial muscle activation, a weaker signal is able to maintain the contraction for longer periods thereafter. The substrate for this function may involve two populations of corticospinal neurons: *Dynamic* neurons produce high output for short time periods and may specify the development of the proper force needed to initiate the movement, whereas *static* neurons fire a less intense signal at a slower rate to maintain the force of contraction.

Interestingly, the red nucleus also exhibits neurons with dynamic and static properties, with the dynamic variety outnumbering their counterpart in the cortex and the static variety proportionally less than that found in the cortex.

Somatosensory Feedback to the Motor Cortex Helps Control the Precision of Muscle Contraction *(p. 672)*

The signals that arise in muscle spindles, Golgi tendon organs, and the skin near joints when movement occurs are relayed to the motor cortex and influence the output of that motor cortex. Generally, the somatosensory input tends to enhance the activity of the motor cortex. For example, as an object is grasped by the fingers, compression of the skin by the object tends to cause further excitement of the muscles and tightening of the fingers around the object.

Stimulation of Spinal Motor Neurons

Large numbers of corticospinal fibers terminate in the cervical and lumbosacral enlargements of the spinal cord; this probably reflects the control over muscles of the upper and lower extremities exerted by this system. Most of the cortical input is focused on the pool of spinal interneurons, but apparently some corticospinal axons synapse directly with ventral horn motor neurons. It is important to recognize that the corticospinal system may carry "command signals" that activate patterns of movement whose composition is determined by aggregates of spinal interneurons. Similarly, it is not necessary for corticospinal signals to inhibit the action of antagonist muscles directly. This can be accomplished by activating the intrinsic cord circuits that produce reciprocal inhibition.

Effect of Lesions in the Motor Cortex or the Corticospinal Pathway—The "Stroke"

A *stroke* is caused by a ruptured blood vessel that bleeds into the brain or by thrombosis of a vessel that produces local ischemia in neighboring brain tissue. When either event involves the primary motor cortex (origin of the corticospinal tract), the resulting motor deficits are characterized by the loss of voluntary control of discrete movements involving the distal portions of the extremities, particularly the fingers and hands. This does not necessarily mean that the muscles are completely paralyzed but, rather, that the control of fine movements is lost. Furthermore, postural movements or gross positioning of the limbs may not be affected. However, hemorrhagic or ischemic cortical strokes typically involve more territory than just the primary motor cortex. When the tissue damage extends beyond the primary cortex and involves neurons that project to the caudate, putamen, or reticular formation, characteristic symptoms such as hyperreflexia, hypertonia, and spasticity occur.

Role of the Brain Stem in Controlling Motor Function

Support of the Body Against Gravity—Roles of the Reticular and Vestibular Nuclei (p. 673)

The pontine and medullary areas of the reticular formation function in opposition to one another through their contributions to the reticulospinal system. The pontine levels tend to excite antigravity muscles, whereas medullary levels inhibit them. Pontine levels are strongly activated by ascending somatosensory fibers, vestibular nuclei, and cerebellar nuclei, and when unopposed by medullary levels, the excitation of antigravity muscles is sufficiently strong to support the body. On the other hand, the inhibitory influence derived from the medullary reticulospinal fibers is strongly influenced by input from the cerebral cortex and the red nucleus. Thus, the pontine and medullary systems can be selectively activated or inactivated to produce the desired excitation or inhibition of antigravity muscles.

Role of the Vestibular Nuclei to Excite the Antigravity Muscles (p. 674)

The lateral vestibular nucleus transmits excitatory signals (mainly by way of the lateral vestibulospinal tract) that strongly excite antigravity muscles. This system is influenced most strongly by the vestibular sensory apparatus and uses the antigravity muscles to maintain balance.

The Decerebrate Animal Develops Spastic Rigidity

When the brain stem is sectioned at about mid-collicular levels, leaving the reticulospinal and vestibulospinal tracts intact, a condition develops known as *decerebrate rigidity*. It is characterized by hyperactivity in the antigravity muscles, primarily in the neck, trunk, and extremities. Activation of the antigravity muscles is unopposed because the corticospinal and rubrospinal tracts have been sectioned, along with the cortical activation of the medullary reticulospinal fibers. Although the cortical drive on the pontine reticulospinal system has also been interrupted, there is sufficient activation remaining from other excitatory inputs such as the ascending somatosensory pathways and cerebellar nuclei. Examination of the antigravity muscles reveals that their stretch reflexes are greatly enhanced, and they are said to exhibit *spasticity*. It is believed that the descending influence from the pontine reticulospinal fibers affects primarily the gamma motor neurons. This is substantiated in animal experiments in which sectioning of the dorsal roots in such a situation eliminates the hyperactivity in the antigravity muscles. The enhanced activation in these muscles is dependent on the action of gamma motor neuron input to muscle spindles and the resultant increased activity of Ia primary afferent fibers.

Vestibular Sensations and Maintenance of Equilibrium

Vestibular Apparatus (p. 674)

The sensory organs for the vestibular sense are located in a system of bony chambers in the petrous portion of the temporal bone. Each bony enclosure houses a membranous chamber or tubular structure that contains the sensory hair cells and the terminal ends of primary sensory fibers of the eighth cranial nerve that lead into the brain. The membranous structures include the three semicircular canals or ducts and two larger chambers, the utricle and saccule.

Function of the Utricle and Saccule in the Maintenance of Static Equilibrium (p. 676)

Within each utricle and saccule is a small specialized structure called the *macula*. It is a flattened area approximately 2 mm in diameter that lies in the horizontal plane on the inferior surface of the utricle and in the vertical plane in the saccule. The surface of each macula is covered by a gelatinous layer in which calcium carbonate crystals called *statoconia* are embedded.

The macula contains supporting cells and sensory hair cells with cilia that protrude upward into the gelatinous layer. Each cell has 50 to 70 stereocilia and one large kinocilium. The latter is always the tallest cilium and is positioned off to one side of the apical surface of the hair cell. The stereocilia become progressively shorter toward the side opposite the kinocilium. Minute filaments connect the tip of each cilium to the next adjacent one and serve to open ion channels in the cilial membrane, which is bathed in endolymphatic fluid. When the stereocilia are bent toward the kinocilium, ion channels are opened, ions enter the cell from the endolymph, and the cell is depolarized. Conversely, movement of the stereocilia away from the kinocilium results in closure of membrane channels and hyperpolarization of the cell. In each macula, groups of hair cell cilia are oriented in specific directions such that some are stimulated and others inhibited with head movement in any direction. The brain recognizes patterns of excitation and inhibition in the sensory fibers and translates that pattern into head orientation. The utricle and saccule are sensitive to *linear acceleration* (but not linear velocity). When the head accelerates in any plane relative to gravity, the statoconia shift and displace hair cell cilia in a specific direction, which depolarizes some cells and hyperpolarizes others.

Detection of Head Rotation by the Semicircular Ducts *(p. 677)*

The three membranous semicircular canals are named the *anterior, posterior,* and *lateral canals;* each is oriented at right angles to the others so they represent the three planes in space. The lateral canal is in the true horizontal plane when the head is tilted forward 30 degrees, whereas the anterior and posterior canals are both in the vertical plane with the anterior canal angled forward at 45 degrees and the posterior canal angled 45 degrees posteriorly. The sensory epithelium in each canal is formed by an *ampulla* composed of ciliated sensory hair cells capped by a small crest called the *crista ampullaris,* which protrudes into an overlying gelatinous mass, the *cupula.* Each canal contains *endolymph,* which is free to move with rotation of the head; as it does, the cupula is deflected, along with the cilia that protrude into it from the hair cells. Movement in one direction is depolarizing; movement in the opposite direction is hyperpolarizing.

When the head begins to rotate (angular acceleration), the endolymph in the canals, because of its inertia, tends to remain stationary and produces relative endolymph flow opposite that of head rotation. The cupula is deflected, the cilia are displaced, and the hair cells are depolarized or hyperpolarized, depending on the direction of cupula deflection. If the head rotation persists in the same direction, the endolymph attains the same direction and velocity as the head rotation, the cupula is no longer deflected, and the hair cells are not stimulated. When the rotation stops, there again is flow of endolymph relative to the cupula (in the direction of rotation); some hair cells depolarize and others hyperpolarize. The semicircular canals do not serve to maintain equilibrium but, rather, signal the beginning (or end) of head rotation; they are thus "predictive" in function.

Vestibular Reflex Actions

- Sudden changes in head orientation result in postural adjustments resulting from activation of receptors in the utricle, saccule, or semicircular canals. The activation of motor responses is achieved by projections from the vestibular nuclei to the lateral vestibulospinal tract.
- When head orientation changes, the eyes must be moved to maintain a stable image on the retina. This correction is accomplished through connections from the semicircular canals to the vestibular nuclei, which then control the motor neurons of the third, fourth, and sixth cranial nerves via projections through the medial longitudinal fasciculus.
- Proprioceptors in muscles and joints of the neck provide input to the vestibular nuclei that counteracts the sensation of dysequilibrium when the neck is bent.
- Input from the visual system, which signals a slight shift in the position of an image on the retina, is effective in maintaining equilibrium when the vestibular system is damaged.

Neuronal Connections of the Vestibular Apparatus with the Central Nervous System (p. 678)

The vestibular nuclei are richly interconnected with components of the brain stem reticular formation. These pathways are used to regulate eye movements via the medial longitudinal fasciculus and to control posture in the trunk and limbs in conjunction with the vestibulospinal tracts. The former connections function to maintain the eyes on a target when head orientation changes. The perception of head and body movement is achieved through vestibular input to the thalamus, which then projects to the cerebral cortex.

Relatively little is known about the anatomy and function of this pathway.

The vestibular system also maintains extensive projections to, and receives projections from, the cerebellum. The cerebellar flocculonodular lobe is related to semicircular canal function and, when affected by lesions, causes a loss of equilibrium during rapid changes in the direction of the head motion. The uvula of the cerebellum plays a similar role in regard to static equilibrium.

CHAPTER 56

Contributions of the Cerebellum and Basal Ganglia to Overall Motor Control

Cerebellum and Its Motor Functions *(p. 681)*

The cerebellum is especially vital to the control of rapid movements. Damage to the cerebellum does not usually produce muscle paralysis but, rather, causes an inability to use the affected muscles in a rapid, smooth, and coordinated manner.

Anatomical Functional Areas of the Cerebellum *(p. 681)*

The cerebellum consists of a three-layered cortex surrounding four pairs of centrally located nuclei. The surface cortex exhibits numerous folds called folia that are similar to the gyri of the cerebral cortex. The cerebellar cortex is divided into three major subdivisions: *anterior, posterior,* and *flocculonodular lobes.* The anterior and posterior lobes are further divided in the sagittal plane into a midline portion, the *vermis;* a slightly more lateral portion with ill-defined borders, the *intermediate zone;* and, most laterally, the large *lateral hemispheres.*

The vermis and the intermediate zone contain a somatotopic map of the body surface that reflects peripheral sensory input from muscles, tendons, joint capsules, and some cutaneous receptors.

The lateral hemispheres receive input primarily from the cerebral cortex via the basilar pontine nuclei, and portions of each hemisphere exhibit a fractured somatotopic organization. This means that some body regions are spatially segregated from their adjoining parts. For example, a lower limb territory might be located adjacent to a portion of the face, and some body regions are represented in more than one location.

The nuclei of the cerebellum include the medial or *fastigial nucleus;* the *globose* and *emboliform* nuclei, which are collectively referred to as interposed nuclei; and the lateral, or *dentate,* nucleus. The output of these nuclei is directed to the cerebral cortex via the thalamus and to the brain stem.

Neuronal Circuit of the Cerebellum *(p. 682)*

Input (Afferent) Pathways to the Cerebellum *(p. 682)*

- The largest afferent projection, the *pontocerebellar system,* originates from cells of the basilar pontine nuclei. Nearly all regions of the cerebral cortex

427

project to cells in the pontine nuclei, which then give rise to pontocerebellar axons. This is the primary route over which cortical information is transmitted to the cerebellum.

- The *olivocerebellar* projections originate from cells in the inferior olivary nuclei.
- *Spinocerebellar* fibers originate in the spinal cord or medulla.
- *Reticulocerebellar* fibers originate from a variety of cell groups in the brain stem.
- *Vestibular* fibers originate from the vestibular nuclei and the vestibular sensory apparatus.

Output (Efferent) Signals from the Cerebellum (p. 683)

- The midline portions (vermis) of the cerebellar cortex project to the fastigial (medial) cerebellar nucleus and then to the vestibular nuclei and reticular formation.
- The cortex of the intermediate zone projects to the globose and emboliform nuclei (interposed nuclei) and then to the ventrolateral and ventral anterior thalamic nuclei. From the thalamus, signals are transmitted to the cerebral cortex and basal ganglia.
- The lateral hemispheres project to the dentate (lateral) cerebellar nucleus and then to the ventrolateral and ventral anterior thalamic nuclei, which project to the cerebral cortex.

Functional Unit of the Cerebellar Cortex—The Purkinje Cell and the Deep Nuclear Cell (p. 684)

The three layers of the cerebellar cortex, beginning nearest the pial surface, are the *molecular layer,* the *Purkinje cell layer,* and the *granular layer.* The fundamental circuit through the cerebellar cortex, which is repeated some 30 million times, is shown in Figure 56–1. The principal cell type is the Purkinje cell, which receives input to its fan-shaped dendritic tree located in the molecular layer. This input comes from two main sources: (1) *climbing fibers* that originate from cells of the inferior olivary complex and (2) *parallel fibers* that represent the axons of granule cells. The granule cells receive synaptic input from *mossy fibers,* which are formed by all the other cerebellar afferent systems. Recently, however, another class of afferent fibers apparently forming synaptic contact with Purkinje cells— *multilayered fibers*—has been shown to originate from

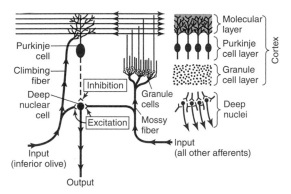

Figure 56–1. The left side of the figure shows the basic neuronal circuit of the cerebellum, with excitatory neurons shown in red and the Purkinje cell (an inhibitory neuron) shown in black. To the right is shown the physical relation of the deep cerebellar nuclei to the cerebellar cortex with its three layers.

biogenic amine cell groups, such as the locus ceruleus, and other nuclei including portions of the hypothalamus.

The fundamental cerebellar circuit is completed by the axon of the Purkinje cell, which forms synaptic contact in one of the cerebellar nuclei, although a few Purkinje axons extend into the vestibular nuclei. The transmission of signals through the fundamental circuit is influenced by three additional considerations:

1. Purkinje cells and cerebellar nuclear cells exhibit a high level of background activity, which can be modulated upward or downward.
2. The cells of the central nuclei receive direct excitatory input from climbing fibers and most mossy fiber systems, whereas the input from Purkinje cells is inhibitory.
3. Three other inhibitory interneurons (basket cells, stellate cells, Golgi cells) in the cerebellar cortex also influence the transmission of signals through the fundamental circuit.

Function of the Cerebellum in Overall Motor Control (p. 686)

The Cerebellum Has a Turn On/Turn Off Function. During nearly every movement, certain muscles must be rapidly turned on and then quickly turned off. Because mossy and climbing fiber afferents can form direct excitatory contact with cerebellar nuclear cells (the cerebellar output neurons), it is possible that such connections establish the turn on signal. However, mossy and climbing fiber afferents also pass through the cerebellar cortex, where they can activate Purkinje cells that inhibit cerebellar nuclear neurons and in this way specify the turn off signal. Such a theory has some merit because cerebellar lesions are known to produce an inability to perform rapid alternating movements (e.g., pronation-supination of the wrist). This deficit is known as *dysdiadochokinesia.*

Purkinje Cells May Learn to Correct Motor Errors. It has been proposed that the role of the climbing fiber input to a Purkinje cell is to modify that cell's sensitivity to parallel fiber input. The climbing fiber input is more vigorous when a mismatch occurs between the anticipated result of a movement and its actual result. Gradually, as the movement is practiced, the mismatch declines and climbing fiber activity begins to return to its previous level of activity. During the time of increased climbing fiber activity, the Purkinje cell can become more or less responsive to parallel fiber input.

The Vestibulocerebellum Joins with the Brain Stem and Spinal Cord to Regulate Equilibrium and Posture. The vestibulocerebellum is a combination of the flocculus and nodulus of the cerebellum and certain of the vestibular nuclei of the brain stem. It is believed that the role of these brain components is to calculate the rate and direction of movement, that is, where the body will be in the next few milliseconds. This computation is the key to moving to the next sequential movement or to maintaining equilibrium. Because the vestibulocerebellar circuitry is associated mainly with axial and girdle muscles, this system seems to be primarily involved in setting and maintaining the posture appropriate for a movement.

The Spinocerebellum Is Involved in the Control of Distal Limb Movements. The spinocerebellum consists of the intermediate zone of the anterior and posterior lobes plus most of the vermis of the anterior and posterior lobes. It is that portion of the cerebellar cortex that receives the bulk of the ascending spinal cord projections (spinocerebellar and cuneocerebellar tracts), particularly the input from muscle spindles, Golgi tendon organs, and joint capsules. It also receives input from the cerebral cortex via the pontine nuclei, so it receives information concerning intended movements as well as ongoing movements.

This part of the cerebellum may be involved in damping movements. For example, when an arm is moved, momentum develops and must be overcome to stop the movement. When lesions affect the spinocerebellum, overshoot develops: That is, the arm might extend past the target in one direction; then, as a correction is made, the arm may overshoot in the opposite direction. This is sometimes interpreted as an *intention* or *action tremor.*

Extremely rapid movements such as the finger movements of a touch-typist are called *ballistic* movements. This implies that the entire movement is preplanned to go into motion, travel a specific distance, and then come to a stop. Saccadic eye movements are also ballistic movements. These types of movements are disrupted when the spinocerebellum is damaged. The movement is slow to be initiated, its force development is weak, and it is slow to be terminated; this results in overshoot or past pointing.

The Cerebrocerebellum Is Involved with the Planning, Sequencing, and Timing of Movement. The lateral cerebellar hemispheres receive the bulk of their input from the cerebral cortex via the pontine nuclei and essentially do not receive any projections directly from the spinal cord. The plan of an intended, sequential movement is thought to be transmitted from the premotor and sensory cortex to the basilar pons and then to the cerebellar nuclei and cortex of the lateral hemisphere. Interestingly, it has been reported that activity in the dentate nucleus reflects the movement that *will be* performed, not the ongoing movement.

When the lateral hemisphere is damaged, the timing of sequential movements is lost; that is, a succeeding movement may begin too early or too late, and complex movements such as writing or running are uncoordinated and do not progress in an orderly sequence from one movement to the next. The timing function involved in estimating the progression of auditory and visual phenomena may also be disrupted. For example, an individual can lose the ability to predict on the basis of sound or sight how rapidly an object is approaching.

Clinical Abnormalities of the Cerebellum *(p. 689)*

- *Dysmetria and ataxia*—movements that overshoot or undershoot the intended target. The effect is called dysmetria, and the abnormal movements are described as ataxic.

- *Past pointing*—failure of a movement signal to be terminated at the proper time, and the limb continues past or beyond its intended target.
- *Dysdiadochokinesia*—inability to perform rapid, alternating movements. The switch that shifts from flexion to extension (or vice versa) is not timed properly.
- *Dysarthria*—speech defect that involves inappropriate progression from one syllable to the next. This is slurred speech in which some syllables are held and others are dropped too quickly.
- *Intention tremor*—a type of tremor present only when a voluntary movement is attempted and that intensifies as the limb nears its target.
- *Cerebellar nystagmus*—in effect, a tremor of the eyes when attempting to fixate on a point in the periphery of the visual field.
- *Hypotonia*—decreased muscle tone in the affected muscles, accompanied by diminished reflexes.

Basal Ganglia—Their Motor Functions (p. 689)

The term basal ganglia refers to the brain region that includes the *caudate nucleus, putamen, globus pallidus, substantia nigra,* and *subthalamic nucleus.* These structures are located deep within the core of each cerebral hemisphere.

Function of the Basal Ganglia in Executing Patterns of Motor Activity—The Putamen Circuit

The circuits that interconnect the structures comprising the basal ganglia are intricate and extremely complex. These connections are represented in Figure 56–2.

In general, functions that involve movement are primarily linked to the putamen rather than to the caudate nucleus. Signals initiated in the premotor and supplementary cortex are transmitted to the putamen and then onto the globus pallidus. The latter structure has internal and external subdivisions that are synaptically linked to one another but also project to different locations. The external segment is reciprocally linked with the subthalamic nucleus, and the internal segment projects to the thalamus and substantia nigra. Motor

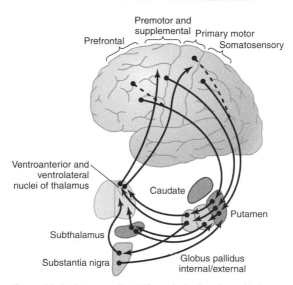

Figure 56–2. Putamen circuit through the basal ganglia for subconscious execution of learned patterns of movement.

nuclei in the thalamus that receive pallidal input project back to premotor and primary motor regions of the cortex.

This set of connections forms a series of loops that link motor cortex to portions of the putamen and globus pallidus. These cells project, in turn, to motor nuclei of the thalamus that transmit signals back to the motor cortex. Within each loop there are two circuits, the so-called *direct* and *indirect* pathways. The direct pathway leads from inhibitory neurons in the putamen to cells in the internal pallidal segment, which then project to thalamic motor nuclei. The neurons in the internal segment form an inhibitory pallidothalamic circuit involving thalamocortical neurons that project to the motor cortex. The end result is that the thalamocortical neurons are disinhibited, and this allows the transmission of excitatory input from thalamus to motor cortex. It is said that the direct pathway *enhances* movement. Conversely, the *indirect pathway* involves a series of inhibitory signals transmitted through the putamen and external pallidal segment that normally result in the disinhibition of cells in the subthalamic nucleus. The subthalamic neurons are "released" and send excitatory signals to neurons of the internal pallidal segment that provide inhibitory input to the thalamic motor nuclei. This results in decreased thalamic activation of motor cortex and slowing of cortically initiated motor activity. However, when this pathway is dysfunctional (as in Huntington disease), neurons in the thalamic motor nuclei are not inhibited from the internal pallidal segment, and this allows thalamocortical neurons to excite motor cortex resulting in the production of involuntary movements—movements that are not willfully initiated by the patient and cannot be stopped. The direct and indirect pathways are both active when a voluntary movement is performed. It is believed that the *direct* pathway leads to the activation of the muscles required to accurately perform the movement, whereas the *indirect* pathway functions to inhibit muscles that would interfere with the intended movement.

In addition to complex connectivity, the basal ganglia synaptic milieu contains an unusually diverse variety of neurotransmitter agents, and individual neurons of the putamen and caudate may express more than one neurotransmitter agent. Consequently, lesions of the basal ganglia give rise to a wide variety of clinical signs and symptoms.

- *Globus pallidus lesion*—writhing movements of the hand and arm or face, called *athetosis*
- *Subthalamic lesion*—flailing movements of an extremity, called *hemiballismus*
- *Putamen lesion*—flicking movements of the hands or face, called *chorea*
- *Substantia nigra dopamine cell degeneration*—Parkinson's disease characterized by bradykinesia (slowing of movement), a shuffling gait, absence of facial expression and a resting (pill rolling) tremor

The Role of the Basal Ganglia for Cognitive Control of Sequences of Motor Patterns—The Caudate Circuit *(p. 691)*

Like the putamen, the caudate nucleus receives dense projections from the cerebral cortex; in this case, however, primarily the cortical association areas are involved rather than the motor cortex. The output from the caudate nucleus sent to the globus pallidus internal segment and thalamus eventually makes its way to the prefrontal, premotor, and supplementary motor cortex; thus it appears that the caudate may function in the control of motor patterns that are linked to memory of previous experience. An example is a situation in which an individual is confronted by a threat. First, he or she recognizes the situation as dangerous on the basis of prior experience. Then a judgment is made to take some course of action in response to the circumstances. When judgment or memory of past experience is associated with movement, it is likely that circuits through the caudate nucleus are involved in controlling the actions.

Function of the Basal Ganglia to Change the Timing and to Scale the Intensity of Movements *(p. 692)*

Two important parameters of any movement are the *speed* and *size* of the movement; they are called timing and scaling functions. Both of these features are disrupted in patients who have basal ganglia lesions, particularly those with lesions that involve the caudate nucleus. This correlates well with the fact that the posterior parietal cortex (especially in the nondominant hemisphere) is the locus for the spatial coordinates of the body and its relationship with the external environment. This part of the cortex projects heavily to the caudate nucleus.

Clinical Syndromes Resulting from Damage to the Basal Ganglia *(p. 693)*

Parkinson's Disease May Be Caused by the Loss of Dopamine-Secreting Nerve Fibers. The disease is characterized by (1) the presence of *rigidity* in many muscle groups, (2) a *tremor present at rest* when no voluntary movement is underway, and (3) difficulty initiating movement (referred to as *akinesia*). Much of this symptomatology is thought to be linked to progressive loss of dopamine-producing cells in the substantia nigra. These neurons are known to project diffusely throughout the caudate and putamen, and the severity of symptoms seems to be proportional to the degree of cell loss in the substantia nigra. The question of why these neurons degenerate remains unanswered at present.

There Are Several Methods for Treating Parkinson's Disease. Because the cell loss results in diminished levels of dopamine, *a dopamine precursor, L-DOPA,* can be administered to increase dopamine availability. This substance can cross the blood-brain barrier, whereas dopamine itself cannot. There are two major problems with this treatment: (1) not all L-DOPA consistently reaches the brain because tissues outside the central nervous system are capable of producing dopamine and (2) as more and more neurons degenerate in the substantia nigra, the required dosage of L-DOPA changes.

- *L-Deprenyl* is an inhibitor of monoamine oxidase, the substance that breaks down dopamine after its release in the brain. It also appears to slow the degeneration of substantia nigra cells; it can be combined with L-DOPA to increase the availability of dopamine.
- *Transplantation of fetal substantia nigra neurons into the caudate and putamen* has been tried in an attempt to increase dopamine levels, but it has had only limited success. The transplanted cells remain viable for only a short time (weeks to months), and the use of aborted fetal tissue creates a potential ethical dilemma. Cultured cell lines (e.g., fibroblasts) that have been genetically altered to produce dopamine are beginning to show promise as a fetal transplantation alternative.
- A procedure called *pallidotomy* is also beginning to show positive results. It has been reasoned that the motor deficits seen in Parkinson's disease patients are the result of abnormal signals transmitted from the globus pallidus to the thalamus. Although the direct effects of dopamine loss appear to be restricted to the caudate and putamen, the output of the latter cell groups in the form of axons projecting to the globus pallidus is still functional but presumably is altered in a major way. One approach has been to position an electrode in the globus pallidus near its output pathways and make a destructive lesion that interrupts the projection to the thalamus. Surprisingly, this is not a technically difficult surgical procedure, and the results thus far look very good. One slight modification has been tried; it was to implant a stimulating electrode in the globus pallidus rather than making a destructive lesion. When activated by the patient, signals generated by the electrode disrupt the flow of impulses from the pallidum to the thalamus; the effect is much the same as a lesion.

Huntington's Disease Is a Genetically Transmitted Disorder (Autosomal Dominant). Typically, Huntington's disease does not appear until the fourth or fifth decade of life. It is characterized by choreiform (flicking) movements at certain joints that gradually progress to the point of involving much of the body. Severe dementia also gradually appears in tandem with the motor deficits. The neural substrate for this disorder is less well understood than Parkinson's disease. It is thought to involve a loss of γ-aminobutyric acid (GABA) neurons in the caudate and putamen and perhaps also a loss of acetylcholine neurons in several parts of the brain including the cerebral cortex. The gene responsible for this defect has been isolated and traced to the short arm of chromosome 4. This determination should eventually facilitate the development of gene therapy for this disorder.

Integration of the Many Parts of the Total Motor Control System *(p. 694)*

- *Spinal cord level.* Organized in the spinal cord are patterns of movement that involve nearly all muscles in the body. These patterns range from the relatively simple withdrawal reflex to coordinated movement of all four extremities.
- *Brain stem (hindbrain) level.* With regard to somatomotor function, neurons in the brain stem play a major role in the control of reflexive eye movements that involve the vestibular sensory apparatus. In addition, the brain stem mediates control over posture and balance, as influenced by the vestibular system, and plays a major role in regulating muscle tone via gamma motor neurons.
- *Corticospinal system.* The output of the motor cortex is delivered to the spinal cord over this vast network of fibers. In general, the motor areas of the cortex can devise a unique and specific motor program that is then sent to the spinal cord, activating various muscle groups. Alternatively, the cortex may select from among the set of motor patterns defined by intrinsic spinal cord circuitry.
- *Cerebellum.* The cerebellum functions at several levels in the motor control hierarchy. At the spinal cord level, it can facilitate stretch reflexes so the ability to manage an unexpected load change or perturbation is enhanced. In the brain stem, the cerebellum is interconnected with the vestibular system to aid in the regulation of posture, equilibrium, and eye movements. The output of the cerebellum is

directed primarily to the thalamus, which then influences the cerebral cortex to provide accessory motor commands or to program in advance the progression from a rapid movement in one direction to a rapid movement in the opposite direction.

- *Basal ganglia.* These neurons and associated cell groups function with motor areas of the cortex to control learned patterns of movement and multiple sequential movements designed to accomplish self-generated or internally guided tasks. Included in this function are the modifications to the motor program needed to regulate the speed and size of the movement—timing and scaling functions.

CHAPTER 57

Cerebral Cortex, Intellectual Functions of the Brain, Learning, and Memory

Physiologic Anatomy of the Cerebral Cortex (p. 697)

The cerebral cortex consists of a relatively thin layer of neurons ranging from 2 to 5 mm in thickness with a total surface area of approximately ¼ square meter and containing about 100 billion neurons.

Most cortical neurons fall into one of three categories: (1) *granular (or stellate)*, (2) *fusiform*, or (3) *pyramidal*. The granule cells are short-axon, local circuit neurons that utilize *glutamate* (excitatory) or *GABA* (inhibitory) as neurotransmitters. In contrast, fusiform and pyramidal neurons have long axons that project at some distance from the cortex. Fusiform cells project to the thalamus, whereas pyramidal neurons project to other locations in the same or opposite hemisphere and to a variety of subcortical locations, such as the red nucleus, basilar pons, and spinal cord.

The neurons of the cerebral cortex are organized into six horizontal layers. Layer IV receives incoming sensory signals from the thalamus, whereas neurons in layer V give rise to long subcortical projections to the brain stem and spinal cord. Corticothalamic fibers originate from cells in layer VI. The corticothalamic interconnections are most significant because damage to the cortex alone seems to result in less dysfunction than occurs when both cortex and thalamus are damaged. Layers I, II, and III are specialized to receive input from and project to other parts of the cortex in the same or opposite hemisphere.

Functions of Specific Cortical Areas (p. 698)

Studies have clearly shown that many areas of the cerebral cortex are specialized for specific functions. Some areas, called *primary* cortex, have direct connections with the spinal cord for controlling movement, whereas other primary regions receive sensory input from various thalamic nuclei that represent each of the special senses (except olfaction) and somatosensation. Secondary cortical areas are called *association* cortex, and they serve to interconnect various portions of the cortex in the same or opposite hemisphere.

Association Areas *(p. 699)*

- *Parieto-occipito-temporal area* includes (1) the posterior parietal area that contains the spatial coordinates for all parts of the contralateral side of the body as well as all contralateral extrapersonal space; (2) the area for language comprehension called *Wernicke's area,* which lies in the superior temporal gyrus; (3) the area for the initial processing of visual language (reading) in the angular gyrus of the inferior parietal lobule; and (4) an area for naming objects located in the anterior part of the occipital lobe.

- *Prefrontal association area* functions in close relation with motor areas of the frontal lobe to plan complex patterns and sequences of movement. Much of its input comes from the parieto-occipito-temporal association cortex, and its principal output is sent to the caudate nucleus for additional processing. It is also involved in nonmotor functions that include memory-related transformations related to problem solving and other internally guided behavior. It contains one specialized region, *Broca's area,* which is involved in the motor aspects of speech and receives input from *Wernicke's area* in the temporal lobe. Broca's area provides output to the nearby motor cortex that controls the muscles required for speech production.

- *Limbic association cortex* includes the anterior pole of the temporal lobe, the ventral aspect of the frontal lobe, and a portion of the cingulate cortex. It is involved with the complex processes of emotional and motivational behavior, and it is connected with limbic system structures such as the hypothalamus, amygdala, and hippocampus.

- *Facial recognition area* is located on the ventromedial surfaces of the occipital and temporal lobes.

Concept of the Dominant Hemisphere *(p. 701)*

The interpretive functions of Wernicke's area, the angular gyrus, and the frontal motor speech areas are more highly developed in one hemisphere, the dominant hemisphere. In approximately 95% of all individuals, the left hemisphere is dominant regardless of handedness. How one hemisphere comes to be dominant is not yet understood.

Wernicke's area is often assigned a *general interpretive function* because damage to this area results in the inability to comprehend spoken or written language even though the individual has no hearing deficit and may be able to read the words on a page. Likewise, damage to the angular gyrus (with Wernicke's area intact) may leave undamaged the ability to understand spoken language, but the ability to comprehend *written* words is lost. This is called *word blindness.*

Interestingly, the area in the nondominant hemisphere that corresponds to *Wernicke's area* is also involved in language function. It is responsible for understanding the emotional content or intonation of spoken language. Similarly, an area in the nondominant frontal lobe corresponds to Broca's area and is responsible for imparting the intonation and inflections that give emotional color or meaning to speech. In a way, these areas are also "dominant" for a particular language function.

Higher Intellectual Functions of the Prefrontal Association Cortex *(p. 702)*

The function of the prefrontal cortex is complex and multifactorial, and it is typically explained by describing the deficits seen in individuals with large lesions in this cortex.

- *Decreased aggressiveness and inappropriate social responses.* This is most apparent when lesions involve the ventral aspect of the prefrontal cortex, the limbic association area.
- *Inability to progress toward goals or to carry through sequential thoughts.* Prefrontal cortex gathers information from widespread areas of the brain to develop solutions to problems, whether they require motor or nonmotor responses. Without this function, thoughts lose their logical progression, and the individual loses the ability to focus attention and becomes highly distractible.
- *Prefrontal cortex as the site of "working memory."* The ability to hold and sort bits of information to be used in a problem-solving function is described as "working memory." By combining these stored bits of information, we can prognosticate, plan for the future, delay a response while further information is gathered, consider the consequences of actions before they are performed, correlate information from many sources, and control actions in accordance with societal or moral laws. All of these actions are considered intellectual functions of the highest order and seem to be definitive for the human experience.

Function of the Brain in Communication—Language Input and Output (p. 703)

There are two aspects to communication: language input (the sensory aspect) and language output (the motor aspect). Some individuals are capable of hearing or identifying written or spoken words, but they do not comprehend the meaning of the words. This is the result of a lesion in Wernicke's area; the condition is known as receptive or *sensory aphasia* and may simply be called *Wernicke's aphasia.* If the lesion extends beyond the confines of Wernicke's area, a total inability to use language communication ensues, termed *global aphasia.*

If an individual is able to formulate verbal language in his or her mind but cannot vocalize the response, the condition is called *motor aphasia.* This indicates a lesion involving Broca's area in the frontal lobe, and the condition can also be referred to as *Broca's aphasia.* The defect is not in control of the musculature needed for speech but, rather, in elaboration of the complex patterns of neural and muscle activation that in effect define the motor aspects of language. Lesions that involve the corresponding language areas in the non-dominant hemisphere cause sensory aprosodia (inability to comprehend the emotional qualities of speech) or motor aprosodia (inability to impart emotional content to speech).

Function of the Corpus Callosum and Anterior Commissure to Transfer Thoughts, Memories, Training, and Other Information between the Two Cerebral Hemispheres (p. 704)

The corpus callosum provides abundant interconnections for most areas of the cerebral hemispheres except for the anterior portion of the temporal lobes, which are connected via the anterior commissure. Some of the more important functional connections mediated by these two fiber bundles are as follows:

• The corpus callosum allows Wernicke's area in the left hemisphere to communicate with the motor cortex in the right hemisphere. In the absence of this connection, voluntary movement of the left side of the body to a communicated command is not possible.

• Visual and somatosensory information from the left side of the body reaches the right hemisphere. Without a corpus callosum, this sensory information cannot extend to Wernicke's area in the left hemisphere.

As a result, such information cannot be used for processing by Wernicke's area, and the left body and left visual field are ignored.

- Without a corpus callosum, only the left half of the brain can understand both the written and spoken word. The right side of the brain can only comprehend the written word, not verbal language. Emotional responses, however, can involve both sides of the brain (and body) if the anterior commissure is intact.

Thoughts, Consciousness, and Memory (p. 705)

The neural substrates for the three processes of thoughts, consciousness, and memory are poorly understood at present. The *holistic theory* suggests that a thought results from patterned stimulation of the cerebral cortex, thalamus, and limbic system; each of these areas contributes its own particular character or quality to the process.

Memory—Roles of Synaptic Facilitation and Synaptic Inhibition (p. 705)

Memories derive from the changes in synaptic transmission between neurons that occur as a result of previous neural activity. These changes cause new pathways, facilitated pathways, or inhibited pathways to develop in the appropriate neural circuitry. The new or altered pathways are called *memory traces.* Although we think of memories as positive collections of previous experiences, probably many are, in a sense, negative memories. Our minds are inundated with sensory information, and an important brain function is the ability to ignore irrelevant or extraneous information. This process is called *habituation.* Conversely, the brain also has the capacity to enhance or store certain memory traces through *facilitation* of synaptic circuits, a mechanism referred to as *memory sensitization.*

It is obvious that some memories last only a few seconds, whereas others last hours, days, months, or years. Consequently, three categories of memories have been described: (1) short-term memories last only seconds or minutes unless they are converted to long-term memory; (2) intermediate long-term memory lasts days to weeks but is eventually lost; and (3) long-term memory, which once stored, can be recalled years later or for a lifetime.

Short-Term Memory. Short-term memory is typified by the memory of a new telephone number recalled for a few seconds or minutes as one continues to think about the number. Several theories concerning the substrate for this mechanism are under investigation: (1) this type of memory is due to continuous neural activity in a reverberating circuit, (2) it occurs as a result of activation of synapses on presynaptic terminals that typically result in prolonged facilitation or inhibition, and (3) the accumulation of calcium in axon terminals may eventually lead to enhanced synaptic output from that terminal.

Intermediate Long-Term Memory. This memory can result from temporary chemical or physical changes in either the presynaptic or postsynaptic membrane that can persist for a few minutes up to several weeks. Some experimental observations on such mechanisms have come from studies in the snail *Aplysia,* as shown in Figure 57–1. Stimulation of a facilitator terminal at the same time as activation of another sensory input causes serotonin to be released at synaptic sites on the sensory terminal. Stimulation of serotonin receptors activates adenyl cyclase in the main sensory terminal, resulting in the formation of cyclic adenosine monophosphate (cAMP), which causes release of a protein kinase and leads to phosphorylation of a protein that blocks potassium channels in the sensory terminal. Decreased potassium conductance causes prolongation of action potentials that reach the sensory terminal, which in turn allows increased calcium to enter the

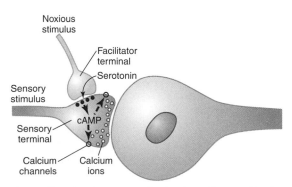

Figure 57–1. Memory system that has been discovered in the snail *Aplysia*.

sensory terminal, resulting in increased neurotransmitter release from the sensory terminal, thereby facilitating transmission at this synapse.

Long-Term Memory. Long-term memory is thought to result from *structural changes* at the synapse that enhance or suppress signal conduction. These structural changes include (1) an increase in the number of synaptic vesicle release sites, (2) an increase in the number of available synaptic vesicles, (3) an increase in the number of synaptic terminals, and (4) changes in the shape or number of postsynaptic spines.

Consolidation of Memory *(p. 708)*

For memories to be converted to long-term memory, they must be *consolidated*; that is, they must initiate the chemical or structural changes that underlie the formation of a long-term memory. In general, 5 to 10 minutes is required for minimal consolidation, whereas 1 hour or more may be needed for strong consolidation. The mechanism of *rehearsal* is thought to represent the consolidation process.

Rehearsal of the same information again and again in the mind potentiates the transfer from short-term to long-term memory. Over time, the important features of sensory experience become progressively more fixed in memory stores. Also during consolidation, memories are codified into various classes of information. For example, new and old experiences relative to a topic are compared for similarities and differences, and it is the latter information that is stored.

Roles of Specific Brain Parts in the Memory Process *(p. 708)*

Lesions of the hippocampus lead to *anterograde amnesia,* or the inability to form or store *new* memories. Memories formed prior to the onset of the lesion are not affected; the reason for this appears to be that the hippocampus (and the dorsomedial thalamic nucleus) is connected to the so-called *punishment and reward* centers. That is, our experiences may be associated in the hippocampus with pleasure or punishment, and that is the substrate for initiating the memory process. The loss of long-term memory occurs with thalamic lesions and, in some instances, with damage to the hippocampus. The hypothesis is that the thalamus may be part of the mechanism that searches the memory stores and "reads" them. Interestingly, individuals with hippocampal lesions do not have difficulty learning physical skills that require only manual repetition and do not involve verbalization or other types of symbolic higher order intelligence. This suggests that memory mechanisms for functions are distributed in more than one brain location.

CHAPTER 58

Behavioral and Motivational Mechanisms of the Brain—The Limbic System and the Hypothalamus

Activating Driving Systems of the Brain (p. 711)

Signals from the brain stem activate the cerebrum in two ways: (1) by stimulating the background level of activity throughout wide areas of the brain and (2) by activating neurohumoral systems that release specific facilitatory or inhibitory hormone-like neurotransmitters into selected areas of the brain.

Control of Cerebral Activity by Continuous Excitatory Signals from the Brain Stem (p. 711)

A *Reticular Excitatory Area* Is Located in the Reticular Formation of the Pons and Midbrain. It forms descending spinal projections to the spinal cord that exert an excitatory influence on motor neurons that innervate antigravity musculature. This same reticular area also sends fibers rostrally to various locations including the thalamus, where neurons distribute to all regions of the cerebral cortex.

The signals that reach the thalamus are of two types. One type arises from the large cholinergic reticular neurons, is rapidly transmitted, and excites the cerebrum for only a few milliseconds. The second type of signal originates from small reticular neurons that generate relatively slow action potentials that terminate mainly in the intralaminar and reticular nuclei of the thalamus. Excitatory signals from the latter input build up slowly and produce a widespread effect that controls the background level of excitability of cortical neurons.

The level of activity in the reticular excitatory area is determined largely by input from ascending somatosensory pathways—the pain pathways, in particular. This was deduced from animal experiments in which the brain stem was transected just rostral to the entry of the trigeminal nerve. This effectively eliminates all ascending somatosensory input, and the excitatory reticular area goes silent as the animal enters a coma-like state. Curiously, the cortex also provides descending excitatory input to the excitatory reticular area, which serves as positive feedback and allows cerebral activity to reinforce the action of the ascending reticular system. The thalamus and cortex are linked by reciprocal connections. Part of the "thinking" process may involve memory formation resulting from the back-and-forth signal transfer between the thalamus and cortex.

The Lower Brain Stem in the Ventromedial Medulla Contains a *Reticular Inhibitory Area*. Like the more rostral excitatory reticular area, this region provides descending spinal projections that inhibit the activity of antigravity muscles. Similarly, the inhibitory reticular area projects rostrally to decrease the excitatory levels of the cerebrum through serotonergic systems (discussed later).

Neurohormonal Control of Brain Activity (p. 712)

A second method for altering the background level of activity in the cerebrum involves projections from cell groups that use excitatory or inhibitory neurotransmitter agents that function similar to hormones; these three agents are *norepinephrine, dopamine,* and *serotonin.*

- The *norepinephrine system* originates from the neurons of the *locus ceruleus,* located in the rostral pons and caudal midbrain. These cells have unusually long, diffusely projecting axons that extend to many areas of the brain, including the thalamus and cerebral cortex. At most of its synaptic targets norepinephrine exerts excitatory effects, although in some regions the receptor to which it binds produces inhibition. Often the effects of norepinephrine are *modulatory.* That is, they might not cause an action potential in the target neuron but, instead, raise the excitability level of the cell and make it more likely to fire action potentials in response to subsequent input.

- Most *dopaminergic neurons* are concentrated in two locations in the midbrain that give rise to the mesostriatal and the mesolimbic systems. Neurons in the compact portion (pars compacta) of the *substantia nigra* represent the important source of dopamine fibers that project rostrally to the caudate and putamen as the *nigrostriatal system.* Dopamine projections can produce either excitation or inhibition. Neurons in some basal ganglion circuits exhibit receptors that cause excitatory postsynaptic potentials when they bind dopamine, whereas other receptors in other circuits produce just the opposite effect (inhibition).

A second group of dopamine-containing neurons is found in the ventral tegmental nucleus located just medial and somewhat posterior to the substantia nigra pars reticulate. These neurons project diffusely to the frontal lobe, ventral striatum, amygdala, and other limbic structures associated with positive reinforcement. Excessive activity in mesocortical dopamine projections to ventral striatum and prefrontal cortex is believed to contribute to the development of schizophrenia.

• The raphe nuclei are relatively small, thin, discontinuous groups of cells located adjacent to the midline at various levels in the brain stem extending from the midbrain to the medulla. Most (but not all) neurons use *serotonin* as a neurotransmitter, and a large number of the serotonin-producing cells project to the thalamus and cortex. When released in the cortex, serotonin nearly always produces inhibitory effects.

A number of other neurotransmitter systems play important functional roles in the thalamus and cerebral cortex, including the enkephalins and endorphins, γ-aminobutyric acid (GABA), glutamate, vasopressin, adrenocorticotropic hormone (ACTH), angiotensin II, vasoactive intestinal peptide, and neurotensin.

Limbic System (p. 714)

The limbic system is the combined neuronal circuitry that controls emotional behavior and motivational drives. This large complex of brain structures is composed of subcortical and cortical components. The *subcortical group* includes the *hypothalamus, septum, paraolfactory area, epithalamus, anterior thalamic nucleus, hippocampus, amygdala,* and portions of the *basal ganglia.* Surrounding the subcortical structures is the limbic cortex, composed of the orbitofrontal cortex, subcallosal gyrus, cingulate gyrus, and parahippocampal gyrus. Among the subcortical structures, the hypothalamus is the most important output source; it communicates with brain stem nuclei through the medial forebrain bundle, which conducts signals in two directions: toward the brain stem and back to the forebrain.

Functional Anatomy of the Limbic System; Key Position of the Hypothalamus (p. 714)

The influence of the hypothalamus extends caudally to the brain stem and rostrally to the diencephalon, limbic cortex, and pituitary gland. The hypothalamus controls (1) vegetative and endocrine functions and (2) behavior and motivation.

Vegetative and Endocrine Control Functions. The hypothalamus can be divided into a number of cell groups responsible for certain functions; however, localization of function is less precise than is suggested by these studies.

- *Cardiovascular regulation* involves control of arterial pressure and heart rate and is focused in general in the posterior and lateral hypothalamic areas, which increase blood pressure and heart rate, or in the preoptic area, which decreases blood pressure and heart rate. These effects are mediated by cardiovascular centers in the pontine and the medullary reticular formation.

- *Body temperature regulation* is controlled by neurons in the preoptic area that are able to sense changes in the temperature of blood flowing through the area. Increases or decreases in temperature signal the appropriate cells to activate body temperature-lowering or temperature-elevating mechanisms.

- *Regulation of body water intake* is controlled by mechanisms that create thirst or control excretion of water into urine. The thirst center is in the lateral hypothalamus; when the concentration of electrolyte levels here is elevated, a desire to "drink" is initiated. The supraoptic nucleus is involved with mechanisms that control urinary excretion of water, and neurons here release antidiuretic hormone (ADH, or vasopressin) into the posterior pituitary gland that then enters the circulation and acts on the collecting ducts in the kidney to cause reabsorption of water, making the urine more concentrated.

- *Uterine contraction and milk ejection* are stimulated by *oxytocin,* which is released by neurons of the paraventricular nucleus.

- *Gastrointestinal and feeding regulation* are controlled by several hypothalamic areas. The lateral hypothalamus is responsible for the desire to seek out food, and damage to this area may result in starvation. In comparison, the ventromedial nucleus is called the satiety center because its activity produces a "stop eating" signal. The mammillary nuclei are involved in certain reflexes related to food intake, such as lip licking and swallowing.

- *Anterior pituitary gland regulation* is achieved by the elaboration of releasing and inhibitory factors from the hypothalamus, which are carried by a portal system to the anterior lobe of the pituitary. Here they act on glandular cells that produce the anterior pituitary hormones. The hypothalamic neurons that produce these factors are found in the periventricular zone, the arcuate nucleus, and the ventromedial nucleus.

Behavioral Control Functions of the Hypothalamus and Associated Limbic Structures. Emotional behavior is affected by stimulation of the hypothalamus or by lesions in the hypothalamus. Stimulation effects include (1) increased general level of activity, leading to rage and aggression; (2) sense of tranquility, pleasure, and reward; (3) fear and feelings of punishment, aversion; and (4) sexual arousal. Effects caused by hypothalamic lesions include (1) extreme passivity and loss of drives and (2) excessive eating and drinking, rage, and violent behavior.

"Reward" and "Punishment" Function of the Limbic System (p. 717)

The major locations that evoke a pleasurable feeling or sense of reward when stimulated are found along the course of the medial forebrain bundle, especially in the lateral and ventromedial hypothalamus. Conversely, areas that when stimulated evoke aversive behavior include the midbrain periaqueductal gray, the periventricular zones of the thalamus and hypothalamus, the amygdala, and the hippocampus.

Rage—Its Association with the Punishment Center (p. 718)

In animals, intense stimulation of aversive centers in the lateral hypothalamus and periventricular zone evokes a rage response. This is characterized by a defense posture, extended claws, elevated tail, hissing and spitting, growling, and piloerection. Normally, the rage reaction is held in check by activity in the ventromedial hypothalamus.

Importance of Reward and Punishment in Behavior (p. 718)

Much of our daily behavior is controlled by punishment and reward. Administration of tranquilizers inhibits both punishment and reward centers and thereby decreases behavioral affect in general. These drugs are not selective, however, and other hypothalamic functions may be depressed as well, thus creating potentially harmful side effects. Also, stimulation that affects either the reward or punishment center tends to build strong memory traces, and the responses to such stimulation are said to be reinforced. Stimulations that are essentially indifferent tend to become habituated.

Specific Functions of Other Parts of the Limbic System (p. 718)

Hippocampus. Stimulation of the hippocampus can evoke rage, passivity, and excessive sexual drive. The hippocampus is hyperexcitable, and weak stimuli can produce epileptic seizures. Lesions of the hippocampus lead to a profound inability to form new memories based on any type of verbal symbolism (language); this is called *anterograde amnesia.* It is suggested that the hippocampus provides the signal for memory consolidation (e.g., transformation from short-term to long-term memory).

Amygdala. This large aggregate of cells is located in the medial, anterior pole of the temporal lobe and consists of two subdivisions: a corticomedial nuclear group and a basolateral group of nuclei. The amygdala output is varied and extensive, reaching the cortex, hippocampus, septum, thalamus, and hypothalamus. Stimulation of the amygdala produces changes in heart rate, arterial pressure, gastrointestinal motility, defecation and urination, pupillary dilation, piloerection, and secretion of anterior pituitary hormones. In addition, involuntary movements can be elicited, including tonic posture, circling movements, clonus, and movements associated with olfaction and eating. Behavior such as rage, fear, escape, and sexual activity can be evoked. Bilateral destruction of the temporal poles leads to the *Klüver-Bucy syndrome,* which includes extreme orality, loss of fear, decreased aggressiveness, tameness, changes in eating behavior, psychic blindness, and excessive sexual drive.

Limbic Cortex. The discrete contributions of various portions of the limbic cortex are poorly understood. Knowledge of their function is derived from lesions that damage the cortex. Bilateral destruction of the anterior temporal cortex leads to the Klüver-Bucy syndrome, as described earlier. Bilateral lesions in the posterior orbitofrontal cortex lead to insomnia and restlessness. Bilateral destruction of the anterior cingulate and subcallosal gyri evokes an extreme rage reaction.

CHAPTER 59

States of Brain Activity—Sleep, Brain Waves, Epilepsy, Psychoses

Sleep (p. 721)

Sleep is defined as a state of unconsciousness from which one can be aroused by sensory stimulation. Investigators now believe that there are two entirely different types of sleep: slow wave sleep and rapid-eye-movement (REM) sleep.

Slow-Wave Sleep. This is the deep, restful type of sleep characterized by decreases in peripheral vascular tone, blood pressure, respiratory rate, and metabolic rate. Dreams can occur during slow-wave sleep, but they are not remembered.

REM Sleep. This is called *paradoxical sleep* because the brain is quite active and skeletal muscle contractions occur. Typically, REM sleep lasts 5 to 30 minutes and repeats at approximately 90-minute intervals. When an individual is extremely tired, REM may be absent but eventually returns as the individual becomes more rested. There are several important features of REM sleep: (1) dreaming occurs and the dream can be recalled, at least in part; (2) waking a person in REM sleep is more difficult, yet in the morning we typically awaken during an REM period; (3) muscle tone is substantially depressed; (4) heart rate and respiration become irregular; (5) despite decreased tone, muscle contractions do occur, especially rapid eye movements; and (6) brain metabolism is increased by as much as 20%, and the electroencephalogram shows brain waves that are characteristic of the waking state.

Basic Theories of Sleep (p. 722)

Initially, the *passive* theory of sleep was in favor; it suggested that sleep occurred when the reticular activating system simply decreased its activity. This concept was called into question by animal experiments that involved transection of the brain stem at midpontine levels, which resulted in an animal that never slept. Now it is believed that sleep is caused by an *active* mechanism that inhibits other parts of the brain.

Neuronal Centers, Neurohumoral Substances, and Mechanisms That Can Cause Sleep—A Possible Specific Role for Serotonin

Sleep can occur by stimulating any one of three brain locations. The most potent site is the *raphe of the caudal pons* and *medulla*. Many of the neurons in the

453

raphe nuclei use *serotonin* as a transmitter, and it is known that drugs that block the formation of serotonin prevent sleep. In addition, stimulation in the nucleus of the solitary tract promotes sleep, but this occurs only if the raphe nuclei are also functional. Activation of the *suprachiasmatic level of the hypothalamus* or the *midline nuclei of the thalamus* produces sleep. Some studies, however, have shown that blood levels of serotonin are lower during sleep than during wakefulness, suggesting that some other substance is responsible for sleep production. One possibility is *muramyl peptide*, which accumulates in cerebrospinal fluid and urine. When microgram amounts of this substance are injected into the third ventricle, sleep is induced within minutes.

REM sleep is enhanced by cholinergic agonists. It is postulated that certain of the projections of cholinergic neurons of the midbrain reticular formation are responsible for the initiation of REM sleep. These projections would activate only neurons that lead to REM sleep activation and avoid those systems that contribute to waking state production and the reticular activating system.

Physiological Effects of Sleep *(p. 723)*

Prolonged wakefulness (absence of sleep) is associated with sluggishness of thought, irritability, and even psychotic behavior. Sleep restores the normal balance of activity in many parts of the brain—from the higher intellectual centers of the cortex to the vegetative and behavioral functions of the hypothalamus and limbic system. The specifics of this process are unknown. Similarly, it is known that sleep deprivation affects other systems in the body that regulate blood pressure, heart rate, peripheral vascular tone, muscle activity, and basal metabolic rate. Again, the mechanisms are not yet defined.

Brain Waves *(p. 723)*

Electrical potentials that originate near the surface of the brain and are recorded from outside the head are called brain waves, and the recording process is *electroencephalography* (EEG). The recorded potentials range from 0 to 200 microvolts, and their frequency ranges from once every few seconds to 50 or more per second. Distinct wave patterns can appear, and some are characteristic for specific brain abnormalities. Four major brain wave patterns have been described: *alpha, beta, theta, and delta waves.*

- *Alpha waves.* These are rhythmical waves with a frequency of 8 to 12 Hz at about 50 microvolts; they are found in normal, awake but resting (eyes closed) individuals.
- *Beta waves.* When the eyes are opened in the light, slightly higher frequency (14 to 80 Hz) *beta* waves appear, with a voltage of less than 50 microvolts. Thalamocortical projections must be intact for these waves to be recorded; presumably, the ascending reticular input to the thalamus also must be functional.
- *Theta waves.* These waves have frequencies in the range of 4 to 7 Hz and occur mainly in the parietal and temporal areas in children, but they can appear in adults during a period of emotional stress. They also appear in association with brain disorders and degenerative brain states.
- *Delta waves.* These are all of the waves below 3.5 Hz and they occur during deep sleep, with serious organic brain disease, and in infants. It appears that they persist in the absence of cortical input from the thalamus and lower brain centers. Because they can be seen during slow-wave sleep, this sleep state is probably due to releasing the cortex from the influence of lower centers.

Effect of Varying Levels of Cerebral Activity on the Frequency of the EEG *(p. 724)*

As one progresses from alert wakefulness to deep sleep, there is a gradual change in brain wave pattern from low-voltage/high-frequency waves (alpha) to high-voltage/low-frequency waves (delta). These changes can also be described as a progression from *desynchronized* activity (alert) to *synchronous* patterns (deep sleep). REM sleep is again paradoxical because it is a sleep state, yet the brain exhibits asynchronous activity characteristic of the waking state.

Epilepsy *(p. 725)*

Epilepsy is characterized by uncontrolled, excessive activity in the nervous system, termed a seizure. Three types of epilepsy are typically described: *grand mal epilepsy, petit mal epilepsy, and focal epilepsy.*

- *Grand mal epilepsy.* This is the most severe variety and seems to be the result of intense discharges in many parts of the brain, including the cortex, thalamus, and brain stem. Initially, generalized tonic seizures affect much of the body followed by alternating tonic-clonic seizures. This activity may persist for 3 to 4 minutes and is followed by postseizure depression of the nervous system, which can leave the individual stuporous, sleepy, and fatigued for several hours. EEG activity during a seizure of this type shows characteristic high-voltage/high-frequency patterns. Grand mal seizures can be precipitated in susceptible individuals by (1) strong emotional stimuli, (2) alkalosis caused by hyperventilation, (3) drugs, (4) fever, or (5) a loud noise or flashing light. In addition, brain trauma and tumors can lead to seizure activity. It is said that grand mal seizures occur in individuals predisposed to abnormal electrogenic circuitry in the brain.

- *Petit mal epilepsy.* This is less severe seizure activity during which the individual loses consciousness for 3 to 30 seconds and exhibits small twitching of muscles around the head or face, especially blinking of the eyes. It is also called an *absence seizure,* and such activity is thought to be limited to abnormal function in the thalamocortical system. On occasion, a petit mal attack progresses to a grand mal seizure.

- *Focal epilepsy.* This type of seizure activity can involve almost any part of the brain and nearly always is caused by some local abnormality, such as scar tissue formation, a tumor, ischemia, or a congenital abnormality. The typical presentation is a focal muscle twitching that progresses to involve adjacent body parts. EEG can often be used to locate the initial focus of abnormal brain activity so it can be surgically removed.

Psychotic Behavior and Dementia—Roles of Specific Neurotransmitter Systems (p. 726)

Depression and Manic-Depressive Psychoses

Depression and manic-depressive psychoses might be the result of decreased production of norepinephrine, serotonin, or both. Drugs that increase the excitatory effects of norepinephrine are effective in treating depression; they include monoamine oxidase inhibitors, tricyclic antidepressants, and drugs that enhance the action of serotonin. Manic-depressive conditions (bipolar disorder) can be treated effectively with lithium compounds that diminish the actions of norepineph-rine and serotonin.

Schizophrenia *(p. 727)*

There are three possible explanations for schizophre-nia, which is diagnosed in individuals who hear voices, have delusions of grandeur, or experience intense fear or paranoia. The explanations are (1) abnormal circuitry in the prefrontal cortex, (2) excessive activity of dopa-mine systems that project to the cortex, or (3) abnormal function of limbic circuitry related to the hippocampus. The excessive dopamine output theory involves mid-brain dopamine neurons (mesolimbic dopamine system) that are distinct from those in the substantia nigra, which are related to Parkinson's disease. Evidence supporting this theory derives from the fact that schizophrenic symptoms are alleviated by drugs such as chlorproma-zine and haloperidol, which diminish dopamine release at axon terminals.

Alzheimer's Disease *(p. 727)*

Alzheimer's disease, seen mostly in the elderly, is char-acterized by the accumulation of *amyloid plaques* and neurofibrillary tangles in widespread areas of the brain, including the cerebral cortex, hippocampus, and basal ganglia. The severe dementia that ensues may be related to the widespread loss of cholinergic input to the cerebral cortex resulting from the loss of neurons in the basal nucleus of Meynert. Many patients also exhibit a genetic abnormality involving apolipoprotein E, a protein that transports cholesterol.

CHAPTER 60

The Autonomic Nervous System and the Adrenal Medulla

The *autonomic nervous system* is the portion of the nervous system that controls the visceral functions of the body. This system acts rapidly to control arterial pressure, gastrointestinal motility and secretion, urinary bladder emptying, sweating, body temperature, and many other activities.

General Organization of the Autonomic Nervous System *(p. 729)*

The central portions of the autonomic nervous system are located in the *hypothalamus, brain stem,* and *spinal cord.* Higher brain centers, such as the *limbic cortex* and portions of the *cerebral cortex,* can influence the activity of the autonomic nervous system by sending signals to the hypothalamus and lower brain areas.

The autonomic nervous system also often operates through *visceral reflexes.* That is, subconscious sensory signals from a visceral organ can enter the autonomic ganglia, the brain stem, or the hypothalamus and then return *subconscious reflex responses* directly back to the visceral organ to control its activities.

The efferent autonomic signals are transmitted to the various organs of the body through two major subdivisions called the *sympathetic nervous system* and the *parasympathetic nervous system.*

The autonomic nervous system is a motor system for the visceral organs, blood vessels, and secretory glands. The cell body of the *preganglionic neuron* is located in either the brain stem or the spinal cord. The axon of this visceral motor neuron projects as a thinly myelinated preganglionic fiber to an *autonomic ganglion.* The postganglionic neuron has its cell body in the ganglia and sends an unmyelinated axon, the *postganglionic fiber,* to visceral effector cells.

In general, *sympathetic ganglia* are located close to the central nervous system, whereas *parasympathetic ganglia* are located close to the effector tissues. Sympathetic pathways have short preganglionic fibers and long postganglionic fibers, whereas parasympathetic pathways have long preganglionic fibers and short postganglionic fibers.

Physiologic Anatomy of the Sympathetic Nervous System

In the sympathetic division of the autonomic nervous system, visceral motor neurons are located in the *intermediolateral horn* of the spinal cord from level T-1 to L-2. The axons of these motor neurons leave the spinal cord via the *ventral root*. From here, the axon can take one of three paths:

1. It can enter the *sympathetic chain* via the *white ramus* and terminate at its level of origin.
2. It can enter the sympathetic chain via the white ramus and ascend or descend before terminating in the sympathetic chain at a different level.
3. It can enter the sympathetic chain through the white ramus and exit without synapsing via a *splanchnic nerve* and terminate in a *prevertebral ganglion*.

The postganglionic neuron originates in one of the sympathetic chain ganglia or prevertebral ganglia. From either source, the postganglionic fibers travel to their destinations.

Preganglionic Sympathetic Nerve Fibers Pass All the Way to the Adrenal Medulla without Synapsing. Preganglionic sympathetic nerve fibers that innervate the adrenal medulla originate in the intermediolateral horn of the spinal cord and pass through the sympathetic chains and splanchnic nerves to reach the adrenal medulla, where they end directly on modified neuronal cells that secrete epinephrine and norepinephrine into the bloodstream. Embryologically, the secretory cells of the adrenal medulla are derived from nervous tissue and are analogous to postganglionic neurons.

Physiologic Anatomy of the Parasympathetic Nervous System

In the parasympathetic division of the autonomic nervous system, visceral motor neurons are located in discrete brain stem nuclei or in sacral spinal cord segments 2 to 4. The axons of these motor neurons leave the brain stem via *cranial nerves III, VII, IX,* and *X* or leave the sacral spinal cord via the *pelvic nerves*.

Parasympathetic fibers in the *third cranial nerve* travel to the pupillary sphincters and ciliary muscles of the eye. Fibers from the *seventh cranial nerve* travel to the lacrimal, nasal, and submandibular glands; and fibers from the *ninth cranial nerve* travel to the parotid gland. About 75% of all parasympathetic nerve fibers are located in the *tenth cranial nerve,* the *vagus nerve.* The vagus nerve supplies parasympathetic input to the heart, lungs, esophagus, stomach, small intestine, proximal half of the colon, liver, gallbladder, pancreas, and upper portions of the ureters.

The *sacral parasympathetic fibers* distribute their fibers to the descending colon, rectum, bladder, and lower portions of the ureters and external genitalia.

Basic Characteristics of Sympathetic and Parasympathetic Function *(p. 731)*

The two primary neurotransmitter substances of the autonomic nervous system are *acetylcholine* and *norepinephrine.* Autonomic neurons that secrete acetylcholine are said to be *cholinergic;* those that secrete norepinephrine are said to be *adrenergic.* All preganglionic neurons in both the sympathetic and parasympathetic divisions of the autonomic nervous system are cholinergic. Acetylcholine and acetylcholine-like substances therefore excite both the sympathetic and parasympathetic postganglionic neurons.

Virtually all postganglionic neurons of the parasympathetic nervous system secrete acetylcholine and are cholinergic. Most postganglionic sympathetic neurons secrete norepinephrine and are adrenergic. A few postganglionic sympathetic nerve fibers, however, are cholinergic. These fibers innervate sweat glands, piloerector muscles, and some blood vessels.

Synthesis and Secretion of Acetylcholine and Norepinephrine by Postganglionic Nerve Endings

Acetylcholine is synthesized in the terminal endings of cholinergic nerve fibers through the combination of *acetyl-coenzyme A* (CoA) with *choline.* Once released by the cholinergic nerve endings, acetylcholine is rapidly degraded by the enzyme *acetylcholinesterase.*

Norepinephrine and epinephrine are synthesized from the amino acid *tyrosine.* Tyrosine is converted to *DOPA,* which is then converted to *dopamine;* dopamine is subsequently converted to norepinephrine. In the adrenal medulla, this reaction proceeds one step further to transform 80% of the norepinephrine to *epinephrine.* The action of norepinephrine is terminated by reuptake into the adrenergic nerve endings or by diffusion from the nerve endings into the surrounding fluids.

Receptors on Effector Organs *(p. 732)*

Cholinergic Receptors Are Subdivided into *Muscarinic* and *Nicotinic* Receptors. Muscarinic receptors are found on all effector cells stimulated by the postganglionic neurons of the parasympathetic nervous system as well as those stimulated by the postganglionic cholinergic neurons of the sympathetic nervous system. Nicotinic receptors are found in the synapses between the preganglionic and postganglionic neurons of both the sympathetic and parasympathetic nervous systems as well as in the skeletal muscle neuromuscular junction.

Adrenergic Receptors Are Subdivided into *Alpha* (α) and *Beta* (β) Receptors. Norepinephrine and epinephrine have somewhat different affinities for the α- and β-adrenergic receptors. Norepinephrine excites mainly α-receptors, although it excites β-receptors to a lesser extent. Epinephrine excites both types of receptor approximately equally. The relative effects of norepinephrine and epinephrine on various effector organs are determined by the types of receptor located on these organs.

The stimulation of α-receptors results in vasoconstriction, dilation of the iris, contraction of the intestinal and bladder sphincters, and contraction of the pilomotor muscles.

The β-receptor is subdivided into β_1-, β_2-, and β_3 receptor subtypes. Stimulation of β_1-receptors causes an increase in heart rate and strength of contraction. Stimulation of β_2-receptors causes skeletal muscle vasodilation, bronchodilation, uterine relaxation, calorigenesis, and glycogenolysis. Stimulation of β_3-receptors induces lipolysis in adipose tissue and the conversion of energy in lipids into heat (thermogenesis).

Excitatory and Inhibitory Actions of Sympathetic and Parasympathetic Stimulation *(p. 733)*

Sympathetic stimulation causes excitatory effects in some organs but inhibitory effects in others. Likewise, parasympathetic stimulation causes excitation in some organs but inhibition in others. Occasionally, the two divisions of the autonomic nervous system act reciprocally in an organ, with one system causing an increase in activity and the other system causing a decrease in activity. Most organs, however, are dominantly controlled by one of the two systems.

Effects of Sympathetic and Parasympathetic Stimulation on Specific Organs (p. 735)

Eyes. Two functions of the eyes are controlled by the autonomic nervous system: *pupillary opening* and *focusing of the lens.* Sympathetic stimulation contracts the *radial dilator muscle* of the iris, resulting in pupillary dilation, whereas parasympathetic stimulation contracts the *sphincter muscle* of the iris, resulting in pupillary constriction. Focusing of the lens is controlled almost entirely by the parasympathetic nervous system. Parasympathetic excitation contracts the ciliary muscle, which releases the tension on the suspensory ligament of the lens and allows it to become more convex. This change allows the eye to focus on close objects.

Glands of the Body. The *nasal, lacrimal, salivary,* and *gastrointestinal glands* are strongly stimulated by the parasympathetic nervous system, resulting in copious quantities of watery secretion. Sympathetic stimulation causes vasoconstriction of blood vessels that supply the glands and in this way often reduces the rate of secretion from these glands. Sympathetic stimulation has a direct effect on glandular cells by causing formation of a concentrated secretion that contains extra enzymes and mucus.

The *sweat glands* secrete large quantities of sweat when the sympathetic nerves are stimulated. Parasympathetic stimulation has no effect on sweat gland secretion. The sympathetic fibers to most sweat glands are cholinergic; almost all other sympathetic fibers are adrenergic.

The *apocrine glands* in the axillae secrete a thick, odoriferous secretion as a result of sympathetic stimulation. These glands do not respond to parasympathetic stimulation. The apocrine glands are controlled by adrenergic fibers rather than by cholinergic fibers.

Intramural Nerve Plexus of the Gastrointestinal System. Sympathetic and parasympathetic stimulation can affect gastrointestinal activity mainly by increasing or decreasing activity on the intestinal *enteric nervous system.* In general, parasympathetic stimulation increases the overall degree of activity of the gastrointestinal tract. Normal function of the gastrointestinal tract is not particularly dependent on sympathetic stimulation. Strong sympathetic stimulation, however, inhibits peristalsis and increases the tone of the various sphincters in the gastrointestinal tract.

Heart. Sympathetic stimulation increases the rate and strength of heart contractions. Parasympathetic stimulation causes the opposite effect.

Systemic Blood Vessels. Sympathetic stimulation causes vasoconstriction of many of the blood vessels of the body, especially the abdominal viscera and the skin on the limbs.

Arterial Pressure. The arterial pressure is determined by two factors: propulsion of blood by the heart and resistance to the flow of this blood through the blood vessels. Sympathetic stimulation increases both propulsion by the heart and resistance to flow, which results in an increase in arterial pressure. Parasympathetic stimulation decreases the pumping ability of the heart but has little effect on peripheral vascular resistance. This change results in a slight fall in arterial pressure.

Other Body Functions. Most of the endodermal structures, such as the ducts of the liver, gallbladder, ureter, urinary bladder, and bronchi, are inhibited by sympathetic stimulation but excited by parasympathetic stimulation. Sympathetic stimulation also has multiple metabolic effects such as release of glucose from the liver, increase in blood glucose concentration, increase in glycogenolysis in both liver and muscle, increase in skeletal muscle strength, increase in basal metabolic rate, and increase in mental activity. The sympathetics and parasympathetics are involved in execution of the male and female sexual acts, as explained in Chapters 80 and 81.

Function of the Adrenal Medullae *(p. 736)*

Stimulation of the sympathetic nerves to the adrenal medulla causes large quantities of epinephrine and norepinephrine to be released into the circulating blood. About 80% of the secretion from the adrenal medulla is epinephrine, and about 20% is norepinephrine. The effect of the epinephrine and norepinephrine released from the adrenal medulla lasts 5 to 10 times longer than when they are released by sympathetic neurons because these hormones are slowly removed from the blood.

The circulating norepinephrine causes vasoconstriction, increased heart rate and contractility, inhibition of the gastrointestinal tract, and dilated pupils. The circulating epinephrine, because of its ability to strongly stimulate the β-receptors, has a greater effect on cardiac performance than does norepinephrine. Epinephrine causes only weak constriction of the blood vessels in muscles, resulting in a slight increase in arterial pressure but a dramatic increase in cardiac output.

Epinephrine and norepinephrine are always released by the adrenal medulla at the same time that organs are directly stimulated by generalized sympathetic activation. This dual mechanism of sympathetic stimulation provides a safety factor to ensure optimal performance when it is needed.

Sympathetic and Parasympathetic "Tone" (p. 737)

The basal rate of activity of the autonomic nervous system is known as *sympathetic* and *parasympathetic tone*. Sympathetic tone and parasympathetic tone allow a single division of the autonomic nervous system to increase or decrease the activity of a visceral organ or to constrict or dilate a vascular bed. Normally, sympathetic tone constricts systemic arterioles to about one half of their maximum diameter, whereas parasympathetic tone maintains normal gastrointestinal motility.

Discrete or Mass Discharges of the Autonomic Nervous System (p. 738)

In some instances, the sympathetic nervous system becomes very active and causes a widespread reaction throughout the body called the *alarm* or *stress response*. At other times, sympathetic activation occurs in isolated areas of the body; for example, local vasodilation and sweating occur in response to a local increase in temperature.

The parasympathetic nervous system is usually responsible for highly specific changes in visceral function, such as changes in salivary and gastric secretion or in bladder and rectal emptying. Also, parasympathetic cardiovascular reflexes usually act only on the heart to increase or decrease its rate of beating and have little effect on vascular resistance.

Widespread activation of the sympathetic nervous system can be brought about by fear, rage, or severe pain. The alarm or stress response that results is often called the *fight or flight reaction*. Widespread sympathetic activation causes increases in arterial pressure, muscle blood flow, metabolic rate, blood glucose concentration, glycogenolysis, and mental alertness and decreases in blood flow to the gastrointestinal tract and kidneys and a shorter coagulation time. These effects allow an individual to perform far more strenuous activity than would otherwise be possible.

Medullary, Pontine, Mesencephalic and Higher Areas of the Brain Control Autonomic Activity (p. 739)

Many neuronal areas in the brain stem reticular substance and along the course of the tractus solitarius of the medulla, pons, and mesencephalon, as well as in many special nuclei control autonomic functions such as arterial pressure, heart rate, glandular secretion in the gastrointestinal tract, gastrointestinal peristalsis, and degree of contraction of the urinary bladder.

Signals from the hypothalamus and even from the cerebrum influence the activities of almost all the brain stem autonomic control centers. For instance, stimulation in appropriate areas mainly of the posterior hypothalamus can activate the medullary cardiovascular control centers strongly enough to increase arterial pressure to more than twice normal. Likewise, other hypothalamic centers control body temperature, increase or decrease salivation and gastrointestinal activity, and cause bladder emptying. To some extent therefore, the autonomic centers in the brain stem act as relay stations for control activities initiated at higher levels of the brain, especially in the hypothalamus.

Pharmacology of the Autonomic Nervous System (p. 739)

Drugs That Act on the Adrenergic Effector Organs— Sympathomimetic Drugs

Drugs that act like norepinephrine and epinephrine at the sympathetic nerve terminal are called *sympathomimetic* or *adrenergic drugs*. There are many drugs in this category and they differ from one another in the degree to which they stimulate the various adrenergic receptors and in their duration of action. Most sympathomimetic drugs have a duration of action of 30 minutes to 2 hours, whereas the action of norepinephrine and epinephrine is only 1 to 2 minutes.

The drug *phenylephrine* specifically stimulates α-receptors. The drug *isoproterenol* stimulates both β_1- and β_2-receptors, and the drug *albuterol* stimulates only β_2-receptors.

Drugs That Release Norepinephrine from Nerve Terminals. Certain drugs have an indirect sympathomimetic action by inducing the release of norepinephrine from storage vesicles in sympathetic nerve endings instead of by directly activating adrenergic receptors.

The drugs *ephedrine, amphetamine,* and *tyramine* belong to this class of compounds.

Drugs That Block Adrenergic Activity. Adrenergic activity can be blocked at several points in the stimulatory process: (1) the synthesis and storage of norepinephrine in sympathetic nerve endings can be blocked by *reserpine;* (2) the release of norepinephrine from sympathetic terminals can be blocked by *guanethidine;* and (3) the adrenergic receptors can be blocked by *phenoxybenzamine* and *phentolamine,* which block α-receptors, or by *propranolol,* which blocks both β_1- and β_2-receptors.

Drugs That Act on Cholinergic Effector Organs

Acetylcholine receptors located on the postganglionic nerve cells of both the sympathetic and parasympathetic nervous systems are the *nicotinic type* of acetylcholine receptor, whereas the acetylcholine receptors located on the parasympathetic effector organs are the *muscarinic type* of acetylcholine receptor. Drugs that act like acetylcholine at the effector organs are therefore called *parasympathomimetic* or *muscarinic* drugs. *Pilocarpine* acts directly on the muscarinic type of cholinergic receptor. The muscarinic action of the drug also stimulates the cholinergic sympathetic fibers that innervate sweat glands, resulting in profuse sweating.

Drugs That Prolong the Activity of Acetylcholine. Some drugs do not have a direct effect on the cholinergic receptors but, rather, prolong the action of acetylcholine by blocking *acetylcholinesterase;* examples of these drugs are *neostigmine, pyridostigmine,* and *ambenonium.*

Drugs That Block Cholinergic Activity. Drugs that block the effect of acetylcholine on the muscarinic type of cholinergic receptors are called *antimuscarinic drugs.* These drugs, which include *atropine, homatropine,* and *scopolamine,* do not affect the nicotinic action of acetylcholine on the postganglionic neurons or skeletal muscle.

Drugs That Stimulate or Block Sympathetic and Parasympathetic Postganglionic Neurons

All postganglionic sympathetic and parasympathetic neurons contain the nicotinic type of acetylcholine receptor. Drugs that stimulate the postganglionic neurons in the same manner as acetylcholine are called *nicotinic drugs.* Nicotine excites both sympathetic and parasympathetic postganglionic neurons at the same

time, which results in a strong sympathetic vasoconstriction and an increase in gastrointestinal activity.

Drugs That Block Impulse Transmission from Preganglionic to Postganglionic Neurons

Drugs that block the effect of acetylcholine to stimulate
the postganglionic neurons in both the sympathetic and
parasympathetic systems simultaneously are called *ganglionic blocking drugs.* The drugs *tetraethyl ammonium,
hexamethonium,* and *pentolinium* are used to block
sympathetic activity but are rarely used to block parasympathetic activity. The effect of sympathetic blockade
far overshadows the effect of parasympathetic blockade
in many tissues. The ganglionic blocking drugs can be
given to reduce arterial pressure in patients with severe
hypertension. These drugs have several side effects,
however, and are difficult to control, which limits
their use.

CHAPTER 61

Cerebral Blood Flow, Cerebrospinal Fluid, and Brain Metabolism

Functioning of the brain is closely tied to the level of cerebral blood flow. Total cessation of blood flow to the brain causes unconsciousness within 5 to 10 seconds because of the decrease in oxygen delivery and the resultant cessation of metabolic activity.

Cerebral Blood Flow (p. 743)

The normal cerebral blood flow in an adult averages 50 to 65 mL/100 g, or about 750 to 900 mL/min; therefore the brain receives approximately 15% the total resting cardiac output.

Cerebral Blood Flow Is Related to the Level of Metabolism. Three metabolic factors—*carbon dioxide, hydrogen ions, oxygen*—have potent effects on cerebral blood flow. Carbon dioxide combines with water to form carbonic acid, which partially dissociates to form hydrogen ions. The hydrogen ions induce cerebral vasodilation in proportion to their concentration in the cerebral blood. Any substance that increases the acidity of the brain, and therefore the hydrogen ion concentration, increases cerebral blood flow; such substances include lactic acid, pyruvic acid, and other acidic compounds that are formed during the course of metabolism. A decrease in cerebral tissue P_{O_2} causes an immediate increase in cerebral blood flow owing to local vasodilation of the cerebral blood vessels.

Measurements of local cerebral blood flow indicate that blood flow in individual segments of the brain changes within seconds in response to local neuronal activity. The act of making a fist with the hand causes an immediate increase in blood flow in the motor cortex of the opposite cerebral hemisphere. The act of reading increases blood flow in the occipital cortex and in the language perception area of the temporal cortex. *Astrocytes* (also called *astroglial cells*), specialized star-shaped nonneuronal cells that support and protect neurons, appear to help couple neuronal activity with local blood flow regulation by releasing vasoactive metabolites in response to stimulation of adjacent neurons.

Cerebral Blood Flow Autoregulation Protects the Brain from Changes in Arterial Pressure. Cerebral blood flow is nearly constant between the limits of 60 and 140 mm Hg mean arterial pressure. Arterial pressure therefore can fall to as low as 60 mm Hg or rise to as high as 140 mm Hg without significant changes occurring in cerebral blood flow. When the arterial pressure falls below 60 mm Hg, cerebral blood flow is usually compromised. If the arterial pressure rises above the limit of autoregulation, blood flow rises rapidly and overstretching or rupture of the cerebral blood vessels can result in brain edema or cerebral hemorrhage.

The Sympathetic Nervous System Has a Role in Regulation of Cerebral Blood Flow. The cerebral circulation has dense sympathetic innervation; under certain conditions, sympathetic stimulation can cause marked constriction of the cerebral arteries. During strenuous exercise or states of enhanced circulatory activity, sympathetic impulses can constrict the large and intermediate-sized arteries and prevent the high pressure from reaching small blood vessels. This mechanism is important for preventing vascular hemorrhage. Under many conditions in which the sympathetic nervous system is moderately activated, however, cerebral blood flow is maintained relatively constant by autoregulatory mechanisms.

Cerebral Microcirculation

The density of capillaries is four times greater in the gray matter of the brain than that in the white matter. The level of blood flow to the gray matter is therefore four times as great as that to the white matter, matching the much higher metabolic needs of gray matter. The brain capillaries are much less "leaky" than capillaries in other portions of the body. Capillaries in the brain are surrounded by "glial feet," which provide physical support to prevent overstretching of the capillaries in the event of exposure to high pressure.

Cerebral "Stroke" Occurs when Cerebral Blood Vessels Are Blocked or Ruptured. Most strokes are caused by arteriosclerotic plaques that occur in one or more of the large arteries of the brain. Plaque material can trigger the clot mechanism, which may result in clot formation, artery blockage, and subsequent loss of function in the brain areas supplied by the vessel. In about one fourth of persons who develop strokes, the cerebral blood vessels rupture as a result of high blood pressure. The resulting hemorrhage compresses the brain tissue, leading to local ischemia and edema.

The neurological effects of a stroke are determined by which brain area is affected. If the middle cerebral artery in the dominant hemisphere is involved, the person is likely to become almost totally debilitated owing to loss of Wernicke's area, which is involved in speech comprehension. In addition, these individuals often become unable to speak because of damage to Broca's motor area for word formation, and loss of other motor control areas of the dominant hemisphere can create spastic paralysis of the muscles of the opposite side of the body.

Cerebrospinal Fluid (CSF) System *(p. 746)*

The entire cavity enclosing the brain and spinal cord has a volume of approximately 1650 mL; about 150 mL of this volume is occupied by CSF, and the remainder is occupied by the brain and spinal cord. This fluid, as shown in Figure 61–1, is found in the *ventricles of the brain,* the *cisterns around the brain,* and the *subarachnoid space* around both the brain and the spinal cord. These chambers are interconnected, and the pressure of the CSF is regulated at a constant level.

CSF Cushions the Brain. The brain and the CSF have about the same specific gravity. The brain therefore essentially floats in the CSF. A blow to the head moves the entire brain simultaneously with the skull, causing no single portion of the brain to be momentarily contorted.

Formation and Absorption of CSF

About 500 mL of CSF is formed each day. Most of this fluid originates from the choroid plexuses of the four ventricles. Additional amounts of fluid are secreted by the ependymal surfaces of the ventricles and the arachnoidal membranes. The choroid plexus is a cauliflower-like growth of blood vessels covered by a thin layer of epithelial cells. This structure projects into the temporal horn of each lateral ventricle, the posterior portion of the third ventricle, and the roof of the fourth ventricle.

The CSF is absorbed by multiple arachnoidal villi that project into the large sagittal venous sinus as well as into other venous sinuses of the cerebrum. The CSF empties into the venous blood through the surfaces of these villi.

The Perivascular Space Functions as a Lymphatic System for the Brain. As the blood vessels that supply the brain penetrate inward, they carry with them a layer of *pia matter.* The pia is only loosely adherent to the vessels, and this creates a space between the pia and the vessels called the *perivascular space.* The perivascular

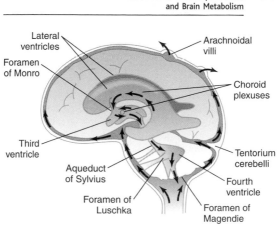

Figure 61–1. Arrows show the pathway of cerebrospinal fluid flow from the choroid plexuses in the lateral ventricles to the arachnoidal villi protruding into the dural sinuses.

space follows both the arteries and veins into the brain as far as the arterioles and venules but not to the level of the capillaries.

Protein that leaks into the interstitial spaces of the brain flows through the perivascular spaces into the subarachnoid space. On reaching the subarachnoid space, the protein flows with the CSF and is absorbed through the arachnoidal villi into the cerebral veins.

CSF Pressure

CSF is formed at a nearly constant rate; therefore, the rate of absorption of this fluid by the arachnoidal villi determines both the quantity of fluid present in the ventricular system and the level of CSF pressure.

The arachnoidal villi function like one-way valves that allow CSF to flow into the blood of the venous sinuses but prevent the flow of blood into the CSF. Normally, the valvelike action of the villi allows CSF to flow into the venous sinuses when the pressure in the fluid is approximately 1.5 mm Hg greater than the pressure of the blood in the venous sinuses. When the villi become blocked by large particulate matter or fibrosis, CSF pressure can rise dramatically.

The normal CSF pressure is 10 mm Hg. Brain tumors, hemorrhage, or infective processes can disrupt the absorptive capacity of the arachnoidal villi and cause CSF pressure to increase to levels three to four times normal.

Obstruction to the Flow of CSF Causes *Hydrocephalus.* This condition is often defined as *communicating hydrocephalus* or *noncommunicating hydrocephalus.* With communicating hydrocephalus fluid flows readily from the ventricular system into the subarachnoid space, whereas with noncommunicating hydrocephalus the flow of fluid out of one or more of the ventricles is blocked.

The communicating type of hydrocephalus is usually caused by blockage of fluid flow into the subarachnoid space around the basal regions of the brain or blockage of the arachnoidal villi themselves. The noncommunicating type of hydrocephalus is usually caused by blockade of the *aqueduct of Sylvius* as a result of a congenital defect or brain tumor. The continual formation of CSF by the choroid plexuses in the two lateral ventricles and the third ventricle causes the volume of these ventricles to increase greatly. This flattens the brain into a thin shell against the skull. In neonates, the increased pressure also causes the entire head to swell because the skull bones have not yet fused.

Blood-CSF and Blood-Brain Barriers *(p. 748)*

The constituents of the CSF are not exactly the same as those of the extracellular fluid elsewhere in the body. Furthermore, many large molecular substances do not pass from the blood into the CSF or into the interstitial fluids of the brain. Barriers called the *blood-CSF barrier* and the *blood-brain barrier* exist between the blood and the CSF and brain fluid. These barriers are highly permeable to water, carbon dioxide, oxygen, most lipid-soluble substances such as alcohol, and most anesthetics; they are slightly permeable to electrolytes such as sodium, chloride, and potassium; and they are almost totally impermeable to plasma proteins and most non–lipid-soluble large organic molecules.

The cause of the low permeability of these barriers is the manner in which the endothelial cells of the capillaries are joined to one another. The membranes of the adjacent endothelial cells are tightly fused with one another rather than having extensive slit pores between them, as is the case with most other capillaries of the body. These barriers often make it impossible to achieve effective concentrations of therapeutic drugs, such as protein antibodies and non–lipid-soluble compounds in the CSF or parenchyma of the brain.

In some areas of the hypothalamus, pineal gland, and area postrema, substances diffuse with greater ease into the tissue spaces. The ease of diffusion in these areas is important because they have sensory receptors that respond to specific changes in the body fluids, such as changes in osmolality and in glucose concentration, as well as receptors for peptide hormones that regulate thirst, such as angiotensin II.

Brain Edema *(p. 749)*

One of the most serious complications of abnormal cerebral hemodynamics and fluid dynamics is the development of brain edema. Because the brain is encased in a solid vault, accumulation of edema fluid compresses the blood vessels, resulting in decreased blood flow and destruction of brain tissue. Brain edema can be caused by greatly increased capillary pressure or by a concussion in which the brain's tissues and capillaries are traumatized and capillary fluid leaks into this tissue.

Once brain edema begins, it sometimes initiates a vicious circle. The edema fluid compresses the vasculature, which in turn decreases the blood flow and causes brain ischemia. The ischemia causes arteriolar dilation with further increases in capillary pressure. The higher capillary pressure causes more edema fluid, and the edema becomes progressively worse. The reduced blood flow also decreases oxygen delivery, which increases the permeability of the capillaries, allowing more fluid leakage. Decreased oxygen delivery depresses brain metabolism, which turns off the sodium pumps of the brain cells, causing them to swell.

Once this process has begun, heroic measures must be taken to prevent total destruction of the brain. One measure is to administer an intravenous infusion of a concentrated osmotic substance such as mannitol. This pulls fluid from the brain tissue through osmosis and breaks the vicious circle. Another procedure is to remove fluid quickly from the lateral ventricles of the brain through ventricular puncture, thereby relieving intracerebral pressure.

Brain Metabolism *(p. 749)*

Under resting conditions, the metabolism of the brain accounts for 15% of the total metabolism of the body even though the mass of the brain is only 2% of the total body mass. Under resting conditions therefore brain metabolism is about 7.5 times the average metabolism of the rest of the body.

The Brain Has Limited Anaerobic Capability. Most tissues of the body can go without oxygen for several minutes. During this time, the cells obtain their energy through anaerobic metabolism. Because of the high metabolic rate of the brain, anaerobic breakdown of glycogen cannot supply the energy needed to sustain neuronal activity. Most neuronal activity therefore depends on the second-by-second delivery of glucose and oxygen from the blood.

Under Normal Conditions, Most Brain Energy Is Supplied by Glucose Derived from the Blood. A special feature of glucose delivery to the neurons is that its transport through the cell membranes of the neurons does not depend on insulin. Even in patients who have serious diabetes glucose diffuses readily into the neurons. When a diabetic patient is overtreated with insulin, the blood glucose concentration can fall to an extremely low level because the excess insulin causes almost all of the glucose in the blood to be transported rapidly into the insulin-sensitive, nonneural cells throughout the body. When this happens, insufficient glucose is left in the blood to supply the neurons, and mental function can become seriously impaired, leading to mental imbalance, psychotic disturbances, and sometimes coma.

Gastrointestinal Physiology

General Principles of Gastrointestinal Function—Motility, Nervous Control, and Blood Circulation

The alimentary tract provides the body with a continual supply of water, electrolytes, vitamins, and nutrients. This requires (1) movement of food through the alimentary tract; (2) secretion of digestive juices and digestion of food; (3) absorption of digestive products, water, electrolytes, and vitamins; (4) circulation of blood to carry away absorbed substances; and (5) nervous and hormonal control of all these functions. The basic principles of function in the entire alimentary tract are discussed in this chapter.

General Principles of Gastrointestinal Motility (p. 753)

Characteristics of the Gastrointestinal Wall

The Motor Functions of the Gut Are Performed by Layers of Smooth Muscle. The intestinal wall is composed of the following layers (from the outer surface inward): (1) *serosa,* (2) *longitudinal smooth muscle layer,* (3) *circular smooth muscle layer,* (4) *submucosa,* and (5) *mucosa.* In addition, a sparse layer of smooth muscle fibers, the muscularis mucosae, lies in the deeper layers of the mucosa.

The Gastrointestinal Smooth Muscle Functions as a Syncytium. The smooth muscle fibers in the longitudinal and circular muscle layers are electrically connected through gap junctions that allow ions to move from one cell to the next. Each muscle layer functions as a syncytium; when an action potential is elicited in the muscle mass, it generally travels in all directions in the muscle. The distance it travels depends on the excitability of the muscle.

Electrical Activity of Gastrointestinal Smooth Muscle (p. 754)

The Rhythm of Most Gastrointestinal Contractions Is Determined by the Frequency of Slow Waves in the Smooth Muscle Membrane Potential. These waves are not action potentials; instead, they are slow, undulating changes in the resting membrane potential. The cause of slow waves is poorly understood, but they may result from slow undulation of the activity of the sodium-potassium pump or rhythmical changes in sodium permeability.

Spike Potentials Are True Action Potentials That Cause Muscle Contraction. They occur when the resting membrane potential becomes more positive than about −40 millivolts (normal resting membrane potential is between −50 and −60 millivolts). The channels responsible for the action potentials allow particularly large numbers of calcium ions to enter along with smaller numbers of sodium ions; they therefore are called *calcium-sodium channels.*

The Basic Level of Resting Membrane Potential of Gastrointestinal Smooth Muscle Can Be Increased or Decreased. The resting membrane potential normally averages about −56 millivolts.

- *Factors that depolarize the membrane* include (1) stretching the muscle, (2) stimulation by acetylcholine, (3) stimulation by parasympathetic nerves that secrete acetylcholine at their endings, and (4) stimulation by gastrointestinal hormones.

- *Factors that hyperpolarize the membrane* include (1) the effect of norepinephrine or epinephrine on the muscle membrane and (2) stimulation of the sympathetic nerves that secrete norepinephrine at their endings.

Neural Control of Gastrointestinal Function: Enteric Nervous System *(p. 755)*

The Gastrointestinal Tract Has Its Own Nervous System, Called the Enteric Nervous System. It lies entirely in the wall of the gut, beginning in the esophagus and extending all the way to the anus. The enteric system is composed mainly of two plexuses:

- The *myenteric plexus,* or *Auerbach's plexus,* is an outer plexus located between the muscle layers. Stimulation causes (1) increased "tone" of the gut wall, (2) increased intensity of rhythmical contractions, (3) increased rate of contraction, and (4) increased velocity of conduction. The myenteric plexus is also useful for inhibiting the pyloric sphincter (which controls emptying of the stomach), the sphincter of the ileocecal valve (which controls emptying of the small intestine into the cecum), and the lower esophageal sphincter (which allows food to enter the stomach).

- The *submucosal plexus,* or *Meissner's plexus,* is an inner plexus that lies in the submucosa. In contrast to the myenteric plexus, it is mainly concerned with controlling function in the inner wall of each minute segment of the intestine. For instance, many sensory signals originate from the gastrointestinal epithelium and are integrated in the submucosal plexus to help control local intestinal secretion, local absorption, and local contraction of the submucosal muscle.

Autonomic Control of the Gastrointestinal Tract (p. 756)

The Parasympathetic Nerves Increase the Activity of the Enteric Nervous System. This in turn enhances the activity of most gastrointestinal functions. The parasympathetic supply to the gut is made up of cranial and sacral divisions:

- The *cranial parasympathetics* innervate, by way of the vagus nerves, the esophagus, stomach, small intestine, pancreas, and first half of the large intestine.
- The *sacral parasympathetics* innervate, by way of the pelvic nerves, the distal half of the large intestine. The sigmoidal, rectal, and anal regions have an especially rich supply of parasympathetic fibers that function in the defecation reflexes.

The Sympathetic Nervous System Usually Inhibits Activity in the Gastrointestinal Tract, Causing Many Effects Opposite to Those of the Parasympathetic System. The sympathetics innervate all portions of the gastrointestinal tract rather than being more extensively supplied to the portions nearest the oral cavity and anus, as is true of the parasympathetics. The sympathetic nerve endings secrete norepinephrine, which exerts its effects in two ways: (1) to a slight extent by a direct action that inhibits smooth muscle, and (2) to a major extent by an inhibitory effect on the neurons of the enteric nervous system.

Gastrointestinal Reflexes (p. 757)

Three Types of Reflexes Are Essential for Gastrointestinal Control

- *Reflexes that occur entirely within the enteric nervous system* control gastrointestinal secretion, peristalsis, mixing contractions, local inhibitory effects, and so forth.

- *Reflexes from the gut to the sympathetic ganglia and then back to the gut* transmit signals for long distances: Signals from the stomach cause evacuation of the colon *(gastrocolic reflex)*; signals from the colon and small intestine inhibit stomach motility and stomach secretion *(enterogastric reflexes)*; and reflexes from the colon inhibit emptying of ileal contents into the colon *(coloileal reflex)*.

- *Reflexes from the gut to the spinal cord or brain stem and then back to the gut* include, in particular: (1) reflexes from the stomach and duodenum to the brain stem and back to the stomach—by way of the vagus nerves—that control gastric motor and secretory activity; (2) pain reflexes that cause general inhibition of the entire gastrointestinal tract; and (3) defecation reflexes that travel to the spinal cord and back again to produce the powerful colonic, rectal, and abdominal contractions required for defecation.

Gastrointestinal Hormones

The Five Major Gastrointestinal Hormones Are Secretin, Gastrin, Cholecystokinin, Gastric Inhibitory Peptide, and Motilin. The gastrointestinal hormones are released into the portal circulation and exert physiological actions on target cells with specific receptors for the hormone. The effects of the hormones persist even after all nervous connections between the site of release and the site of action have been severed. Table 62–1 outlines the actions of each gastrointestinal hormone as well as the stimulus for secretion and site at which secretion takes place.

Functional Movements in the Gastrointestinal Tract *(p. 759)*

Two types of movement occur in the gastrointestinal tract: *propulsive movements* and *mixing movements.*

Peristalsis Is the Basic Propulsive Movement of the Gastrointestinal Tract. Distention of the intestinal tract causes a contractile ring to appear around the gut, which moves analward a few centimeters before ending. At the same time, the gut sometimes relaxes several centimeters down toward the anus, which is called *receptive relaxation,* allowing the food to be propelled more easily toward the anus. This complex pattern does not occur in the absence of the myenteric plexus; therefore the complex is called the *myenteric*

Table 62–1. Gastrointestinal Hormone Actions, Stimuli for Secretion, and Site of Secretion

Hormone	Stimuli for Secretion	Site of Secretion	Actions
Secretin	Acid Fat	S-cells of the duodenum, jejunum, and ileum	Stimulates pepsin secretion, pancreatic bicarbonate secretion, biliary bicarbonate secretion, growth of exocrine pancreas Inhibits gastric acid secretion
Gastrin	Protein Distention Nerve (Acid inhibits release)	G-cells of the antrum, duodenum, and jejunum	Stimulates gastric acid secretion, mucosal growth
Cholecystokinin	Protein Fat Acid	I-cells of the duodenum, jejunum, and ileum	Stimulates pancreatic enzyme secretion, pancreatic bicarbonate secretion, gallbladder contraction, growth of exocrine pancreas Inhibits gastric emptying
Gastric inhibitory peptide	Protein Fat Carbohydrate	K-cells of the duodenum and jejunum	Stimulates insulin release Inhibits gastric acid secretion
Motilin	Fat Acid Nerve	M-cells of the duodenum and jejunum	Stimulates gastric motility, intestinal motility

reflex, or *peristaltic reflex.* The peristaltic reflex plus the direction of movement toward the anus is called the *law of the gut.*

Peristalsis and Local Constrictive Contractions Cause Mixing in the Alimentary Tract. In some areas, the peristaltic contractions themselves cause most of the mixing. This is especially true when forward progression of the intestinal contents is blocked by a sphincter, so a peristaltic wave can only churn the intestinal contents, rather than propel them forward. At other times, local constrictive contractions called segmental contractions occur every few centimeters in the gut wall. These constrictions usually last for only a few seconds; then new constrictions occur at other points in the gut, mixing the contents of the intestine.

Gastrointestinal Blood Flow: Splanchnic Circulation (p. 759)

The Blood Vessels of the Gastrointestinal Tract Are Part of the Splanchnic Circulation. The splanchnic circulation includes blood flow through the gut itself plus blood flow through the spleen, pancreas, and liver. The blood that courses through the splanchnic circulation flows immediately into the liver by way of the portal vein. In the liver, the blood passes through liver sinusoids and finally leaves the liver by way of hepatic veins.

Gastrointestinal Blood Flow Usually Is Proportional to the Level of Local Activity. For instance, during active absorption of nutrients, blood flow in the villi and adjacent regions of the submucosa is greatly increased. Likewise, blood flow in the muscle layers of the intestinal wall is greater with increased motor activity in the gut. Although the precise cause or causes of increased blood flow during increased gastrointestinal activity are still unclear, some facts are known.

- Vasodilator substances are released from the mucosa during the digestive process. Most of them are peptide hormones, including cholecystokinin, gastrin, and secretin.
- Some of the gastrointestinal glands also release two kinins, kallidin and bradykinin, into the gut wall. These kinins are powerful vasodilators.
- Decreased oxygenation of the gut wall can increase intestinal blood flow by at least 50%; therefore, tissue hypoxia resulting from greater gut activity probably causes much of the vasodilation.

Nervous Control of Gastrointestinal Blood Flow
(p. 762)

Parasympathetic Stimulation Increases Blood Flow. Stimulation of the parasympathetic nerves to the stomach and lower colon increases local blood flow and increases glandular secretion. This greater flow probably results secondarily from the greater glandular activity.

Sympathetic Stimulation Decreases Blood Flow. After a few minutes of sympathetic-induced vasoconstriction, the flow often returns almost to normal by means of *autoregulatory escape:* The local metabolic vasodilator mechanisms that are elicited by ischemia become prepotent over the sympathetic vasoconstriction and therefore redilate the arterioles.

Sympathetic Vasoconstriction Is Important When Other Parts of the Body Need Extra Blood Flow. A major value of sympathetic vasoconstriction in the gut is that it allows the shutting off of gastrointestinal and other splanchnic blood flow for short periods during heavy exercise and during circulatory shock when increased flow is needed elsewhere.

CHAPTER 63

Propulsion and Mixing of Food in the Alimentary Tract

For food to be processed optimally in the alimentary tract, the length of time it remains in each part of the tract is critical, and appropriate mixing must also occur. The purpose of this chapter is to discuss these movements and the mechanisms that control them.

Ingestion of Food *(p. 763)*

The Pharyngeal Stage of Swallowing Is Involuntary and Constitutes the Passage of Food through the Pharynx into the Esophagus. When the food is ready for swallowing, it is voluntarily pushed into the pharynx by the tongue, which constitutes the voluntary stage of swallowing. The bolus of food stimulates swallowing receptors, and impulses from these receptors pass to the brain stem to initiate a series of automatic pharyngeal muscle contractions as follows:

- The soft palate is pulled upward, preventing reflux of food into the nasal cavities.
- The palatopharyngeal folds on either side of the pharynx are pulled medially, forming a sagittal slit that impedes the passage of large objects into the posterior pharynx.
- The vocal cords are strongly approximated, the larynx is pulled upward and anteriorly by the neck muscles, and the epiglottis swings backward over the opening of the larynx. These effects prevent passage of food into the trachea.
- The upper esophageal sphincter relaxes, allowing food to move into the upper esophagus.
- A fast peristaltic wave originating in the pharynx forces the bolus of food into the upper esophagus.

The Esophagus Exhibits Two Types of Peristaltic Movement: Primary Peristalsis and Secondary Peristalsis

- *Primary peristalsis* is a continuation of the peristaltic wave that begins in the pharynx. This wave, mediated by the vagus nerves, passes all the way from the pharynx to the stomach.
- *Secondary peristalsis* results from distention of the esophagus when the primary peristaltic wave fails to move the food into the stomach: it does not require vagal innervation.

The Lower Esophageal Sphincter Relaxes ahead of the Peristaltic Wave. At the lower end of the esophagus, the esophageal circular muscle functions as a lower esophageal sphincter. It remains tonically constricted until a peristaltic swallowing wave passes down the esophagus. The sphincter then relaxes ahead of the peristaltic wave, allowing propulsion of food into the stomach.

Motor Functions of the Stomach (p. 765)

There Are Three Motor Functions of the Stomach

- Storage of food until the food can be processed in the duodenum.
- Mixing of food with gastric secretions until it forms a semifluid mixture called *chyme*.
- Emptying of food into the small intestine at a rate suitable for proper digestion and absorption.

The Stomach Relaxes when Food Enters It. Normally, when food enters the stomach, a "vagovagal reflex" from the stomach to the brain stem and then back to the stomach reduces the tone in the muscular wall of the stomach. The wall can bulge progressively outward, accommodating about 1.5 L in the completely relaxed stomach.

"Retropulsion" Is an Important Mixing Mechanism of the Stomach. Each time a peristaltic wave passes over the antrum toward the pylorus, the pyloric muscle contracts, which further impedes emptying through the pylorus. Most of the antral contents are squirted backward through the peristaltic ring toward the body of the stomach.

The Pyloric Sphincter Is Important for Controlling Stomach Emptying. The pyloric sphincter remains slightly contracted most of the time. The constriction normally prevents passage of food particles until they have become mixed in the chyme to an almost fluid consistency.

Gastric Emptying Is Inhibited by Enterogastric Reflexes from the Duodenum. When food enters the duodenum, multiple nervous reflexes are initiated from its wall that pass back to the stomach and slow or even stop stomach emptying as the volume of chyme in the duodenum becomes too much. Factors that can excite the enterogastric reflexes include the following:

- Degree of distention of the duodenum
- Presence of any degree of irritation of the duodenal mucosa

- Degree of acidity of the duodenal chyme
- Degree of osmolality of the chyme
- Presence of breakdown products of proteins

Cholecystokinin Inhibits Gastric Emptying. Cholecystokinin is released from the mucosa of the duodenum and jejunum in response to fatty substances in the chyme. The contents of the stomach are therefore released very slowly after ingestion of a fatty meal.

Movements of the Small Intestine *(p. 768)*

Distention of the Small Intestine Elicits Mixing Contractions Called *Segmentation Contractions*. These are concentric contractions that have the appearance of a chain of sausages. These segmentation contractions usually "chop" the chyme about two or three times a minute, promoting progressive mixing of the solid food particles with the secretions of the small intestine.

Chyme is Propelled through the Small Intestine by Peristaltic Waves. They move toward the anus at a velocity of 0.5 to 2.0 cm/sec. Movement of chyme along the small intestine averages only 1 cm/min. About 3 to 5 hours are required for passage of chyme from the pylorus to the ileocecal valve.

Peristalsis Is Controlled by Nervous and Hormonal Signals. Peristaltic activity of the small intestine is greatly increased after a meal for the following reasons:

- *Nervous signals.* These are caused in part by the entry of chyme into the duodenum and in part by a so-called *gastroenteric reflex* that is initiated by distention of the stomach and conducted principally through the myenteric plexus along the wall of the small intestine.
- *Hormonal signals.* Gastrin, cholecystokinin, and insulin are released after a meal and can enhance intestinal motility. Secretin and glucagon inhibit small intestinal motility.

The Ileocecal Valve Prevents Backflow of Fecal Contents from the Colon into the Small Intestine. The lips of the ileocecal valve protrude into the lumen of the cecum and are forcefully closed when excess pressure builds up in the cecum and the cecal contents push backward against the lips. The wall of the ileum near the ileocecal valve has a thickened muscular coat called the *ileocecal sphincter*. This sphincter normally remains mildly constricted and slows the emptying of ileal contents into the cecum, except immediately after a meal.

The Ileocecal Sphincter and the Intensity of Peristalsis in the Terminal Ileum Are Controlled by Reflexes from the Cecum. Whenever the cecum is distended, the contraction of the ileocecal sphincter is intensified, and ileal peristalsis is inhibited, which greatly delays emptying of additional chyme from the ileum. Any irritant in the cecum delays emptying. These reflexes from the cecum to the ileocecal sphincter and ileum are mediated by way of the myenteric plexus in the gut wall itself and through extrinsic nerves, especially reflexes by way of the prevertebral sympathetic ganglia.

Movements of the Colon (p. 770)

The principal functions of the colon are (1) absorption of water and electrolytes from chyme and (2) storage of fecal matter until it can be expelled. The proximal half of the colon is concerned principally with absorption, and the distal half is concerned with storage.

Contraction of Circular and Longitudinal Muscles in the Large Intestine Causes Haustrations to Develop. These combined contractions cause the unstimulated portion of the large intestine to bulge outward into bag-like sacs called *haustrations.* The haustral contractions perform two main functions:

- *Propulsion.* Haustral contractions at times move slowly toward the anus during their period of contraction and thereby provide forward propulsion of the colonic contents.
- *Mixing.* Haustral contractions dig into and roll over the fecal material in the large intestine. In this way, all the fecal material is gradually exposed to the surface of the large intestine, and fluid and dissolved substances are progressively absorbed.

Mass Movements Are Important for Propelling the Fecal Contents through the Large Intestine. A mass movement is characterized by the following sequence of events: A constrictive ring occurs at a distended or irritated point in the colon, and then the colon distal to the constriction contracts as a unit, forcing the fecal material in this segment en masse through the colon. When a mass of feces has been forced into the rectum, the desire for defecation is felt.

The Appearance of Mass Movements after Meals Is Facilitated by Gastrocolic and Duodenocolic Reflexes. These reflexes result from distention of the stomach and duodenum. The reflexes are conducted through the extrinsic nerves of the autonomic nervous system. Mass movements can also be initiated by intense stimulation of the parasympathetic nervous system or by overdistention of a segment of the colon.

Defecation Can Be Initiated by an Intrinsic Reflex Mediated by the Local Enteric Nervous System. When feces enter the rectum, distention of the rectal wall initiates afferent signals that spread through the myenteric plexus to initiate peristaltic waves in the descending colon, sigmoid, and rectum, forcing feces toward the anus. As the peristaltic wave approaches the anus, the internal anal sphincter is relaxed by inhibitory signals from the myenteric plexus; if the external anal sphincter is consciously relaxed at the same time, defecation occurs.

The Intrinsic Defecation Reflex Functioning by Itself Is Relatively Weak. To be effective in causing defecation, the reflex usually must be fortified by a parasympathetic defecation reflex that involves the sacral segments of the spinal cord. Parasympathetic signals greatly intensify the peristaltic waves, relax the internal anal sphincter, and thus convert the intrinsic defecation reflex from a weak movement into a powerful process of defecation.

CHAPTER 64

Secretory Functions of the Alimentary Tract

Secretory glands serve two primary functions in the alimentary tract: (1) digestive enzymes are secreted in most areas and (2) mucous glands provide mucus for lubrication and protection of all parts of the alimentary tract. The purpose of this chapter is to describe the alimentary secretions and their functions as well as the regulation of their production.

General Principles of Alimentary Tract Secretion (p. 773)

Contact of Food with the Epithelium Stimulates Secretion. Direct mechanical stimulation of glandular cells by food causes the local glands to secrete digestive juices. In addition, epithelial stimulation activates the enteric nervous system of the gut wall. The stimuli that accomplish this are (1) tactile stimulation, (2) chemical irritation, and (3) gut wall distention.

Parasympathetic Stimulation Increases the Rate of Glandular Secretion. This is true of salivary glands, esophageal glands, gastric glands, the pancreas, Brunner's glands in the duodenum, and the glands in the distal portion of the large intestine. Secretion in the remainder of the small intestine and in the first two thirds of the large intestine occurs mainly in response to local neural and hormonal stimuli.

Sympathetic Stimulation Can Have a Dual Effect on Glandular Secretion. Sympathetic stimulation may increase or decrease glandular secretion, depending on the existing secretory activity of the gland. This dual effect can be explained as follows:

- Sympathetic stimulation alone usually slightly increases secretion.
- If secretion has already increased, superimposed sympathetic stimulation usually reduces the secretion because it reduces blood flow to the gland.

Secretion of Saliva (p. 775)

Saliva Contains a Serous Secretion and a Mucous Secretion

- The *serous secretion* contains ptyalin (an α-amylase), which is an enzyme for digesting starches.

- The *mucous secretion* contains mucin for lubrication and for surface protection.

Saliva Contains High Concentrations of Potassium and Bicarbonate Ions and Low Concentrations of Sodium and Chloride Ions. Salivary secretion is a two-stage operation: The primary secretion from the acini contains ptyalin and/or mucin in a solution with an ionic composition similar to that of extracellular fluid. The primary secretion is then modified in the ducts, as follows:

- Sodium ions are actively reabsorbed and potassium ions are actively secreted into the ducts. An excess of sodium reabsorption creates a negative charge in the salivary ducts, causing chloride ions to be reabsorbed passively.
- Bicarbonate ions are secreted into the ducts caused in part by exchange of bicarbonate for chloride ions but also by an active secretory process.

Salivation Is Controlled Mainly by Parasympathetic Nervous Signals. The salivatory nuclei in the brain stem are excited by taste and tactile stimuli from the tongue, mouth, and pharynx. Salivation can also be affected by higher centers of the brain (e.g., salivation increases when a person smells favorite foods).

Gastric Secretion (p. 777)

The Stomach Mucosa Has Two Important Types of Tubular Gland

- The *oxyntic (acid-forming) glands* are located in the body and fundus. They contain three types of cells: *mucous neck cells,* which secrete mainly mucus but also some pepsinogen; *peptic (chief) cells,* which secrete pepsinogen; and *parietal (oxyntic) cells,* which secrete hydrochloric acid and intrinsic factor.
- The *pyloric glands,* which are located in the antrum, secrete mainly mucus for protection of the pyloric mucosa but also some pepsinogen and, importantly, the hormone gastrin.

Gastric Acid Is Secreted by Parietal Cells. When these cells secrete their acidic juice, the membranes of the canaliculi empty their secretion directly into the lumen of the oxyntic gland. The final secretion entering the canaliculus contains concentrated hydrochloric acid (155 mEq/L), potassium chloride (15 mEq/L), and small amounts of sodium chloride.

Hydrochloric Acid Is as Necessary as Pepsin for Protein Digestion in the Stomach. The pepsinogens have no digestive activity when they are first secreted; however, as soon as they come into contact with hydrochloric acid and especially when they come into contact with previously formed pepsin plus the hydrochloric acid, they are changed to form active pepsin.

Parietal Cells Also Secrete "Intrinsic Factor." Intrinsic factor is essential for absorption of vitamin B_{12} in the ileum. When the acid-producing cells of the stomach are destroyed, which often occurs with chronic gastritis, the person develops not only achlorhydria but often also pernicious anemia owing to failure of the red blood cells to mature.

Basic Factors That Stimulate Gastric Secretion Are Acetylcholine, Gastrin, and Histamine. Acetylcholine excites secretion of pepsinogen by peptic cells, hydrochloric acid by parietal cells, and mucus by mucous cells. In comparison, both gastrin and histamine strongly stimulate secretion of acid by parietal cells but have little effect on the other cells.

Acid Secretion Is Stimulated by Gastrin. Nerve signals from the vagus nerves and local enteric reflexes cause gastrin cells (G-cells) in the antral mucosa to secrete gastrin. Gastrin is carried by blood to the oxyntic glands, where it strongly stimulates parietal cells and peptic cells to a lesser extent.

Histamine Stimulates Acid Secretion by Parietal Cells. Whenever acetylcholine and gastrin stimulate the parietal cells at the same time, histamine can enhance acid secretion. Thus histamine is a cofactor for stimulating acid secretion.

Pepsinogen Secretion Is Stimulated by Acetylcholine and Gastric Acid. Acetylcholine is released from vagus nerves or other enteric nerves. Gastric acid probably does not stimulate peptic cells directly but elicits additional enteric reflexes. When the ability to secrete normal amounts of acid is lost, the pepsinogen level is low even though the peptic cells are normal.

Gastric Secretion Is Inhibited by Excess Acid in the Stomach. When the pH of gastric juice falls below 3.0, gastrin secretion is decreased for two reasons: (1) the high acidity stimulates the release of somatostatin from delta cells, which in turn depresses gastrin secretion by the G-cells, and (2) the acid causes an inhibitory nervous reflex that inhibits gastric secretion. This mechanism protects the stomach.

There Are Three Phases of Gastric Secretion

- The *cephalic phase* accounts for 30% of the response to a meal and is initiated by the anticipation of eating and the odor and taste of food. It is mediated entirely by the vagus nerve.
- The *gastric phase* accounts for 60% of the acid response to a meal. It is initiated by distention of the stomach, which leads to nervous stimulation of gastric secretion. In addition, partial digestion products of proteins in the stomach cause *gastrin* to be released from the antral mucosa. The gastrin then causes secretion of a highly acidic gastric juice.
- The *intestinal phase* (10% of the response) is initiated by nervous stimuli associated with distention of the small intestine. The presence of digestion products of proteins in the small intestine can also stimulate gastric secretion via a humoral mechanism.

Chyme in the Small Intestine Inhibits Secretion During the Gastric Phase. This inhibition results from at least two influences:

- *Enterogastric reflex.* The presence of food in the small intestine initiates this reflex, which is transmitted through the enteric nervous system and through the extrinsic sympathetic and vagus nerves; it inhibits stomach secretion. The reflex can be initiated by distention of the small bowel, the presence of acid in the upper intestine, the presence of protein breakdown products, or irritation of the mucosa.
- *Hormones.* The presence of chyme in the upper small intestine causes the release of several intestinal hormones. Secretin and gastric inhibitory peptide are especially important for inhibition of gastric secretion.

Pancreatic Secretion (p. 780)

Digestive Enzymes Are Secreted by the Pancreatic Acini

- The more important enzymes for digestion of proteins are trypsin, chymotrypsin, and carboxypolypeptidase, which are secreted in the inactive forms trypsinogen, chymotrypsinogen, and procarboxypolypeptidase.
- The pancreatic digestive enzyme for carbohydrates is pancreatic amylase, which hydrolyzes starches, glycogen, and most other carbohydrates (except cellulose) to form disaccharides and a few trisaccharides.

- The main enzyme for fat digestion is pancreatic lipase, which hydrolyzes triglycerides into fatty acids and monoglycerides; cholesterol esterase, which causes hydrolysis of cholesterol esters; and phospholipase, which splits fatty acids from phospholipids.

Bicarbonate Ions and Water Are Secreted by Epithelial Cells of the Ductules and Ducts. Bicarbonate ion in the pancreatic juice serves to neutralize acid emptied into the duodenum from the stomach.

Pancreatic Secretion Is Stimulated by Acetylcholine, Cholecystokinin, and Secretin

- *Acetylcholine*, which is released from nerve endings, mainly stimulates secretion of digestive enzymes.
- *Cholecystokinin*, which is secreted mainly by the duodenal and jejunal mucosae, mainly stimulates secretion of digestive enzymes.
- *Secretin*, which is secreted by the duodenal and jejunal mucosae when highly acidic food enters the small intestine, mainly stimulates secretion of sodium bicarbonate.

Pancreatic Secretion Occurs in Three Phases

- *Cephalic phase*. The nervous signals that cause gastric secretion also cause acetylcholine release by vagal nerve endings in the pancreas; this accounts for about 20% of the pancreatic enzymes after a meal.
- *Gastric phase*. The nervous stimulation of enzyme secretion continues, accounting for another 5% to 10% of the enzymes secreted after a meal.
- *Intestinal phase*. After chyme enters the small intestine, pancreatic secretion becomes copious, mainly in response to the hormone secretion. In addition, cholecystokinin causes still much more increase in the secretion of enzymes.

Secretin Stimulates Secretion of Bicarbonate, Which Neutralizes Acidic Chyme. When acid chyme enters the duodenum from the stomach, the hydrochloric acid causes the release of prosecretin and activation to secretin, which is subsequently absorbed into the blood. Secretin in turn causes the pancreas to secrete large quantities of fluid that contain a high concentration of bicarbonate ion.

Cholecystokinin Stimulates Enzyme Secretion by the Pancreas. The presence of food in the upper small intestine also causes cholecystokinin to be released from cells called I-cells in the mucosa of the duodenum, jejunum, and upper ileum. This effect results in particular from the presence of proteases and peptones (which are products of partial protein digestion) and of long-chain fatty acids; hydrochloric acid from the stomach juices also causes cholecystokinin release in smaller quantities.

Secretion of Bile by the Liver; Functions of the Biliary Tree *(p. 783)*

Bile Is Important for (1) Fat Digestion and Absorption and (2) Waste Product Removal from the Blood

- *Fat digestion and absorption.* Bile salts help emulsify the large fat particles into minute particles that can be attacked by the lipase enzyme secreted in pancreatic juice. They also aid in the transport and absorption of the digested fat end products to and through the intestinal mucosal membrane.
- *Waste product removal.* Bile serves as a means for excretion of several important waste products from the blood, especially bilirubin, an end product of hemoglobin destruction, and excess cholesterol synthesized by the liver cells.

Bile Is Secreted in Two Stages by the Liver

- The initial portion, which is secreted by liver hepatocytes, contains large amounts of bile acids, cholesterols, and other organic constituents. It is secreted into the minute bile canaliculi that lie between the hepatic cells in the hepatic plates.
- A watery solution of sodium and bicarbonate ions is added to the bile as it flows through the bile ducts. This second secretion is stimulated by secretin, causing increased quantities of bicarbonate ions that supplement pancreatic secretions for neutralizing gastric acid.

Bile Is Concentrated in the Gallbladder. Active transport of sodium through the gallbladder epithelium is followed by secondary absorption of chloride ions, water, and most other soluble constituents. Bile is normally concentrated about fivefold in this way.

Cholecystokinin Stimulates Contraction of the Gallbladder. Fatty foods that enter the duodenum cause cholecystokinin to be released from the local I-cells. Cholecystokinin causes rhythmical contractions of the gallbladder and simultaneous relaxation of the *sphincter of Oddi*, which guards the exit of the common bile duct into the duodenum.

Secretions of the Small Intestine (p. 786)

Brunner's Glands Secrete Alkaline Mucus in the Small Intestine. Secretion of mucus is stimulated by the following:

• Tactile stimuli or irritating stimuli of the overlying mucosa
• Vagal stimulation, which causes secretion concurrently with an increase in stomach secretion
• Gastrointestinal hormones, especially secretin

Mucus Protects the Duodenal Wall from Digestion by Gastric Juice. Brunner's glands respond rapidly and intensely to irritating stimuli. In addition, secretin-stimulated secretion by the glands contains a large excess of bicarbonate ions, which add to the bicarbonate ions from pancreatic secretion and liver bile in neutralizing acid that enters the duodenum.

Intestinal Digestive Juices Are Secreted by the Crypts of Lieberkühn. The crypts of Lieberkühn lie between the intestinal villi, and the intestinal surfaces of both crypts and villi are covered by an epithelium composed of two cell types.

• *Goblet cells* secrete mucus, which provides its usual functions of lubrication and protection of the intestinal mucosa.
• *Enterocytes* secrete large quantities of water and electrolytes in the crypts. They also reabsorb the water and electrolytes along with the end products of digestion over the surfaces of the villi.

Secretions of the Large Intestine (p. 787)

Most of the Secretion in the Large Intestine Is Mucus. The mucus protects the large intestine wall against excoriation, provides the adherent medium for fecal matter, protects the intestinal wall from bacterial activity, and provides a barrier to keep acids from attacking the intestinal wall.

CHAPTER 65

Digestion and Absorption in the Gastrointestinal Tract

The primary foods on which the body lives can be classified as *carbohydrates*, *fats*, and *proteins*. This chapter discusses (1) the digestion of carbohydrates, fats, and proteins and (2) the mechanisms by which the end products of digestion as well as water, electrolytes, and other substances are absorbed.

Digestion of Various Foods by Hydrolysis

Digestion of Carbohydrates (p. 789)

The Digestion of Carbohydrates Begins in the Mouth and Stomach. Saliva contains the enzyme ptyalin (an α-amylase), which hydrolyzes starch into maltose and other small polymers of glucose. Less than 5% of the starch content of a meal is hydrolyzed before swallowing. However, digestion can continue in the stomach for about 1 hour before the activity of salivary amylase is blocked by gastric acid. Nevertheless, α-amylase hydrolyzes as much as 30% to 40% of the starches to maltose.

Pancreatic Secretion, Like Saliva, Contains a Large Quantity of α-Amylase. The function of pancreatic α-amylase is almost identical to that of the α-amylase in saliva but is several times as powerful; therefore, soon after chyme empties into the duodenum and mixes with pancreatic juice, virtually all the starches are digested.

Disaccharides and Small Glucose Polymers Are Hydrolyzed to Monosaccharides by Intestinal Epithelial Enzymes. The microvilli brush border contains enzymes that split the disaccharides lactose, sucrose, and maltose as well as small glucose polymers into their constituent monosaccharides. Glucose usually represents more than 80% of the final products of carbohydrate digestion.

- *Lactose* splits into a molecule of *galactose* and a molecule of glucose.
- *Sucrose* splits into a molecule of *fructose* and a molecule of glucose.
- *Maltose* and the other small glucose polymers all split into molecules of *glucose*.

Digestion of Proteins (p. 790)

Protein Digestion Begins in the Stomach. The ability of pepsin to digest collagen is especially important because the collagen fibers must be digested for enzymes to penetrate meats and digest cellular proteins.

Most Protein Digestion Results from Actions of Pancreatic Proteolytic Enzymes. Proteins leaving the stomach in the form of proteoses, peptones, and large polypeptides are digested into dipeptides, tripeptides, and some larger peptides by proteolytic pancreatic enzymes; only a small percentage of proteins are digested by pancreatic juices to form amino acids.

- *Trypsin and chymotrypsin* split protein molecules into small polypeptides.
- *Carboxypolypeptidase* cleaves amino acids from the carboxyl ends of the polypeptides.
- *Proelastase* gives rise to elastase, which in turn digests the elastin fibers that hold meat together.

Amino Acids Represent More Than 99% of Protein Digestive Products. The last digestion of proteins in the intestinal lumen is achieved by enterocytes that line the villi.

- *Digestion at the brush border.* Aminopolypeptidase and several dipeptidases succeed in splitting larger polypeptides into tripeptides, dipeptides, and some amino acids. These are transported into the enterocyte.
- *Digestion inside the enterocyte.* The enterocyte contains multiple peptidases that are specific for linkages between the various amino acids. Within minutes, virtually all of the last dipeptides and tripeptides are digested to amino acids, which then enter the blood.

Digestion of Fats *(p. 791)*

The First Step in Fat Digestion Is Emulsification by Bile Acids and Lecithin. Emulsification is the process by which fat globules are broken into smaller pieces by the detergent actions of bile salts and especially lecithin. The emulsification process increases the total surface area of the fats. The lipases are water-soluble enzymes and can attack fat globules only on their surfaces. Consequently, it can be readily understood how important this detergent action of bile salts and lecithin is for the digestion of fats.

Triglycerides Are Digested by Pancreatic Lipase. The most important enzyme for digestion of triglycerides is pancreatic lipase. This is present in such enormous quantities in pancreatic juice that all triglycerides are digested into free fatty acids and 2-monoglycerides within a few minutes.

Bile Salts Form Micelles That Accelerate Fat Digestion. The hydrolysis of triglycerides is highly reversible; therefore, accumulation of monoglycerides and free fatty acids in the vicinity of digesting fats quickly blocks further digestion. Bile salts form micelles that remove monoglycerides and free fatty acids from the vicinity of the digesting fat globules. Micelles are composed of a central fat globule (containing monoglycerides and free fatty acids) with molecules of bile salt projecting outward to cover the surface of the micelle. The bile salt micelles also carry monoglycerides and free fatty acids to the brush borders of the intestinal epithelial cells.

Basic Principles of Gastrointestinal Absorption (p. 793)

The Folds of Kerckring, Villi, and Microvilli Increase the Mucosal Absorptive Area by Nearly 1000-Fold. The total area of the small intestinal mucosa is 250 square meters or more—about the surface area of a tennis court.

- *Folds of Kerckring* increase the surface area of the absorptive mucosa by about threefold.
- *Villi* project about 1 mm from the surface of the mucosa, increasing the absorptive area by an additional 10-fold.
- *Microvilli* covering the villar surface (brush border) increase the surface area exposed to the intestinal contents by at least an additional 20-fold.

Absorption in the Small Intestine (p. 794)

Absorption of Water

Water Is Transported through the Intestinal Membrane by Diffusion. It is absorbed from the gut when the chyme is dilute and moves into the intestine when hyperosmotic solutions enter the duodenum. As dissolved substances are absorbed from the gut, the osmotic pressure of the chyme tends to decrease, but water diffuses so readily through the intestinal membrane that it almost instantaneously "follows" the absorbed substances into the blood. Thus the intestinal contents are always isotonic with the extracellular fluid.

Absorption of Ions (p. 794)

Sodium Is Actively Transported through the Intestinal Membrane. Sodium is actively transported from inside the intestinal epithelial cells through the basal and side walls (basolateral membrane) of these cells into the paracellular spaces, which decreases the intracellular sodium concentration. This low concentration of sodium provides a steep electrochemical gradient for sodium movement from the chyme through the brush border into the epithelial cell cytoplasm. The osmotic gradient created by the high concentration of ions in the paracellular space causes water to move by osmosis through the tight junctions between the apical borders of the epithelial cells and, finally, into the circulating blood of the villi.

Aldosterone Greatly Enhances Sodium Absorption. Dehydration leads to aldosterone secretion by the adrenal glands, which greatly enhances sodium absorption by the intestinal epithelial cells. The increased sodium absorption then causes secondary increased absorption of chloride ions, water, and some other substances. This effect of aldosterone is especially important in the colon.

Cholera Causes Extreme Secretion of Chloride Ions, Sodium Ions, and Water from the Crypts of Lieberkühn. The toxins of cholera and some other diarrheal bacteria can stimulate secretion of sodium chloride and water so greatly that as much as 5 to 10 L of water and salt can be lost each day as diarrhea. In most instances, the life of the cholera victim can be saved by simply administering large amounts of sodium chloride solution to make up for the losses.

Calcium, Iron, Potassium, Magnesium, and Phosphate Ions Are Actively Absorbed

- *Calcium ions* are actively absorbed in relation to the need of the body for calcium. Calcium absorption is controlled by parathyroid hormone and vitamin D; the parathyroid hormone activates vitamin D in the kidneys, and the activated vitamin D in turn greatly enhances calcium absorption.
- *Iron ions* are also actively absorbed from the small intestine, as discussed in Chapter 32.
- *Potassium, magnesium, phosphate,* and probably *other ions* can also be actively absorbed through the mucosa.

Absorption of Carbohydrates *(p. 796)*

Essentially All Carbohydrates Are Absorbed in the Form of Monosaccharides. The most abundant of the absorbed monosaccharides is glucose, usually accounting for more than 80% of the absorbed carbohydrate calories.

Glucose is the final digestion product of our most abundant carbohydrate food, the starches.

Glucose Is Transported by a Sodium Co-Transport Mechanism. Active transport of sodium through the basolateral membranes into the paracellular spaces depletes the sodium inside the cells. This decrease causes sodium to move through the brush border of the enterocyte to its interior by secondary active cotransport. The sodium combines with a transport protein that requires another substance, such as glucose, to bind simultaneously. When intestinal glucose combines with the transport protein, sodium and glucose are transported into the cell at the same time.

Other Monosaccharides Are Transported. *Galactose* is transported by the exact same mechanism as glucose. In contrast, *fructose* is transported by facilitated diffusion all the way through the enterocyte but is not coupled with sodium transport. Much of the fructose is converted to glucose within the enterocyte and finally is transported to blood in the form of glucose.

Absorption of Proteins *(p. 797)*

Most Proteins Are Absorbed through the Luminal Membranes of the Intestinal Epithelial Cells in the Form of Dipeptides, Tripeptides, and Free Amino Acids. The energy for most of this transport is supplied by sodium co-transport mechanisms in the same way that sodium co-transport of glucose and galactose occurs. A few amino acids do not require this sodium co-transport mechanism but, instead, are transported by special membrane transport proteins in the same way that fructose is transported—via facilitated diffusion.

Absorption of Fats *(p. 797)*

Monoglycerides and Fatty Acids Diffuse Passively through the Enterocyte Cell Membrane to the Interior of the Enterocyte. Lipids are soluble in the enterocyte membrane. After entering the enterocyte, the fatty acids and monoglycerides are mainly recombined to form new triglycerides. A few of the monoglycerides are further digested into glycerol and fatty acids by an intracellular lipase. Triglycerides themselves cannot pass through the enterocyte membrane.

Chylomicrons Are Excreted from the Enterocytes by Exocytosis. The reconstituted triglycerides aggregate within the Golgi apparatus into globules that contain cholesterol and phospholipids. The phospholipids arrange themselves with the fatty portions toward the center and the polar portions on the surface, providing an electrically charged surface that makes the globules miscible with water. The globules are released from the Golgi apparatus and are excreted by exocytosis into the basolateral spaces; from there, they pass into the lymph in the central lacteal of the villi. These globules are then called *chylomicrons*.

Chylomicrons Are Transported in the Lymph. From the basolateral surfaces of the enterocytes, the chylomicrons wind their way into the central lacteals of the villi and are then propelled, along with the lymph, upward through the thoracic duct to be emptied into the great veins of the neck.

Absorption in the Large Intestine: Formation of Feces (p. 797)

The Proximal Half of the Colon Is Important for Absorption of Electrolytes and Water. The mucosa of the large intestine has a high capability for active absorption of sodium, and the electrical potential created by absorption of sodium causes chloride absorption as well. The tight junctions between the epithelial cells are tighter than those of the small intestine, which decreases back-diffusion of ions through these junctions. This allows the large intestinal mucosa to absorb sodium ions against a higher concentration gradient than can occur in the small intestine. The absorption of sodium and chloride ions creates an osmotic gradient across the large intestinal mucosa, which in turn causes absorption of water.

The Large Intestine Can Absorb a Maximum of about 5 to 7 L of Fluid and Electrolytes Each Day. When the total quantity entering the large intestine through the ileocecal valve or by way of large intestine secretion exceeds this maximum absorptive capacity, the excess appears in the feces as diarrhea.

The Feces Normally Are about Three-Fourths Water and One-Fourth Solid Matter. The solid matter is composed of about 30% dead bacteria, 10% to 20% fat, 10% to 20% inorganic matter, 2% to 3% protein, and 30% undigested roughage of the food and dried constituents of digestive juices, such as bile pigment and sloughed epithelial cells. The brown color of feces is caused by stercobilin and urobilin, which are derivatives of bilirubin. The odor is caused principally by indole, skatole, mercaptan, and hydrogen sulfide.

CHAPTER 66

Physiology of Gastrointestinal Disorders

The logical therapy of most gastrointestinal disorders depends on a basic knowledge of gastrointestinal physiology. In this chapter, we discuss a few representative types of malfunction that have special physiological bases or consequences.

Disorders of Swallowing and the Esophagus (p. 799)

Paralysis of the Swallowing Mechanism Can Result from Nerve Damage, Brain Damage, or Muscle Dysfunction

- *Nerve damage.* Damage to the fifth, ninth, or tenth cranial nerve can cause paralysis of the swallowing mechanism.
- *Brain damage.* Diseases such as poliomyelitis and encephalitis can prevent normal swallowing by damaging the swallowing center in the brain stem.
- *Muscle dysfunction.* Paralysis of the swallowing muscles, as occurs with muscular dystrophy or with failure of neuromuscular transmission in patients with myasthenia gravis or botulism, can also prevent normal swallowing.

Achalasia is a Condition in Which the Lower Esophageal Sphincter Fails to Relax. Swallowed material builds up, stretching the esophagus; and over months and years the esophagus becomes markedly enlarged, a condition called *megaesophagus.*

Disorders of the Stomach (p. 799)

***Gastritis* Means Inflammation of the Gastric Mucosa.** The inflammation can penetrate the gastric mucosa, causing atrophy. Gastritis can be acute and severe, with ulcerative excoriation of the stomach mucosa. It may be caused by chronic bacterial infection of the gastric mucosa; in addition, irritant substances, such as alcohol and aspirin, can damage the protective gastric mucosal barrier.

The Stomach Is Protected by the Gastric Mucosal Barrier. Absorption from the stomach is normally low for two reasons: (1) the gastric mucosa is lined with mucous cells that secrete viscid, adherent mucus and (2) the mucosa has tight junctions between adjacent epithelial cells. These impediments to gastric absorption are called the *gastric mucosal barrier.* During gastritis this barrier becomes leaky, allowing hydrogen ions to back diffuse into the stomach epithelium. A vicious circle of progressive mucosal damage and atrophy can develop, making the mucosa susceptible to peptic digestion, often resulting in gastric ulcer.

Chronic Gastritis Can Lead to Hypochlorhydria or Achlorhydria. Chronic gastritis can cause atrophy of the gastric mucosal glandular function.

- *Achlorhydria* means simply that the stomach fails to secrete hydrochloric acid.
- *Hypochlorhydria* means diminished acid secretion.

Pernicious Anemia Is a Common Accompaniment of Achlorhydria and Gastric Atrophy. Intrinsic factor is secreted by parietal cells. It combines with vitamin B_{12} in the intestine to protect it from being destroyed in the gut. When the intrinsic factor–vitamin B_{12} complex reaches the terminal ileum, the intrinsic factor binds with receptors on the ileal epithelial surface, making it possible for the vitamin B_{12} to be absorbed.

Peptic Ulcer Is an Excoriated Area of the Mucosa Caused by the Digestive Action of Gastric Juice. A peptic ulcer can result from one of two situations:

- Excess secretion of acid and pepsin by the gastric mucosa
- Diminished ability of the gastroduodenal mucosal barrier to protect against the digestive properties of the acid–pepsin complex

Bacterial Infection by *Helicobacter Pylori* Breaks Down the Gastroduodenal Mucosal Barrier and Stimulates Gastric Acid Secretion. At least 75% of peptic ulcer patients have recently been found to have chronic infection of the gastric and duodenal mucosa by the bacterium *H. pylori.* The bacterium produces ammonium that liquefies the gastric mucosal barrier, and also stimulates the secretion hydrochloric acid, thereby allowing gastric secretions to digest the epithelial cells, which leads to peptic ulceration.

Disorders of the Small Intestine *(p. 801)*

Abnormal Digestion Results from Failure of the Pancreas to Secrete its Juice. The loss of pancreatic juice means the loss of many digestive enzymes. As a result, large portions of the ingested food are not used for nutrition, and copious, fatty feces are excreted. The lack of pancreatic secretion often occurs in the following instances:

- Pancreatitis (discussed later)
- When the pancreatic duct is blocked by a gallstone at the papilla of Vater
- After the head of the pancreas has been removed because of malignancy

Pancreatitis **Means Inflammation of the Pancreas.** Ninety percent of all cases are caused by excess alcohol ingestion (chronic pancreatitis) or blockage of the papilla of Vater by a gallstone (acute pancreatitis). When the main secretory duct is blocked by a gallstone, the pancreatic enzymes are dammed up in the pancreas. These enzymes rapidly digest large portions of the pancreas.

Disorders of the Large Intestine *(p. 802)*

Severe Constipation Can Lead to Megacolon. When large quantities of fecal matter accumulate in the colon for an extended time, the colon can distend to a diameter of 3 to 4 inches. This condition is called *megacolon*. *Hirschsprung's disease*, the most frequent cause of megacolon, results from a lack or deficiency of ganglion cells in the myenteric plexus, usually in a segment of the sigmoid colon of newborns.

Diarrhea Often Results from the Rapid Movement of Fecal Matter through the Large Intestine. The following are some of the causes of diarrhea:

- *Enteritis.* This is infection in the intestinal tract, most often occurring in the large intestine. The result is increased motility and increased rate of secretion by the irritated mucosa, both of which contribute to diarrhea.
- *Psychogenic diarrhea.* This type of diarrhea is caused by parasympathetic stimulation, which excites both the motility and secretion of mucus in the distal colon.
- *Ulcerative colitis.* This is a disease in which the walls of the large intestine become inflamed and ulcerated. The motility of the ulcerated colon is often so great that mass movements occur most of the time. In addition, the secretions of the colon are greatly increased.

General Disorders of the Gastrointestinal Tract (p. 803)

The Vomiting Act Results from a Squeezing Action of Abdominal Muscles with Sudden Opening of the Esophageal Sphincters. Once the vomiting center has been stimulated and the vomiting act is instituted, the first effects are (1) a deep breath, (2) raising of the hyoid bone and larynx to pull open the upper esophageal sphincter, (3) closing of the glottis, and (4) lifting of the soft palate to close the posterior nares. Next, the diaphragm and abdominal muscles contract simultaneously, building the intragastric pressure to a high level. Finally, the lower esophageal sphincter relaxes, allowing expulsion of gastric contents.

The Abnormal Consequences of Obstruction Depend on the Point in the Gastrointestinal Tract That Becomes Obstructed

- *If the obstruction occurs at the pylorus*, which often results from fibrotic constriction after peptic ulceration, persistent vomiting of stomach contents occurs. This depresses bodily nutrition; it also causes excessive loss of hydrogen ions and can result in metabolic alkalosis.

- *If the obstruction is beyond the stomach*, antiperistaltic reflux from the small intestine causes intestinal juices to flow into the stomach, and these juices are vomited along with the stomach secretions. The person becomes severely dehydrated, but the loss of acids and bases may be approximately equal, so there is little change in the acid-base balance.

- *If the obstruction is near the lower end of the small intestine*, it is possible to vomit more basic than acidic substances; in this case, metabolic acidosis may result. In addition, after a few days of obstruction, the vomitus becomes fecal in character.

- *If the obstruction is near the distal end of the large intestine*, feces can accumulate in the colon for several weeks. The patient develops an intense feeling of constipation, but it finally becomes impossible for additional chyme to move from the small intestine into the large intestine. At this point severe vomiting begins.

XIII

Metabolism and Temperature Regulation

CHAPTER 67

Metabolism of Carbohydrates, and Formation of Adenosine Triphosphate

The next few chapters deal with the chemical processes that make it possible for cells to continue living.

Adenosine Triphosphate Is the "Energy Currency" of the Body. A great proportion of the chemical reactions in cells are concerned with making the energy in foods available to the various physiological systems of the cell. The substance *adenosine triphosphate* (ATP) plays a key role in making the energy of the foods available for this purpose. ATP is a labile chemical compound containing two high-energy phosphate bonds. The amount of free energy in each of these phosphate bonds is approximately 12,000 calories under conditions found in the body.

The ATP is present in the cytoplasm and nucleoplasm of all cells. Essentially all of the physiological mechanisms that require energy for operation obtain this energy directly from ATP (or other, similar high-energy compounds, such as *guanosine triphosphate*). In turn, the food in the cells is gradually oxidized, and the released energy is used to re-form the ATP so a supply of this substance is continually maintained. The main purpose of this chapter is to explain how the energy from carbohydrates can be used to form ATP in the cells. Normally, 90% or more of all the carbohydrates used by the body are used for this purpose.

Transport of Glucose through the Cell Membrane *(p. 810)*

The final products of carbohydrate digestion in the alimentary tract are almost entirely *glucose, fructose*, and *galactose*. These monosaccharides cannot diffuse through the usual pores in the cell membrane. To enter the cell, these monosaccharides combine with protein carriers in the membrane that allow them to pass through the membrane via facilitated diffusion into the cell, as discussed in Chapter 4. After passing through the membrane, the monosaccharides become dissociated from the carriers.

Insulin Facilitates Diffusion of Glucose. The rate of glucose transport through the cell membranes is greatly increased by *insulin*. The amount of glucose that can diffuse into the cells of the body in the absence of insulin, with the exception of the liver and brain, is too little to supply the amount of glucose normally required for energy metabolism; therefore, the rate of carbohydrate utilization by the body is controlled mainly by the rate of insulin secretion from the pancreas.

Glucose Is Phosphorylated in the Cell by the Enzyme Glucokinase. The phosphorylation of glucose is almost completely irreversible, except in liver cells, renal tubular epithelium, and intestinal epithelial cells, where *glucose phosphatase* is available for reversing the reaction. In most tissues of the body, phosphorylation serves to capture glucose in the cell. Once in the cell, the glucose does not diffuse out except from special cells that have the necessary phosphatase.

Storage of Glycogen in Liver and Muscle (p. 811)

After absorption into cells, glucose can be used immediately for energy or stored in the form of *glycogen*, a large polymer of glucose. All cells of the body are capable of storing some glycogen, but liver and muscle cells can store large quantities of it. The glycogen molecule can be polymerized to form very large molecules with an average molecular weight of 5 million. These large glycogen molecules precipitate to form solid granules.

Glycogenesis Is the Process of Glycogen Formation. *Glycogenolysis* is the process of glycogen breakdown to re-form glucose; it is not the reverse process of glycogenesis. In glycogenolysis, the glucose molecule on each branch of the glycogen polymer is split away by the process of phosphorylation catalyzed by the enzyme *phosphorylase.*

Under resting conditions, the phosphorylase enzyme is in an inactive form. When it is required to re-form glucose from glycogen, phosphorylase can be activated by the hormones *epinephrine* and *glucagon.* The initial effect of each of these hormones is to increase the formation of *cyclic adenosine monophosphate* (cAMP). The cAMP initiates a cascade of chemical reactions that activates the phosphorylase.

Release of Energy from Glucose Molecules by the Glycolytic Pathway (p. 812)

The complete oxidation of 1 mole of glucose releases 686,000 calories of energy, but only 12,000 calories of energy are required to form 1 mole of ATP. It would be an extreme waste of energy if glucose decomposed to water and carbon dioxide while forming only a single molecule of ATP. Fortunately, cells contain an extensive series of enzymes that cause the glucose molecule to split a little at a time in many successive steps. The energy in glucose is released in small packets to form one molecule of ATP at a time. A total of 38 moles of ATP is formed for each mole of glucose used by the cells.

Glycolysis Is the Splitting of Glucose to Form Pyruvic Acid. During glycolysis the glucose molecule is split to form two molecules of pyruvic acid. This process occurs in 10 successive steps, with each step being catalyzed by at least one specific enzyme.

Despite the many chemical reactions in the glycolytic series, only 2 moles of ATP are formed for each mole of glucose used; this amounts to 24,000 calories of energy stored in the form of ATP. The total amount of energy lost from the original glucose molecule is 56,000 calories, so the overall efficiency for ATP formation during glycolysis is 43%. The remaining 57% of the energy is lost in the form of heat.

Pyruvic Acid Is Converted to *Acetyl-Coenzyme* A (Acetyl-CoA). The next stage in the degradation of glucose is conversion of the two molecules of pyruvic acid to two molecules of acetyl-CoA. During this reaction, two carbon dioxide molecules and four hydrogen atoms are released. No ATP is formed. Six molecules of ATP are produced, however, when the four hydrogen atoms are later oxidized via the process of *oxidative phosphorylation.*

Continued Degradation of the Glucose Molecule Occurs in the Citric Acid Cycle. This is a sequence of chemical reactions in which the acetyl portion of acetyl-CoA is degraded to carbon dioxide and hydrogen atoms. These reactions occur *in the matrix of the mitochondrion.* The hydrogen atoms released are subsequently oxidized, liberating tremendous amounts of energy to form ATP. No large amount of energy is released during the citric acid cycle however: For each molecule of glucose metabolized, two molecules of ATP are formed.

Formation of ATP by Oxidation of Hydrogen: The Process of Oxidative Phosphorylation (p. 814)

Despite the complexities of glycolysis and the citric acid cycle, only small amounts of ATP are formed during these processes. Two ATP molecules are formed in the glycolytic scheme, and another two molecules are formed in the citric acid cycle. Almost 95% of the total amount of ATP is formed during subsequent oxidation of the hydrogen atoms released during these early stages of glucose degradation. The principal function of these earlier stages is to make the hydrogen of the glucose molecule available in a form that can be used for oxidation.

Oxidative phosphorylation is accomplished through a series of enzyme-catalyzed reactions in the mitochondria (Fig. 67–1). During this process, the hydrogen atoms are converted to hydrogen ions and electrons. The electrons eventually combine with the dissolved oxygen of the fluids to form hydroxyl ions. The hydrogen and hydroxyl ions combine with each other to form water. During this sequence of oxidative reactions, tremendous quantities of energy are released to form ATP; this is called *oxidative phosphorylation.*

Figure 67–1. Mitochondrial chemiosmotic mechanism of oxidative phosphorylation used to form large quantities of ATP. This figure shows the relationship of the oxidative and phosphorylation steps at the outer and inner membranes of the mitochondrion.

This process occurs entirely in the mitochondria via a highly specialized process called the *chemiosmotic mechanism*.

The electrons removed from the hydrogen atoms enter an electron transport chain that is an integral component of the inner membrane of the mitochondria. This transport chain consists of a series of electron acceptors that can be reversibly reduced or oxidized by accepting or giving up electrons. The important members of the electron transport chain include *flavoprotein*, several *iron sulfide proteins*, *ubiquinone*, and *cytochromes B, C_1, C, A, and A_3*. Each electron is shuttled from one of the acceptors to the next until it reaches cytochrome A_3. Cytochrome A_3 is called *cytochrome oxidase* because by giving up two electrons it is capable of causing elemental oxygen to combine with hydrogen ions to form water. During the transport of these electrons through the electron transport chain, energy is released and used to synthesize ATP.

Conversion of ADP to ATP. The energy released as the electrons pass through the electron transport chain is used to create a gradient of hydrogen ions across the inner membrane of the mitochondria. The high concentration of hydrogen ions across this space creates a large electrical potential difference across the membrane, which causes hydrogen ions to flow into the mitochondrial matrix through a molecule called *ATP synthetase*. The energy derived from the hydrogen ions is used by the ATP synthetase to convert adenosine diphosphate (ADP) to ATP. For each two hydrogen atoms ionized by the electron transport chain, up to three molecules of ATP are synthesized.

Summary of ATP Formation during Breakdown of Glucose *(p. 815)*

- During glycolysis four molecules of ATP are formed, but two are expended to initially phosphorylate the glucose, giving a net gain of two molecules of ATP.
- Two molecules of ATP are formed during the citric acid cycle.
- A total of 34 molecules of ATP are formed during oxidative phosphorylation.
- Adding all the ATP molecules together results in 38 ATP molecules formed for each molecule of glucose.

Therefore, 456,000 calories of energy are stored in the form of ATP, whereas 686,000 calories are released during the complete oxidation of each mole of glucose; this represents an overall efficiency of 66%. The remaining 34% of the energy becomes heat.

Glycolysis and Glucose Oxidation Are Regulated. Continuous release of energy from glucose when the energy is not needed by the cells would be an extremely wasteful process. Glycolysis and the subsequent oxidation of hydrogen atoms are continually controlled in accordance with the needs of the cell for ATP. This control is accomplished by a feedback mechanism related to the concentrations of both ADP and ATP.

One important way in which ATP helps control energy metabolism is allosteric inhibition of the enzyme *phosphofructokinase.* This enzyme promotes the formation of fructose-1,6-diphosphate during the initial steps of the glycolytic series. The net effect of excess cellular ATP is to stop glycolysis, which in turn stops most carbohydrate metabolism. Conversely, ADP causes the opposite allosteric change in this enzyme, greatly increasing its activity. Whenever ATP is used by the tissues for energy, ATP inhibition of the enzyme is reduced, but at the same time its activity is increased as a result of the ADP formed. The glycolytic process is thus set in motion. When cellular stores of ATP are replenished, the enzyme is again inhibited.

Anaerobic Release of Energy—"Anaerobic Glycolysis" (p. 815)

If oxygen becomes either unavailable or insufficient, cellular oxidation of glucose cannot take place. Under these conditions, a small amount of energy can still be released to the cells through glycolysis because the chemical reactions in the glycolytic breakdown of glucose to pyruvic acid do not require oxygen. The process of *anaerobic glycolysis* is extremely wasteful of glucose because only 24,000 calories of energy are used to form ATP for each mole of glucose. This represents a little over 3% of the total energy in the glucose molecule; however, this release of glycolytic energy to the cells can be a lifesaving measure for a few minutes when oxygen is unavailable.

The Formation of *Lactic Acid* during Anaerobic Glycolysis Allows the Release of Extra Anaerobic Energy. The end products of the glycolytic reactions—pyruvic acid and nicotinamide adenine dinucleotide (NADH)—combine under the influence of the enzyme *lactic dehydrogenase* to form lactic acid and NAD^+. This prevents the build-up of pyruvic acid and NADH, which would inhibit the glycolytic reactions. The lactic acid formed readily diffuses out of the cells into the extracellular fluids. Lactic acid represents a "sinkhole" into which the glycolytic end products can disappear, allowing glycolysis to proceed far longer than would otherwise be possible.

Release of Energy from Glucose by the Pentose Phosphate Pathway (p. 816)

As much as 30% of glucose breakdown in the liver and fat cells is accomplished independent of glycolysis and the citric acid cycle. The pentose phosphate pathway is a cyclic process that removes one carbon atom from a glucose molecule to produce carbon dioxide and hydrogen during each turn of the cycle. The hydrogen produced eventually enters the oxidative phosphorylation pathway to form ATP. This pathway provides the cell with another mechanism of glucose utilization in the event of enzymatic abnormalities.

Formation of Carbohydrates from Proteins and Fats—Gluconeogenesis (p. 817)

When body stores of carbohydrates decrease below normal levels, moderate quantities of glucose can be formed from amino acids and the glycerol portion of fat through the process of gluconeogenesis. Approximately 60% of the amino acids in body proteins can be easily converted to carbohydrates; each amino acid is converted to glucose through a slightly different chemical process. A low level of carbohydrates in the cells and a decrease in blood glucose are the basic stimuli that increase the rate of gluconeogenesis.

CHAPTER 68

Lipid Metabolism

Several chemical compounds in food and in the body are classified as lipids, including (1) *neutral fat,* or *triglycerides,* (2) *phospholipids,* and (3) *cholesterol.* Chemically, the basic lipid moiety of the triglycerides and phospholipids is fatty acids, which are simply long-chain hydrocarbon organic acids. Although cholesterol does not contain fatty acids, its sterol nucleus is synthesized from degradation products of fatty acid molecules, giving it many of the physical and chemical properties of other lipid substances.

The triglycerides are mainly used in the body to provide energy for the various metabolic processes, a function shared almost equally with the carbohydrates. Some lipids, especially cholesterol, phospholipids, and derivatives of these compounds, are used throughout the body to perform other intracellular functions.

Transport of Lipids in Body Fluids *(p. 819)*

Chylomicrons Transport Lipids from the Gastrointestinal Tract to the Blood Via Lymph. Essentially all fats in the diet are absorbed into the lymph in the form of chylomicrons. The chylomicrons are transported in the thoracic duct and emptied into venous blood. They are removed from the plasma as they pass through the capillaries of adipose and liver tissue. The membranes of the adipose and liver cells contain large quantities of an enzyme called *lipoprotein lipase;* this enzyme hydrolyzes the triglycerides of the chylomicrons into fatty acids and glycerol. The fatty acids immediately diffuse into the cells; once inside, they are resynthesized into triglycerides.

"Free Fatty Acids" Released from Adipose Tissue Are Transported in the Blood in Combination with Albumin. When the fat that has been stored in fat cells is to be used elsewhere in the body, it must be transported to other tissues; it is mainly transported in the form of *free fatty acids.* On leaving the fat cells, the fatty acids ionize strongly in the plasma and immediately combine loosely with the albumin of the plasma proteins. The fatty acid bound with proteins in this manner is called *free fatty acid* to distinguish it from other fatty acids in the plasma that exist in the form of esters of glycerol, cholesterol, or other substances.

Lipoproteins Transport Cholesterol, Phospholipids, and Triglycerides. Lipoproteins are particles that are much smaller than chylomicrons but similar in composition; they contain mixtures of triglycerides, phospholipids, cholesterols, and proteins. The three major classes of lipoproteins are (1) *very low density lipoproteins (VLDLs)*, which contain high concentrations of triglycerides and moderate concentrations of both phospholipids, and cholesterol; (2) *low-density lipoproteins (LDLs)*, which contain relatively few triglycerides but a very high concentration of cholesterol; and (3) *high-density lipoproteins (HDLs)*, which contain about 50% protein with smaller concentrations of lipids.

Almost All of the Lipoproteins Are Formed in the Liver. The principal function of the various lipoproteins in the plasma is to transport a specific type of lipid throughout the body. Triglycerides are synthesized in the liver mainly from carbohydrates and transported to adipose and other peripheral tissue in the VLDLs. The LDLs are residuals of the VLDLs after they have delivered most of their triglycerides to the adipose tissue and left behind large concentrations of cholesterol and phospholipids in the LDLs. The HDLs transport cholesterol away from the peripheral tissues to the liver; this type of lipoprotein plays a very important role in preventing the development of atherosclerosis.

Fat Deposits *(p. 821)*

Large Quantities of Lipids Are Stored in Fat Cells (Adipocytes). The major function of adipose tissue is to store triglycerides until they are needed to provide energy elsewhere in the body. A secondary function of adipose tissue is to provide insulation for the body.

Fat cells of the adipose tissue are modified fibroblasts that are capable of storing almost pure triglycerides in quantities equal to 80% to 95% of their volume. Large quantities of lipases are present in adipose tissue. Some of these enzymes catalyze the deposition of triglycerides derived from chylomicrons and other lipoproteins. Others, when activated by hormones, cause splitting of the triglycerides in the fat cells to release free fatty acids. Because of the rapid exchange of the fatty acids, the triglycerides in the fat cells are renewed approximately once every 2 to 3 weeks, making fat a dynamic tissue.

The Liver Contains Large Quantities of Triglycerides, Phospholipids, and Cholesterol. The liver has multiple functions in lipid metabolism: (1) to degrade fatty acids into smaller compounds that can be used for energy;

(2) to synthesize triglycerides, mainly from carbohydrates and proteins; and (3) to synthesize other lipids from fatty acids, especially cholesterol and phospholipids.

When large quantities of triglycerides are mobilized from adipose tissue, which occurs during starvation or with diabetes mellitus, the triglycerides are redeposited in the liver, where the initial stages of fat degradation begin. Under normal physiologic conditions, the amount of triglycerides present in the liver is determined by the rate at which lipids are being used for energy.

Use of Triglycerides for Energy *(p. 822)*

The dietary intake of fat varies in persons of different cultures, averaging as little as 10% to 15% of energy intake in some Asian populations to as much as 35% to 50% of the caloric intake in many Western populations. The first stage in conversion of fats to energy is hydrolysis of the triglycerides into fatty acids and glycerol. The fatty acids and glycerol are then transported to active tissues, where they are oxidized to release energy. Almost all cells, with some exceptions such as brain tissue and red blood cells, can use fatty acids almost interchangeably with glucose for energy.

Degradation and oxidation of fatty acids occur only in the mitochondria, and the first step in the metabolism of fatty acids is their transport into the mitochondria. This is a carrier-mediated process that employs carnitine as a carrier substance. Once inside the mitochondria, the fatty acids split away from the carnitine and are degraded and oxidized.

Fatty acids are degraded in the mitochondria by *β-oxidation*, which releases two-carbon segments to form *acetyl-coenzyme A* (acetyl-CoA), which enters the citric acid cycle and is degraded to carbon dioxide and hydrogen atoms. The hydrogen is subsequently oxidized by the oxidative enzymes of the mitochondria and is used to form ATP.

Acetoacetic Acid Is Formed in the Liver. A large share of the degradation of fatty acids into acetyl-CoA occurs in the liver, but the liver uses only a small portion of the acetyl-CoA for its own intrinsic metabolic processes. Instead, pairs of acetyl-CoA condense to form molecules of *acetoacetic acid.* A large part of the acetoacetic acid is converted to *β-hydroxybutyric acid* and minute quantities of *acetone.* The acetoacetic acid and β-hydroxybutyric acid freely diffuse through the liver cell membranes and are transported by the blood to peripheral tissues. In the peripheral tissue, these compounds diffuse into the cells in which reverse reactions occur and acetyl-CoA molecules are re-formed. These molecules enter the citric acid cycle of the cells and are oxidized for energy.

Synthesis of Triglycerides from Carbohydrates (p. 824)

Whenever quantities of carbohydrates enter the body that are greater than can be used immediately for energy or stored as glycogen, the excess is rapidly converted to triglyceride, which is stored in adipose tissue. Most triglyceride synthesis occurs in the liver, but a small amount occurs in fat cells. The triglycerides formed in the liver are mainly transported by the lipoproteins to fat cells of the adipose tissue and stored until needed for energy.

Carbohydrates Are Converted to Fatty Acids. The first step in the synthesis of triglycerides from carbohydrates is conversion of the carbohydrates to acetyl-CoA; this occurs during the normal degradation of glucose by the glycolytic system. Fatty acids are actually large polymers of the acetyl portion of acetyl-CoA, so it is not difficult to understand how acetyl-CoA can be converted to fatty acids.

Fatty Acids Combine with α-glycerophosphate to Form Triglycerides. Once the synthesized fatty acid chains have grown to contain 14 to 18 carbon atoms, they automatically bind with glycerol to form triglycerides. The glycerol portion of the triglyceride is furnished by α-glycerophosphate, which is also a product of the glycolytic breakdown of glucose. The importance of this mechanism in the formation of triglycerides is that the final combination of fatty acids with glycerol is controlled mainly by the concentration of α-glycerophosphate, which in turn is determined by the availability of carbohydrates. When carbohydrates form large quantities of α-glycerophosphate, the equilibrium shifts to promote formation and storage of triglycerides. When carbohydrates are not available, the process shifts in the opposite direction; the excess fatty acids become available to substitute for the lack of carbohydrate metabolism.

Fat Synthesis from Carbohydrates Is Important. Fat synthesis from carbohydrates is especially important because the various cells of the body have limited capacity for storing carbohydrates in the form of glycogen. The average person has about 150 times as much energy stored as fat as is stored as carbohydrate. Storage of energy in the form of fat is also important because each gram of fat contains approximately two and a half times as many calories of usable energy as each gram of glycogen. For a given weight gain, a person can store far more energy in the form of fat than in the form of carbohydrate.

Synthesis of Triglycerides from Proteins *(p. 825)*

Many amino acids can be converted to acetyl-CoA, which subsequently can be converted to triglycerides. When more protein is available in the diet than can be used as protein or directly for energy, a large share of the excess energy is stored as fat.

Regulation of Energy Release from Triglycerides *(p. 825)*

Carbohydrates Are Preferred Over Fats for Energy when Excess Carbohydrates Are Available. Excess carbohydrates in the diet have a "fat-sparing" effect and are used preferentially for energy. One reason for this is that excess carbohydrates result in increased *α-glycerophosphate*, which binds the free fatty acids and increases stored triglycerides. Metabolism of excess carbohydrates also results in increased synthesis of acetyl-CoA, which is converted to fatty acids. Thus excess amounts of dietary carbohydrates not only have a fat-sparing effect, they also increase fat stores.

Conversely, when carbohydrates are not available, fat is mobilized from adipocytes and used in place of carbohydrates.

Hormonal Regulation of Fat Utilization. Several hormones secreted by the endocrine system, in addition to *insulin* (discussed elsewhere), have marked effects on fat utilization:

- *Epinephrine* and *norepinephrine* released by the adrenal medulla dramatically increase fat utilization during heavy exercise. These two hormones directly activate *hormone-sensitive triglyceride lipase*, which is present in abundance in fat cells. The activated hormone causes rapid breakdown of triglycerides and mobilization of fatty acids. Other stressors that activate the sympathetic nervous system similarly increase fatty acid mobilization and utilization.

- *Corticotropin* is released by the anterior pituitary gland in response to stress and causes the adrenal cortex to secrete *glucocorticoids (cortisol)*. Both corticotropin and the glucocorticoids activate hormone-sensitive triglyceride lipase, which increases the release of fatty acids from the fat tissue.

- *Growth hormone* has an effect similar to, but less effective than, that of corticotropin and glucocorticoids in activating the hormone-sensitive lipases. Growth hormone can also have a mild fat-mobilizing effect. A lack of *insulin* activates hormone-sensitive lipase and causes rapid mobilization of fatty acids. When carbohydrates are not available in the diet, insulin secretion diminishes; this promotes fatty acid metabolism.

- *Thyroid hormone* causes rapid mobilization of fat. This process is believed to result indirectly from an increased rate of energy metabolism in all the cells of the body under the influence of this hormone.

Phospholipids and Cholesterol *(p. 826)*

Phospholipids. The three major types of phospholipid in the body are *lecithins, cephalins,* and *sphingomyelins.* Phospholipids are used throughout the body for various structural purposes; they are an important constituent of lipoproteins in the blood and are essential for the formation and function of these compounds. The absence of phospholipids can cause serious abnormalities in the transport of cholesterol and other lipids. Thromboplastin, which is needed to initiate the clotting process, is composed mainly of one of the cephalins. Large quantities of sphingomyelins are present in the nervous system. This substance acts as an insulator in the myelin sheath around the nerve fibers. Perhaps the most important function of the phospholipids is participation in the formation of the structural elements, mainly membranes, in cells throughout the body.

   Cholesterol. Cholesterol is present in all diets and is absorbed slowly from the gastrointestinal tract into the intestinal lymph. In addition to the cholesterol absorbed each day from the gastrointestinal tract *(exogenous cholesterol)*, a large quantity is formed in the cells of the body *(endogenous cholesterol)*. Essentially all of the endogenous cholesterol that circulates in lipoproteins in the plasma is formed by the liver. Cholesterol is a structural component in cell membranes.

By far the most abundant nonmembranous use of cholesterol in the body is for the formation of *cholic acid* in the liver; about 80% of the cholesterol is converted to cholic acid. Cholic acid is conjugated with other substances to form bile salts, which promote digestion and absorption of fats.

A small quantity of cholesterol is used by the (1) adrenal glands to form *adrenal cortical hormones,* (2) the ovaries to form *progesterone* and *estrogen,* and (3) the testes to form *testosterone.*

Atherosclerosis *(p. 827)*

Atherosclerosis is a disease of the large and intermediate-sized arteries in which fatty lesions called *atheromatous plaques* develop on the inside surfaces of the arterial walls. *Arteriosclerosis,* in contrast, is a general term that refers to thickened and stiffened blood vessels of all sizes.

Damage to the vascular endothelial cells occurs early in atherosclerosis, decreasing their ability to release nitric oxide and other substances that help prevent adhesion of macromolecules, platelets, and monocytes to the endothelium. After damage of the vascular endothelium, circulating monocytes and lipids (mostly LDLs) begin to accumulate at the site of injury. The monocytes cross the endothelium and differentiate to become *macrophages,* which then ingest and oxidize the accumulated lipoproteins, giving the macrophages a foamlike appearance. These *macrophage foam cells* then aggregate on the blood vessel and form a visible *fatty streak.*

As the fatty streaks grow larger, the surrounding fibrous and smooth muscle tissues proliferate to form larger plaques, a process exacerbated by release of *inflammatory substances* from the macrophages. As the plaque bulges into the lumen of the artery it can greatly reduce blood flow, sometimes even causing complete vessel occlusion. Even without occlusion, the fibroblasts of the plaque eventually deposit such extensive amounts of dense connective tissue that *sclerosis* (fibrosis) is severe and the arteries become stiff and unyielding.

Increased Blood LDLs Can Cause Atherosclerosis. An important factor causing atherosclerosis is a high blood plasma concentration of cholesterol in the form of LDLs. The plasma concentration of these high cholesterol

LDLs is increased by several factors including eating highly saturated fat in the daily diet, obesity, and physical inactivity.

Familial Hypercholesterolemia Can Cause Atherosclerosis. When a person inherits defective genes for the formation of LDL receptors on the membrane surfaces of the body's cells, the liver cannot absorb either the intermediate density lipoproteins or the LDLs. Without this absorption, the cholesterol machinery of the liver cells goes on a rampage of producing new cholesterol and VLDLs, which are released into the plasma.

HDL Helps Prevent Atherosclerosis. HDLs are believed to absorb cholesterol crystals that are beginning to deposit in the arterial walls. Consequently, when a person has a high *ratio* of HDL/LDL, the likelihood of developing atherosclerosis is greatly reduced.

Other Major Risk Factors for Atherosclerosis. Some of the factors known to predispose to atherosclerosis are (1) *physical inactivity and obesity,* (2) *diabetes mellitus,* (3) *hypertension,* (4) *hyperlipidemia,* and (5) *cigarette smoking.*

Several of these risk factors occur together in many overweight and obese patients, greatly increasing their risk for atherosclerosis, which in turn may lead to heart attack, stroke, and kidney disease. Some of these factors cause atherosclerosis by increasing the concentration of LDLs in the plasma. Others, such as hypertension, lead to atherosclerosis by causing damage to the vascular endothelium and other changes in the vascular tissues that predispose to cholesterol deposition.

Prevention of Atherosclerosis. The most important measures for reducing the risk of developing atherosclerosis and its progression to serious vascular disease are (1) maintaining a healthy weight, being physically active, and eating a diet that contains mainly unsaturated fat with low cholesterol content; (2) preventing hypertension or effectively controlling blood pressure with antihypertensive drugs if hypertension does develop; (3) effectively controlling blood glucose with insulin treatment or other drugs if diabetes develops; (4) avoiding cigarette smoking.

Several drugs that lower plasma lipids and cholesterol have also proved valuable for preventing atherosclerosis. One group of drugs, called *statins,* competitively inhibit *hydroxymethylglutaryl-coenzyme A (HMG-CoA) reductase,* a rate-limiting enzyme in the synthesis of cholesterol. This inhibition decreases cholesterol synthesis and increases LDL receptors in the liver, usually causing a 25% to 50% reduction in the plasma levels of LDLs. Studies generally show that for each 1 mg/dL decrease in LDL cholesterol in the plasma there is about a 2% decrease in mortality from atherosclerotic heart disease. Therefore, appropriate preventive measures are valuable for decreasing the risk for serious vascular disease.

CHAPTER 69

Protein Metabolism

About three fourths of the body solids are proteins, including *structural proteins, enzymes, proteins that transport oxygen, proteins of the muscle that causes contraction,* and many other types that perform specific intracellular and extracellular functions both.

The principal constituents of proteins are amino acids, 20 of which are present in the body in significant quantities. The amino acids are aggregated into long chains by means of *peptide linkages.* A complicated protein molecule may have as many as 100,000 amino acids. Some protein molecules are composed of several peptide chains rather than a single chain; these chains may be linked by hydrogen bonding, electrostatic forces, or sulfhydryl, phenolic, or salt entities.

Transport and Storage of Amino Acids (p. 831)

The normal concentration of amino acids in the blood is between 35 and 65 mg/dL. Recall that the end products of protein digestion in the gastrointestinal tract are almost entirely amino acids and polypeptides or protein molecules are only rarely absorbed into the blood. After a meal, the amino acids entering the blood are absorbed within 5 to 10 minutes by cells throughout the entire body.

The molecules of essentially all the amino acids are much too large to diffuse through the pores of the cell membranes; therefore amino acids are transported through the membrane only by active transport or facilitated diffusion using a carrier mechanism.

Amino Acids Are Stored as Proteins in the Cells. Almost immediately after entry into the cells, amino acids are conjugated under the influence of intracellular enzymes with cellular proteins, so the concentration of free amino acids inside the cells almost always remains low. The amino acids are stored mainly in the form of proteins. Many intracellular proteins can be rapidly decomposed into amino acids under the influence of intracellular lysosomal digestive enzymes; and these amino acids can then be transported back into the blood. Special exceptions are proteins in the chromosomes of the nucleus and structural proteins such as collagen and muscle contractile proteins; these proteins do not participate significantly in this reversible storage of amino acids.

Whenever the plasma amino acid concentration falls below the normal level, amino acids are transported out of the cell to replenish the supply in the plasma. Simultaneously, intracellular proteins are degraded into amino acids.

Each cell type has an upper limit to the amount of protein it can store. After the cells have reached their limits, the excess amino acids in the circulation are degraded to other products and used for energy or converted to fat or glycogen and stored.

Functional Roles of the Plasma Proteins (p. 833)

The major proteins present in the plasma are *albumin, globulin,* and *fibrinogen.* The principal function of albumin is to provide colloid osmotic pressure in the plasma. The globulins are mainly responsible for immunity against invading organisms. Fibrinogen polymerizes into long, branching fibrin threads during blood coagulation, thereby forming blood clots that help repair leaks in the circulatory system.

Plasma Proteins Form in the Liver. Essentially all of the albumin and fibrinogen and 50% to 80% of the globulins are formed in the liver. The remaining globulins (mainly γ-globulins in antibodies) are formed in lymphoid tissue. The rate of plasma protein formation by the liver can be as much as 30 g per day. The rapid production of plasma proteins by the liver is valuable in preventing death from conditions such as those found with severe burns, which cause the loss of many liters of plasma through the denuded areas of the skin, and severe renal disease, in which as much as 20 g of plasma protein per day can be lost in urine.

When the tissues become depleted of proteins, the plasma proteins can act as a source for rapid replacement. Whole plasma proteins can be absorbed by the liver, split into amino acids, transported back into the blood, and used throughout the body to build cellular proteins. In this way, the plasma proteins function as a labile storage medium and represent a rapidly available source of amino acids.

Essential and Nonessential Amino Acids. Of the 20 amino acids normally present in animal proteins, 10 can be synthesized in the cells; the other 10 amino acids either cannot be synthesized or are synthesized in quantities too small to supply the needs of the body. The latter amino acids are called *essential amino acids* because they must be supplied in the diet. Synthesis of the nonessential amino acids depends on the formation of the appropriate α-*keto acid* precursor of the respective amino acid. Pyruvic acid, which is formed in large quantities during the glycolytic breakdown of glucose, is the α-keto acid precursor of the amino acid *alanine.*

Proteins Can Be Used for Energy. Once the protein stores of the cell are full, additional amino acids in the body fluids are degraded and used for energy or stored mainly as fat or glycogen. This degradation occurs almost entirely in the liver. The first step in the degradation process is the removal of amino groups through the process of deamination. This generates the specific α-keto acid that can enter into the citric acid cycle. The amount of adenosine triphosphate (ATP) formed from each gram of protein oxidized is slightly less than that formed from each gram of glucose. The ammonia released during the deamination process is removed from the blood almost entirely through conversion to *urea* by the liver. In the absence of the liver or with severe liver disease, ammonia accumulates in the blood. The ammonia is highly toxic, especially to the brain, and often leads to the state of *hepatic coma.*

Obligatory Degradation of Proteins Can Occur. When the diet contains no proteins, a certain proportion of the proteins of the body continue to be degraded into amino acids. These amino acids are deaminated and oxidized; the process involves 20 to 30 g of protein per day and is called the *obligatory loss of proteins.* To prevent a net loss of proteins from the body, one must ingest at least 20 to 30 g of protein per day. The minimum recommended amount of protein in the diet is 60 to 75 g per day.

Hormonal Regulation of Protein Metabolism (p. 835)

Growth Hormone Increases the Rate of Synthesis of Cellular Proteins, Causing the Tissue Proteins to Increase. The mechanism of action of growth hormone on protein synthesis is not known, but growth hormone is believed to enhance the transport of amino acids through the cell membrane and accelerate DNA and RNA transcription and translation processes for protein synthesis. Part of the action might also result from the effect of growth hormone on fat metabolism. Growth hormone causes an increased rate of fat liberation from fat depots, which reduces the rate of oxidation of amino acids and subsequently increases the quantity of amino acids available for synthesis into proteins.

Insulin Accelerates the Transport of Amino Acids into Cells. Insulin deficiency reduces protein synthesis to almost zero. It also increases the availability of glucose to cells, so use of amino acids for energy is correspondingly reduced.

Glucocorticoids Decrease the Quantity of Proteins in Most Tissues and Increase the Amino Acid Concentration in the Plasma. It is believed that glucocorticoids act by increasing the rate of breakdown of extrahepatic proteins, making larger quantities of amino acid available in the body fluids. The effects of glucocorticoids on protein metabolism are especially important for promoting ketogenesis and gluconeogenesis.

Testosterone Increases the Deposition of Protein in Tissues throughout the Body, Especially Muscle. The mechanism of this effect is not known, but it is different from the effect of growth hormone. Growth hormone causes tissues to continue growing almost indefinitely, whereas testosterone causes the muscles and other protein tissues to enlarge only for several months. Beyond this time, despite the continued administration of testosterone, further protein deposition ceases.

Estrogen Causes Slight Deposition of Protein. The effect of estrogen is relatively insignificant compared with that of testosterone.

Thyroxine Increases the Rate of Metabolism in All Cells and Indirectly Affects Protein Metabolism. If insufficient carbohydrates and fats are available for energy, thyroxine causes rapid degradation of proteins for energy. If adequate quantities of carbohydrates and fats are available, the excess amino acids are used to increase the rate of protein synthesis.

A deficiency of thyroxine causes growth to be greatly inhibited because of a lack of protein synthesis. It is believed that thyroxine has little specific direct effect on protein metabolism but does have an important general effect on increasing the rates of both normal anabolic and normal catabolic protein reactions.

CHAPTER 70

The Liver as an Organ

The liver performs many interrelated functions, including the following basic functions:

- Filtration and storage of blood
- Metabolism of carbohydrates, fats, proteins, hormones, and xenobiotics
- Formation and excretion of bile
- Storage of vitamins and iron
- Formation of coagulation factors

Hepatic Vascular and Lymph Systems (p. 837)

The Rate of Blood Flow to the Liver Is High, and the Vascular Resistance Is Low. The rate of blood flow from the portal vein to the liver is approximately 1050 mL/min. An additional 300 mL/min enters the liver through the hepatic artery, so the rate of total blood flow to the liver is 1350 mL/min, or about 27% of the cardiac output. Under normal conditions, resistance to blood flow through the liver is low, as demonstrated by a 9 mm Hg pressure drop from the portal vein (average pressure 9 mm Hg) to the vena cava (average pressure 0 mm Hg). Under certain pathological conditions, such as cirrhosis (development of fibrous tissue in the liver) or blood clots in the portal vein, blood flow through the liver can be greatly impeded. The rise in vascular resistance in the liver can lead to a rise in capillary pressure throughout the splanchnic circulation, causing significant fluid loss from the capillaries of the intestinal tract, ascites, and possibly death.

Lymph Flow Rate from the Liver Is Very High. The pores of the hepatic sinusoids are extremely permeable, readily allowing passage of both proteins and fluids into the lymphatic system. The protein concentration in the lymph from the liver is approximately 6 g/dL (slightly less than the plasma protein concentration). The relatively high permeability of the liver sinusoidal epithelium allows leakage of large amounts of protein, causing large quantities of lymph to form. About half of all lymph formed in the body under normal conditions comes from the liver.

A rise in hepatic pressure (resulting from cirrhosis or congestive heart failure) causes a corresponding rise in liver lymph flow. A rise in vena cava pressure from 0 mm Hg to 15 mm Hg can increase liver lymph flow to as much as 20 times the normal rate. Under certain pathological conditions, the excess amount of lymph formed can begin to transude through the outer surface of the liver directly into the abdominal cavity, resulting in ascites.

Metabolic Functions of the Liver *(p. 839)*

Taken together, the hepatic cells comprise a large chemically reactant pool that share substrates and energy from myriad metabolic systems. The liver processes and synthesizes multiple substances that are transported to and from other areas of the body.

Carbohydrate Metabolism. The liver performs the following functions for carbohydrate metabolism:

- Stores large quantities of glycogen
- Converts galactose and fructose to glucose
- Acts as the primary site for gluconeogenesis
- Produces intermediate products of carbohydrate metabolism.

One of the major functions of the liver in carbohydrate metabolism is maintaining a normal blood glucose concentration. The liver can remove excess glucose from the blood and store it in the form of glycogen. When blood glucose levels begin to fall, the liver can convert the glycogen back to glucose; this is called the *glucose buffer function* of the liver. When the blood glucose concentration falls below normal, the liver begins to convert amino acids and glycerol to glucose through the process of gluconeogenesis in an effort to maintain a normal blood glucose concentration.

Fat Metabolism. Although almost all cells in the body metabolize fat, certain aspects of fat metabolism occur mainly in the liver:

- *β-Oxidation of fats to acetyl-coenzyme A (acetyl-CoA) occurs rapidly in the liver.* The excess acetyl-CoA formed is converted to acetoacetic acid, a highly soluble molecule that can be transported to other tissues, where it can be reconverted to acetyl-CoA and used for energy.
- *The liver synthesizes large quantities of cholesterol, phospholipids, and most lipoproteins.* About 80% of the cholesterol synthesized in the liver is converted to bile salts; the remainder is transported by lipoproteins to the tissues of the body. Phospholipids are also transported in the blood by lipoproteins. Both

cholesterol and phospholipids are used by various cells of the body to form membranes and intracellular structures.

- *Almost all of the fat synthesis from carbohydrates and proteins occurs in the liver.* The fat synthesized in this way is transported by the lipoproteins to adipose tissue for storage.

Protein Metabolism. The body cannot dispense with the services of the liver in protein metabolism for more than a few days without death ensuing. The most important functions of the liver in protein metabolism are as follows:

- *Deamination of amino acids,* which is required before they can be used for energy or converted to carbohydrates or fats. Almost all deamination of amino acids takes place in the liver.
- *Formation of urea,* which removes ammonia from the body fluids. Large amounts of ammonia are formed by the deamination process and produced by the action of gut bacteria. In the absence of this function in the liver, the plasma ammonia concentration can rise rapidly.
- *Formation of plasma proteins.* Essentially all plasma proteins are formed in the liver (with the exception of the γ-globulins, which are formed in lymphoid tissues).
- *Interconversion of the various amino acids and synthesis of metabolic compounds from amino acids.* An important function of the liver is to synthesize the nonessential amino acids and to convert amino acids into other metabolically important compounds.

Other Metabolic Functions of the Liver *(p. 840)*

The Liver Stores Vitamins and Iron. The liver has a propensity for storing vitamins and iron. It stores a sufficient quantity of vitamin D to prevent vitamin D deficiency for about 4 months, sufficient vitamin A to prevent vitamin A deficiency for approximately 10 months, and sufficient vitamin B_{12} to prevent vitamin B_{12} deficiency for 1 year.

When iron is available in extra quantities in body fluids, it combines with the protein apoferritin to form ferritin and is stored in this form in hepatic cells.

The Liver Forms Clotting Factors. The liver forms the following substances needed during the coagulation process: *fibrinogen, prothrombin, accelerator globulin,* and *factor VII.* Therefore, liver dysfunction can lead to blood coagulation abnormalities.

The Liver Metabolizes Hormones and Xenobiotics. The liver is well known for its ability to detoxify and excrete many drugs and hormones, such as estrogen, cortisol, and aldosterone. Liver damage can lead to the accumulation of drugs and hormones in the body.

Measurement of Bilirubin in Bile as a Clinical Diagnostic Tool *(p. 840)*

Bilirubin is a toxic end product of hemoglobin metabolism that is excreted in bile. When the heme portion of hemoglobin is metabolized, a substance called *biliverdin* is formed; this substance is rapidly reduced to *bilirubin,* which immediately combines with plasma albumin. This combination of plasma albumin and bilirubin is called *free bilirubin.*

Free bilirubin is absorbed by hepatic cells, where it is released from plasma albumin and conjugated with either glucuronide to form *bilirubin glucuronide* or sulfate to form *bilirubin sulfate.* The conjugated forms of bilirubin are excreted in bile into the intestine, where they are converted through bacterial action to *urobilinogen.* Urobilinogen is highly soluble, and some of the urobilinogen is reabsorbed by the intestinal mucosa into the blood. About 5% of the urobilinogen absorbed in this way is excreted in urine by the kidneys; the remaining urobilinogen is re-excreted by the liver (Fig. 70–1).

Jaundice Represents an Excess of Either Free or Conjugated Bilirubin in the Extracellular Fluid. Jaundice can be caused by (1) increased destruction of red blood cells (i.e., hemolytic jaundice) or (2) obstruction of the bile ducts or damage to the liver cells so bilirubin cannot be excreted into the gastrointestinal tract (i.e., obstructive jaundice).

With *hemolytic jaundice,* the excretory function of the liver is not impaired, but red blood cells are hemolyzed so rapidly the hepatic cells cannot excrete the bilirubin as fast as it is formed. The plasma concentration of free bilirubin rises to levels much above normal. With *obstructive jaundice* bile ducts may be obstructed by gallstones or cancer, or the hepatic cells may be damaged, as with hepatitis. The rate of bilirubin formation and the conjugation of bilirubin by the liver are

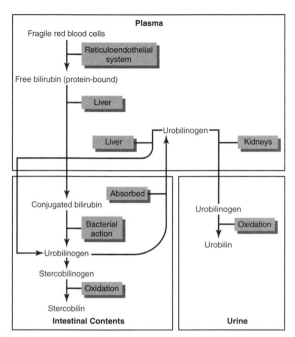

Figure 70–1. Bilirubin formation and excretion.

near normal, but conjugated bilirubin cannot pass into the intestines. With obstructive jaundice the level of conjugated bilirubin in the blood rises, so most of the bilirubin in the plasma is the conjugated form rather than the free form.

CHAPTER 71

Dietary Balances; Regulation of Feeding; Obesity and Starvation; Vitamins and Minerals

Energy Intake and Output Are Balanced Under Steady-State Conditions. Intake of carbohydrates, proteins, and fats provides energy that can be used to perform various functions in the body or stored for later use. The stability of body composition over long periods of time requires that energy intake be balanced with energy expenditure. When a person is overfed and intake of energy persistently exceeds expenditure, most of the excess energy is stored as fat, and the body weight increases; conversely, loss of body mass and starvation occur when energy intake is insufficient to meet the body's metabolic needs.

Energy Is Available in Carbohydrates, Fats, and Proteins. The approximate energy liberated from each gram of carbohydrate as it is oxidized to carbon dioxide and water is 4.1 calories. The amount of energy liberated from fat is 9.3 calories per gram and from protein 4.35 calories per gram.

Average Americans receive about 15% of their energy from protein, 40%, and 45% from carbohydrates. In non-Western diets most of the energy comes from carbohydrates; proteins and fats comprise only 15% to 20% of the total energy consumed.

The Average Daily Protein Requirement is 30 to 50 g. About 20 to 30 g of protein per day are degraded by the body to manufacture other compounds, so all cells must continue to form new proteins to take the place of those being destroyed. *The average person can maintain normal protein stores when consuming 30 to 50 g of protein per day.*

Some proteins have inadequate amounts of certain *essential amino acids* and cannot replace the degraded proteins. Proteins that lack the essential amino acids are called *partial proteins*. For example, cornmeal lacks the amino acid *tryptophan.* A person consuming cornmeal as the only source of protein develops a protein-deficient syndrome called *kwashiorkor,* which consists of failure to grow, depressed mentality, and low plasma protein that, in turn, leads to severe edema.

Methods for Determining Utilization of Nutrients by the Body (p. 844)

The Respiratory Quotient Is the Carbon Dioxide Output to Oxygen Utilization Ratio. When carbohydrates are metabolized with oxygen, one carbon dioxide molecule is formed for every molecule of oxygen consumed. For carbohydrates, the respiratory quotient is 1.0. When fat is metabolized with oxygen, 7 carbon dioxide molecules are formed for every 10 molecules of oxygen consumed, so the respiratory quotient for fat metabolism is 0.70. For proteins, the respiratory quotient is 0.80.

The respiratory quotient can be an index of the relative utilization of various foods by the body. A person metabolizing mostly fat would have a respiratory quotient close to 0.70, whereas a person metabolizing mostly carbohydrates would have a respiratory quotient close to 1.0.

Nitrogen Balance Is an Index of the Quantity of Protein Breakdown Each Day. The average protein contains about 16% nitrogen. During protein metabolism, about 90% of this nitrogen is excreted in urine in the form of *urea* and *creatinine*. The remaining 10% is excreted in feces. The amount of protein breakdown (in grams) can be estimated by measuring the amount of nitrogen in urine, adding 10% for fecal excretion, and multiplying by 6.25 (100/16). Therefore, excretion of 8 g of nitrogen in the urine each day means that there has been about 55 g of protein breakdown.

If the daily intake of protein is less than the daily breakdown of protein, the person is said to have a *negative nitrogen balance*. This indicates that the body stores of protein are decreasing.

Regulation of Food Intake and Energy Storage (p. 845)

Only about 27% of the energy ingested normally reaches the functional systems of the cells, and much of this is eventually converted to heat generated by protein metabolism, muscle activity, and activities of the various organs and tissues of the body. Energy intake in excess of that needed to perform body functions is stored mainly as fat or glycogen. A deficit of energy intake will cause consumption of stored energy until the energy expenditure equals energy intake—or death occurs. Maintenance of an adequate energy supply in the body is so critical that there are multiple short-term and long-term control systems that regulate not only food intake but also energy expenditure and energy stores.

Neural Centers Regulate Food Intake (p. 845)

- *Hunger* is the intrinsic desire for food. It is associated with several physiological effects, such as rhythmic contractions of the stomach and restlessness.
- *Appetite* is the desire for a particular type of food. It is useful for helping a person choose the quality of food to be eaten.
- *Satiety* is the opposite of hunger. It is the feeling of fullness after intake of food.

The Hypothalamus Contains Hunger and Satiety Centers. Stimulation of the *lateral hypothalamic nuclei* induces eating behaviors; this area is referred to as the *feeding center*. Stimulation of the *ventromedial hypothalamic nuclei* induces satiety, making this area of the hypothalamus the *satiety center*. Lesions of these areas produce voracious and continued eating until the animal becomes extremely obese. Other areas of the brain, especially the paraventricular, dorsomedial, and arcuate nuclei of the hypothalamus, also play a major role in regulating food intake, and there is considerable chemical cross-talk among the neurons of the hypothalamus.

The hypothalamus receives neural signals from the gastrointestinal tract that provide sensory information about stomach filling, chemical signals from nutrients in the blood (glucose, amino acids, fatty acids) that signify satiety, signals from gastrointestinal hormones, signals from hormones released by adipose tissue, and signals from the cerebral cortex (sight, smell, taste) that influence feeding behavior (Fig. 71–1).

Neurons and Neurotransmitters in the Hypothalamus Can Stimulate or Inhibit Feeding. There are two distinct types of neuron in the arcuate nuclei of the hypothalamus that are especially important as controllers of appetite as well as energy expenditure: (1) *pro-opiomelanocortin (POMC) neurons* that produce α-melanocyte-stimulating hormone (α-MSH) together with cocaine- and amphetamine-related transcript (CART) and (2) *neurons that produce neuropeptide Y* (NPY) and *agouti-related*

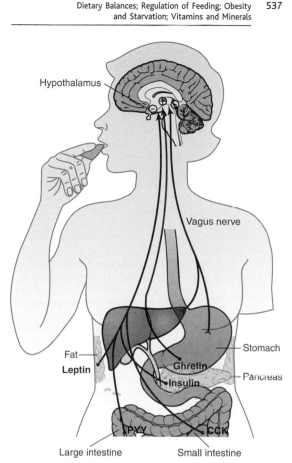

Figure 71–1. Feedback mechanisms for controlling food intake. Stretch receptors in the stomach activate sensory afferent pathways in the vagus nerve and inhibit food intake. Peptide YY (PYY), cholecystokinin (CCK), and insulin are gastrointestinal hormones that are released by the ingestion of food and suppress further feeding. Ghrelin is released by the stomach, especially during fasting, and stimulates appetite. Leptin is a hormone produced in increasing amounts by fat cells as they increase in size. It inhibits food intake.

protein (AGRP). Activation of the POMC neurons decreases food intake and increases energy expenditure, whereas activation of the NPY/AGRP neurons increases food intake and reduces energy expenditure. These neurons are major targets for the actions of several hormones that regulate appetite, including *leptin, insulin, cholecystokinin* (CCK), and *ghrelin* (Table 71–1).

The hypothalamic POMC neurons play a powerful role in regulating energy stores of the body, and defective signaling of the melanocortin pathway is associated with extreme obesity. In fact, mutations of the *MCR-4* represent the most common known monogenic (single gene) cause of human obesity, and some studies suggest that *MCR-4* mutations account for as much as 5% to 6% of early-onset severe obesity in children.

NPY, released from neurons of the arcuate nuclei when energy stores of the body are low, stimulates appetite. At the same time, firing of the POMC neurons is reduced, thereby reducing activity of the melanocortin pathway and further stimulating appetite.

Neural Centers Control the Mechanical Process of Feeding. Another important aspect of feeding is the mechanical act of the feeding process itself. The mechanics of feeding, such as chewing, swallowing, and salivating, are controlled by centers in the brain stem.

Table 71–1. Neurotransmitters and Hormones That Influence Feeding and Satiety Centers in the Hypothalamus

Decrease Feeding (Anorexogenic)	Increase Feeding (Orexogenic)
α-MSH	Neuropeptide Y (NPY)
Leptin	Agouti-related protein (AGRP)
Serotonin	Melanin-concentrating hormone (MCH)
Norepinephrine	Orexins A and B
Corticotropin-releasing hormone	Endorphins
Insulin	Galanin (GAL)
Cholecystokinin (CCK)	Amino acids (glutamate and γ-aminobutyric acid)
Glucagon-like peptide (GLP)	Cortisol
Cocaine and amphetamine regulated transcript (CART)	Ghrelin
Peptide YY (PYY)	Endocannabinoids

α-MSH = α-melanocyte-stimulating hormone.

The function of the higher centers in feeding is to control the quantity of food intake and to stimulate the lower feeding mechanics centers to activity.

The *prefrontal cortex* and *amygdala* are also thought to play important roles in the control of appetite. The activities of these centers are closely coupled with those of the hypothalamus. Bilateral destruction of the amygdala produces a "psychic blindness" in the choice of foods and an inability to control the type or quality of the food consumed.

Factors That Regulate Quantity of Food Intake (p. 848)

Regulation of quantity of food intake can be divided into *short-term regulation,* which is concerned with the prevention of overeating at each meal, and *long-term regulation,* which is concerned with the long-term maintenance of normal quantities of energy stores in the body.

Short-Term Regulation of Food Intake Is Accomplished through Several Feedback Signals from the Alimentary Tract. Distention of the stomach and duodenum causes inhibitory signals to be transmitted to the feeding center by way of the *vagi,* reducing the desire for food. The gastrointestinal hormone *cholecystokinin* (CCK), which is released in response to fat entering the duodenum, activates receptors on local sensory nerves in the duodenum, sending messages to the brain, via the vagus nerve, that contribute to satiation and meal cessation. The effect of CCK is short-lived and chronic administration of CCK by itself has no major effect on body weight. Therefore, CCK functions mainly to prevent overeating during meals but may not play a major role in the frequency of meals or the total energy consumed.

Intermediate-Term and Long-Term Regulation of Food Intake May Be Related to the Concentration of Glucose, Lipids, and Amino Acids in the Blood and the Hormones Released from Adipose Tissue. An increase or a decrease in the blood concentration of nutrients causes a corresponding decrease or increase in food intake. Our knowledge of the long-term regulation of food intake is imprecise, but in general when energy stores of the body fall below normal the feeding centers become active. When energy stores are adequate (mainly the fat store), the satiety centers become active, and a person loses the desire for food.

Experimental studies suggest that the hypothalamus senses energy storage through the actions of *leptin*, a peptide hormone released from adipocytes. When the amount of adipose tissue increases (signaling excess energy storage), the adipocytes produce increased amounts of leptin, which is released into the blood and acts at multiple sites in the hypothalamus. Leptin especially activates the POMC neurons and inhibits NPY neurons of the arcuate nuclei, and both of these actions reduce food intake. In mice or humans with mutations that render their fat cells unable to produce leptin or mutations that cause defective leptin receptors in the hypothalamus, marked hyperphagia and morbid obesity occur. However, leptin gene mutations are rare and most obese persons have high levels of leptin. Therefore failure of elevated leptin levels to suppress appetite in obese persons has been suggested to be related, at least partially, to "resistance" of the hypothalamus to leptin's anorexogenic actions.

Obesity (p. 850)

Obesity can be defined as an excess of body fat. A surrogate marker for body fat content is the body mass index (BMI), which is calculated as: BMI = weight (kg)/height (m^2). In clinical terms, a person with a BMI between 25.0 and 29.9 kg/m^2 is called overweight, and one with a BMI greater than 30 kg/m^2 is considered to be obese. However, BMI is not a direct estimate of adiposity and does not take into account the fact that some individuals may have a high BMI resulting from a large muscle mass.

Obesity Results from a Greater Energy Intake Than Energy Expenditure. The excess caloric intake results in an increase in fat stores and a corresponding increase in body weight. For each 9.3 calories of excess energy that enters the body, 1 g of fat is stored. Once a person becomes obese and a stable weight is obtained, energy intake once again equals energy output. For a person to reduce body weight, energy intake must be *less* than the energy expenditure.

The causes of obesity are complex and poorly understood. Although genes play an important role in determining food intake or energy metabolism, low physical activity caused by a sedentary lifestyle and other environmental factors may play the dominant role in many obese people, as evidenced by the rapid increase in the prevalence of obesity during the past 20 to 30 years.

Inanition, Anorexia, Cachexia, Starvation (p. 851)

Inanition is the opposite of obesity and is characterized by extreme weight loss. It can be caused by inadequate food availability or by pathophysiological conditions that greatly decrease the desire for food, including psychogenic disturbances, hypothalamic abnormalities, and factors released from peripheral tissues. With serious diseases such as cancer, the reduced desire for food may be associated with increased energy expenditure, causing serious weight loss.

Anorexia is a reduction in food intake caused primarily by diminished appetite. This can occur with diseases such as cancer where other common problems, such as pain and nausea, may cause a person to consume less food. *Anorexia nervosa* is an abnormal psychic state in which a person loses all desire for food and even becomes nauseated by it; as a result, severe inanition occurs.

Cachexia is a metabolic disorder of increased energy expenditure leading to weight loss greater than that caused by reduced food intake alone. Anorexia and cachexia often occur together with many types of cancer or with the "wasting syndrome" observed in patients with acquired immunodeficiency syndrome (AIDS) and chronic inflammatory disorders.

Central neural and peripheral factors are believed to contribute to cancer-induced anorexia and cachexia. For example, inflammatory cytokines, such as *tumor necrosis factor-α*, released by cancerous tissues, cause anorexia and cachexia in part by activation of POMC neurons in the hypothalamus.

Starvation results when food intake is chronically insufficient to meet the metabolic needs of the body. During starvation, the energy stores of the body are depleted at different rates. Carbohydrate stores (glycogen) are depleted within 12 to 24 hours. Fat is the main source of energy during starvation, and it is depleted at a constant rate. Proteins are used rapidly at first as they are converted to glucose through the process of gluconeogenesis. As starvation continues and the readily available stores of protein are exhausted, the rate of gluconeogenesis is reduced to about one fourth its previous rate, and the rate of protein depletion is greatly reduced.

When almost all the available fat stores become depleted, the rate of protein utilization increases, as the proteins become the only remaining energy source. Because proteins are essential to the maintenance of cellular function, death ordinarily occurs when the body's proteins are depleted to about one half their normal level.

Vitamins (p. 852)

Vitamins are organic compounds that are needed in small quantities for normal metabolism. Vitamins cannot be synthesized in the cells of the body and therefore must be supplied in the diet. Vitamin deficiency causes specific metabolic deficits.

Vitamin A Occurs in Animal Tissues as Retinol. Vitamin A does not occur in foods of vegetable origin, although provitamins for the formation of vitamin A occur in abundance in many vegetables. These provitamins can be converted to vitamin A in the liver. The basic function of vitamin A in metabolism is not clear except in relation to its use in the formation of retinal pigments in the eye. Vitamin A deficiency causes (1) night blindness, (2) scaliness of the skin and acne, (3) failure of skeletal growth in young animals, and (4) failure of reproduction.

Thiamine (Vitamin B$_1$) Is Needed for the Final Metabolism of Carbohydrates and Many Amino Acids. Thiamine operates in metabolic systems of the body as a co-carboxylase in conjunction with a protein decarboxylase for decarboxylation of pyruvic acid and other α-keto acids. Thiamine deficiency *(beriberi)* causes decreased utilization of pyruvate and some amino acids by the tissues; it can affect the central nervous system, cardiovascular system, and gastrointestinal tract.

Niacin (Nicotinic Acid) Functions in the Body as a Hydrogen Acceptor. Niacin in the form of *nicotinamide adenine dinucleotide* (NAD) and *nicotinamide adenine dinucleotide phosphate* (NADP) functions as a coenzyme in the metabolic cascades. When a niacin deficiency exists, the normal rate of dehydrogenation cannot be maintained. Oxidative delivery of energy from food to the functional elements of the cells cannot occur at normal rates. Niacin deficiency *(pellagra)* causes lesions of the central nervous system, irritation and inflammation of the mucous membranes, muscle weakness, poor glandular secretion, and gastrointestinal hemorrhage.

Riboflavin (Vitamin B_2) Functions as a Hydrogen Carrier. Riboflavin combines with phosphoric acid to form *flavin adenine dinucleotide* (FAD), which operates as a hydrogen carrier of the important oxidative systems of the body. Riboflavin deficiencies can cause many of the same effects as a lack of niacin in the diet. These debilities result from a generalized depression of the oxidative process in the cells.

Vitamin B_{12} Functions as a Hydrogen Acceptor Coenzyme. Perhaps the most important function of vitamin B_{12} is its ability to act as a coenzyme for reducing ribonucleotides to deoxyribonucleotides, a step necessary for the replication of genes. Vitamin B_{12} is important for red blood cell formation, growth, and maturation. Vitamin B_{12} deficiency leads to poor growth and *pernicious anemia,* a type of anemia caused by failure of red blood cell maturation.

Vitamin B_{12} deficiency is not caused by lack of this substance in foods but, rather, by a deficiency of *intrinsic factor.* Intrinsic factor is normally secreted by the parietal cells of the gastric glands and is essential to the absorption of vitamin B_{12} by the ileal mucosa.

Folic Acid (Pteroylglutamic Acid) Is a Potent Promoter of Growth and Maturation of Red Blood Cells. One of the significant effects of folic acid deficiency is the development of *macrocytic anemia,* an anemia almost identical to pernicious anemia.

Pyridoxine (Vitamin B_6) Is a Coenzyme for Many Chemical Reactions Related to Amino Acid and Protein Metabolism. The most important role of pyridoxine is that of a coenzyme in the transamination process for the synthesis of amino acids. Pyridoxine deficiency can cause dermatitis, decreased rate of growth, development of a fatty liver, anemia, and evidence of mental deterioration.

Pantothenic Acid Is Incorporated in the Body into *Coenzyme A* (CoA). A lack of pantothenic acid can lead to depressed metabolism of both carbohydrates and fats.

Ascorbic Acid (Vitamin C) Is Essential for Collagen Formation. Ascorbic acid activates the enzyme *prolyl hydroxylase,* which promotes the hydroxylation step in the formation of *hydroxyproline,* an integral component of collagen. Without ascorbic acid, the collagen fibers are defective and weak. This vitamin is essential for the growth and strength of collagen fibers in subcutaneous tissue, cartilage, bone, and teeth. Deficiency of ascorbic acid *(scurvy)* results in failure of wounds to heal, inhibition of bone growth, and petechial hemorrhages throughout the body.

Vitamin D Increases Calcium Absorption from the Gastrointestinal Tract and Helps Control Calcium Deposition in Bone. Vitamin D promotes active transport of calcium through the epithelium of the ileum. Vitamin D deficiency *(rickets)* causes abnormalities of calcium metabolism, which can affect the strength and growth of bones.

Vitamin E Prevents Oxidation of Unsaturated Fats. In the absence of vitamin E, the quantity of unsaturated fats in cells becomes diminished, causing abnormal structure and function of the mitochondria, lysosomes, and cell membranes.

Vitamin K Is Necessary for the Formation of Clotting Factors. Synthesis of *prothrombin, factor VII, factor IX,* and *factor X* in the liver requires vitamin K. Deficiency of vitamin K causes retardation of blood clotting. Vitamin K is normally synthesized by bacteria in the colon and absorbed by the colonic epithelium.

Mineral Metabolism *(p. 855)*

The functions of minerals such as sodium, potassium, and chloride are presented in other parts of the book. Only a few minerals, including magnesium, calcium, phosphorus, and iron, are discussed in this chapter.

- *Magnesium* is required as a catalyst for many intracellular enzymatic reactions, particularly those related to carbohydrate metabolism.
- *Calcium* is present in the body mainly in the form of calcium phosphate in the bone.
- *Phosphorus* is the major anion of extracellular fluids. *Phosphates* have the ability to combine reversibly with many of the coenzyme systems necessary for operation of the metabolic processes.
- *Iron* functions in the body as a carrier of oxygen and as an electron acceptor; it is absolutely essential to both the transport of oxygen to tissues and the operation of oxidative systems in tissue cells.

Trace Elements. *Iodine, zinc,* and *fluorine* are present in the body in such small quantities that they are called *trace elements.* Iodine is important for the formation and function of thyroid hormone. Zinc is an important component of *carbonic anhydrase,* the enzyme responsible for the rapid combination of carbon dioxide and water in the blood, gastrointestinal mucosa, and kidney tubules. Zinc also is a component of *lactic dehydrogenase*, which is important for the interconversions of pyruvic acid and lactic acid. Fluorine does not seem to be necessary for metabolism but does function to prevent tooth decay.

CHAPTER 72

Energetics and Metabolic Rate

The intracellular substance used to energize almost all cellular functions is *adenosine triphosphate* (ATP). ATP is often referred to as the "energy currency" of metabolism. It energizes the synthesis of cellular components, muscle contraction, active transport across membranes, glandular secretions, and nerve conduction.

Phosphocreatine Serves as an "ATP Buffer." Phosphocreatine, another substance that contains high-energy phosphate bonds, is present in cells in quantities several times as great as ATP. Phosphocreatine cannot act in the same manner as ATP as a direct coupling agent for the transfer of energy between food substances and functional cellular systems; however, phosphocreatine can transfer energy interchangeably with ATP. Phosphocreatine is synthesized when extra amounts of ATP are available; this builds a storehouse of energy in the form of phosphocreatine. When ATP utilization increases, the energy in phosphocreatine is transferred rapidly back to ATP. This effect keeps the concentration of ATP at an almost constant level for as long as any phosphocreatine remains.

Anaerobic Versus Aerobic Energy *(p. 860)*

Anaerobic energy is energy derived from food without using oxygen. Aerobic energy is energy derived from food by oxidative metabolism. Under anaerobic conditions, carbohydrates are the only significant source of energy. In fact, glycogen is the best source of energy under anaerobic conditions because it is already phosphorylated, whereas glucose must be phosphorylated (a step requiring expenditure of energy) before it can be used.

Anaerobic Energy Is Used during Strenuous Bursts of Activity. Oxidative processes are too slow to provide the energy required for a strenuous burst of activity. Such energy must be supplied from (1) the ATP already present in muscle cells, (2) phosphocreatine, and (3) glycolytic breakdown of glycogen to lactic acid.

Extra Oxygen Consumption "Repays" the Oxygen Debt after Completion of Strenuous Activity. After a period of strenuous exercise, a person continues to breathe hard and consume extra amounts of oxygen for a few minutes. This excess oxygen is used to (1) reconvert the accumulated lactic acid back to glucose, (2) reconvert adenosine monophosphate (AMP) and adenosine diphosphate (ADP) to ATP, (3) re-establish phosphocreatine levels, (4) re-establish normal concentrations of oxygen bound to hemoglobin and myoglobin, and (5) increase the oxygen concentration in the lungs back to normal levels.

Metabolic Rate *(p. 862)*

The metabolic rate is normally expressed in terms of the rate of heat liberation during the chemical reactions in all cells of the body. Heat is the end product of almost all of the energy released in the body. On the average, 35% of the energy in foods becomes heat during ATP formation. More energy becomes heat as it is transferred from ATP to the functional systems of the body. Under the best conditions, approximately 27% of all the energy from food is used by the functional systems, and almost all of this energy eventually becomes heat. The only significant exception is when muscles are used to perform some form of work outside the body, such as elevating an object or walking up steps. In these cases, energy is created by elevating the object (or mass) against gravity. When external expenditure of energy is not taking place, it is safe to assume that all the energy released by the metabolic processes eventually becomes body heat.

The *calorie* is the unit used for expressing the quantity of energy released from foods or expended by the functional processes of the body. The *gram calorie* is the quantity of heat required to increase the temperature of 1 g of water 1° C. The gram calorie is much too small a unit for ease of expression when speaking of energy in the body, so the "large calorie" (sometimes spelled with a capital "C" and often called the *kilocalorie,* which is equivalent to 1000 calories) is the unit ordinarily used when discussing energy metabolism.

Measurement of Metabolic Rate. Because a person is ordinarily not performing external work, the whole body metabolic rate can be determined by measuring the total quantity of heat liberated from the body within a given time. *Direct calorimetry,* which measures the quantity of heat liberated in a specially constructed chamber, is difficult to perform and is used mainly for research purposes. Other indirect methods are therefore used to determine the metabolic rate. One of the most accurate indirect methods is to determine the rate of oxygen utilization. For the average diet, the quantity of energy liberated per liter of oxygen consumed in the body is about 4.825 Calories. This is called the *energy equivalent* of oxygen. With this equivalent, one can calculate, with a high degree of precision, the rate of heat liberated in the body from the quantity of oxygen used during a given period of time.

Basal Metabolic Rate Is the Minimum Energy Expenditure Required for the Body to Exist. The basal metabolic rate is a measure of the inherent metabolic rate of the tissues independent of exercise or other extraneous factors; it is the rate of energy utilization in the body during absolute rest while the person is awake. The usual method for determining the basal metabolic rate is to measure the rate of oxygen utilization during a given period of time. The basal metabolic rate is then calculated in terms of calories per hour. The basal metabolic rate normally averages about 60 Calories/hour in young men and about 53 Calories/hour in young women. To correct for body size, the basal metabolic rate is normally expressed in proportion to the body surface area; this allows comparison of basal metabolic rates among individuals of different sizes.

Factors That Affect the Metabolic Rate

When an average 70-kg man lies in bed all day, he uses approximately 1650 Calories of energy. The performance of other basic functions, such as sitting in a chair and eating, increases the amount of energy used. The daily energy requirement for simply existing (i.e., performing essential functions only) is about 2000 Calories/day.

Several factors can raise or lower the metabolic rate. The metabolic rate increases after a meal is ingested; this is mainly the result of the stimulatory effect of amino acids derived from the proteins of the ingested food on the chemical processes in the cell. Thyroid hormone, male sex hormone, growth hormone, sympathetic stimulation, and fever all increase the metabolic rate. Sleep, malnutrition, and age all decrease the metabolic rate.

CHAPTER 73

Body Temperature Regulation, and Fever

Normal Body Temperatures *(p. 867)*

The temperature of the deep tissues of the body (core temperature) remains constant within $\pm 1°$ F ($\pm 0.6°$ C) despite large fluctuations in the environmental temperature. The average normal body temperature is generally thought to be between 98.0° F and 98.6° F when measured orally and about 1° F higher rectally.

Body Temperature Is Controlled by the Balance between Heat Production and Heat Loss. Heat production is a byproduct of metabolism. Extra heat can be generated by muscle contraction (shivering) in the short term or by an increase in thyroxine in the long term. Most of the heat produced in the body is generated in the deep tissues. The rate of heat loss is determined by the rate of heat conduction to the skin and the rate of heat conduction from the skin to the surroundings.

Blood Flow to the Skin from the Body Core Provides Heat Transfer. Blood vessels are distributed profusely immediately underneath the skin. An increase in blood flow to these vessels causes more heat loss, and a decrease in blood flow to these vessels causes less heat loss. The rate of flow to these vessels can vary from 0% to 30% of the cardiac output. The skin is a highly effective "heat radiator" system for transferring heat from the body core to the skin.

Heat Loss

Heat loss from the skin to the surroundings occurs by *radiation, conduction, convection,* and *evaporation.*

Radiation Causes Loss of Heat in the Form of Infrared Rays. All objects above absolute zero radiate infrared waves in all directions. If the body temperature is greater than that of the surroundings, the body radiates heat to the surroundings. Conversely, if the body temperature is lower than that of the surroundings, the surroundings radiate heat to the body. About 60% of body heat is normally lost through radiation.

Conductive Heat Loss Occurs by Direct Contact with an Object. The body usually loses about 3% of its heat by conduction to objects. An additional 15% of body heat is lost by conduction to air; the air in contact with the surface of the skin warms to near body temperature. This warm air has a tendency to rise away from the skin.

Convective Heat Loss Results from Air Movement.
The air next to the skin surface is warmed by conduction. When this warm air is removed, the skin conducts heat to the "new" layer of unwarmed air.

Convective heat loss is the mechanism for the cooling effect of wind. The cooling effect of water is similar. Because water has such a high specific heat, however, the skin cannot warm a thin layer of water next to the body. As a consequence, heat is continuously removed from the body if the water is below body temperature.

Evaporation Is a Necessary Mechanism of Heat Loss at Very High Temperatures. As water evaporates, 0.58 calorie of heat is lost for each gram of water converted to the gaseous state. The energy to change water from a liquid to a gas is derived from the body temperature.

Evaporation usually accounts for 22% of the heat lost by the body; evaporation of water through the skin (insensible water loss) accounts for about 16 to 19 calories of heat loss per hour.

Evaporative heat loss is very important when the environmental temperatures are at or near body temperature. Under these conditions, heat loss by radiation diminishes greatly. Evaporative heat loss becomes the only way to cool the body when environmental temperatures are high.

Air movement across the skin increases the rate of evaporation and as a result increases the effectiveness of evaporative heat loss (e.g., the cooling effect of a fan).

Sweating and Its Regulation by the Autonomic Nervous System (p. 870)

Sweat glands contain a deep, coiled glandular portion and a straight ductal portion that exits on the surface of the skin. A *primary secretion* similar to plasma but without plasma proteins is formed by the glandular portion of the sweat gland. As the solution moves up the duct toward the surface of the skin, most of the electrolytes are reabsorbed, leaving a dilute, watery secretion.

Sweat glands are innervated by *sympathetic cholinergic fibers.* When sweat glands are stimulated, the rate of precursor solution secretion is increased. The reabsorption of electrolytes occurs at a constant rate. If large volumes of precursor solution are secreted and at the same time electrolyte reabsorption remains constant, more electrolytes (primarily sodium chloride) are lost in the sweat.

The Sweating Mechanism Can Adapt to Meet Environmental Needs. Exposure to a hot climate causes an
increase in the maximum rate of sweat production
from about 1 L/hr in the nonacclimatized person to as
much as 2 to 3 L/hr in the acclimatized individual. This
larger amount of sweat increases the rate of evaporative
heat loss and helps maintain normal body temperature.
Associated with an increase in the rate of sweat production is a decrease in the sodium chloride content
of the sweat; this allows better conservation of body
salt. The decline in the sodium chloride content of
the sweat is primarily the result of increased secretion
of *aldosterone,* which enhances sodium reabsorption
from the ductal portion of the sweat gland.

Regulation of Body Temperature—Role of the Hypothalamus *(p. 871)*

The *anterior hypothalamic-preoptic area* contains large
numbers of heat-sensitive neurons; the septum and reticular substance of the midbrain contain large numbers of
cold-sensitive neurons. When the temperature centers
detect that the body is either too hot or too cold, these
areas institute appropriate and familiar temperature-
increasing or temperature-decreasing procedures.

Temperature-Decreasing Mechanisms. Three important mechanisms are used to cool the body:

- *Vasodilatation* of the blood vessels of the skin can
  increase the amount of heat transfer to the skin by
  as much as eightfold.
- *Sweating* increases the rate of evaporative heat loss. A
  1° C increase in body temperature induces sufficient
  sweating to remove 10 times the basal rate of heat
  production.
- *Strong inhibition of mechanisms that increase heat
  production takes place,* such as shivering and chemical thermogenesis.

Temperature-Increasing   Mechanisms. When   the
body is too cold, the temperature control systems initiate mechanisms to reduce heat loss and increase heat
production:

- *Vasoconstriction* of the blood vessels of the skin,
  which decreases transfer of heat from the core of
  the body
- *Piloerection,* which raises the hair to trap air next to
  the skin and create a layer of warm air that acts as

an insulator. This mechanism works best in animals that have a complete layer of fur. The vestiges of this system are present in humans (goosebumps), but the effectiveness of this mechanism in humans is limited because of the relative sparseness of body hair.

- *Greater heat production by metabolic systems* such as sympathetic excitation of heat production, increased thyroxine secretion, and shivering. Shivering can increase the rate of heat production by four- to five-fold. The primary *motor center for shivering* is located in the dorsomedial portion of the posterior hypothalamus; this area is inhibited by an increase in body temperature and stimulated by a decrease in body temperature. The output signals from this area are not rhythmic and do not cause the actual muscle shaking; instead, the output signals from this area cause a generalized increase in muscle tone. The greater muscle tone sets up an oscillation in the muscle spindle reflex, which leads to muscle shaking. During maximum shivering, body heat production can rise to four to five times normal.

Set Point for Temperature Control. The body maintains a critical core temperature of 37.1° C. When body temperature increases above this level, heat-losing mechanisms are initiated. When body temperature falls below this level, heat-generating mechanisms are initiated. This critical temperature is called the *set point* of the temperature control system. All temperature control mechanisms continually attempt to bring the body temperature back to this level.

Behavioral Control of Body Temperature

The body has another temperature-control mechanism—*behavioral control of temperature*, which can be explained as follows: Whenever the internal body temperature becomes too high, the temperature-controlling areas in the brain give the person a psychic sensation of being overheated. Conversely, whenever the body becomes too cold, signals from the skin and from some deep body receptors elicit the feeling of cold discomfort. Therefore the person makes appropriate environmental adjustments to re-establish comfort, such as moving into a heated room or wearing well-insulated clothing in freezing weather. This is a powerful system of body temperature control and is the only really effective mechanism to maintain body heat control in severely cold environments.

Abnormalities of Body Temperature Regulation (p. 875)

Fever Is a Body Temperature above Normal. An elevation in body temperature may be caused by an abnormality in the brain itself or by toxic substances that affect the temperature-regulating centers. Fever results from a resetting of the set point for temperature control; this resetting can be the result of proteins, protein breakdown products, or bacterial toxins (lipopolysaccharides), collectively called *pyrogens.* Some pyrogens act directly on the temperature control center, but most act indirectly.

When bacterial or viral particles are present in the body, they are phagocytized by *leukocytes, tissue macrophages,* and *large granular killer lymphocytes.* In response to the phagocytized particles, these cells release *cytokines,* a diverse group of peptide signaling molecules involved in the innate and adaptive immune responses. One of the most important of these cytokines in causing fever is *interleukin-1.* Interleukin-1 induces the formation of prostaglandin E2, which acts on the hypothalamus to elicit the fever reaction. When prostaglandin formation is blocked by drugs, the fever is completely abrogated or at least reduced. This is the proposed mechanism of action for *aspirin* and other antipyretics to reduce the level of fever, and it explains why these compounds do not lower the body temperature in a normal, healthy person (who does not have elevated levels of interleukin-1).

When the interleukin-1 mechanism resets the set point for temperature control, body temperature is maintained at a higher level. Raising the set point of body temperature induces the subjective sensations of being cold, and nervous mechanisms initiate shivering and piloerection. Once the body temperature has reached the new set point, the individual no longer has the subjective sensation of being cold, and body temperature is elevated above normal. When the pyrogens have been cleared from the body, the set point for temperature control returns to normal levels. At this point, the body temperature is too warm, which induces the subjective sensations of being too hot, and nervous mechanisms initiate vasodilatation of the skin blood vessels and sweating. This sudden change of events in a febrile state is known as the "crisis" or, more appropriately, the "flush" and typically signals that the temperature will soon be decreasing.

Endocrinology and Reproduction

CHAPTER 74

Introduction to Endocrinology

Coordination of Body Functions by Chemical Messengers *(p. 881)*

The types of intercellular communication by chemical messengers in the extracellular fluid include the following:

- *Neural,* in which neurotransmitters are released at synaptic junctions and act locally
- *Endocrine,* in which hormones released from specialized glands or cells reach the circulating blood and influence the function of target cells some distance away
- *Neuroendocrine (neurocrine),* in which secretion products from neurons *(neurohormones)* reach the circulating blood and influence the function of target cells some distance away
- *Paracrine,* in which cell secretion products diffuse into the extracellular fluid and affect neighboring target cells
- *Autocrine,* in which cell secretion products affect the function of the same cell by binding to cell surface receptors
- *Cytokine,* in which secreted cell proteins function as autocrines, paracrines, or endocrines and often act on a broad spectrum of target cells

Maintenance of Homeostasis and Regulation of Body Processes

In many instances, neural and endocrine control of body processes is achieved through interactions between these two systems. These systems are linked by *neuroendocrine cells* located in the hypothalamus whose axons terminate in the posterior pituitary gland and median eminence. The *neurohormones* secreted from these neuroendocrine cells include *antidiuretic hormone* (ADH), *oxytocin,* and *hypophysiotropic hormones* (which control secretion of the anterior pituitary hormones). Hormones and neurohormones play a critical role in the regulation of almost all aspects of body function, including metabolism, growth and development, water and electrolyte balance, reproduction, and behavior.

Chemistry, Synthesis, Storage, and Secretion of Hormones *(p. 881)*

Hormones Classified According to Chemical Structure

Chemically, hormones and neurohormones are of three types:

- *Proteins and peptides.* Included in this group are peptides ranging from as small as three amino acids (thyrotropin-releasing hormone) to proteins almost 200 amino acids long (growth hormone and prolactin).
- *Steroids.* These are derivatives of cholesterol and include the adrenocortical (cortisol, aldosterone) and gonadal (testosterone, estrogen, progesterone) hormones.
- *Derivatives of the amino acid tyrosine.* Included in this group are hormones from the thyroid gland (thyroxine, triiodothyronine) and adrenal medulla (epinephrine and norepinephrine).

Synthesis, Storage, and Secretion of Hormones

Protein/Peptide Hormones Are Synthesized Like Most Proteins. Protein/peptide hormones are synthesized on the rough endoplasmic reticulum in the same fashion as most other proteins. Typically, the initial protein formed by the endoplasmic reticulum is larger than the active hormone and is called a *preprohormone.* The signal sequence of this large protein is cleaved in the endoplasmic reticulum to form a prohormone. Subsequently, in the Golgi apparatus the prohormone is packaged in secretion granules along with proteolytic enzymes that cleave the prohormone into active hormone and other fragments. When the endocrine cell is stimulated, the secretion granules migrate from the cytoplasm to the cell membrane. Free hormone and co-peptides are then released into the extracellular fluid by exocytosis.

Steroid Hormones Are Synthesized from Cholesterol. In contrast to protein/peptide hormones, there is little hormone storage in steroid-producing endocrine cells. Typically, there are large stores of cholesterol esters in cytoplasmic vacuoles that can be rapidly mobilized for synthesis of steroid hormones after stimulation of the steroid-producing cell. Once the steroid hormone appears in the cytoplasm, storage does not take place, and the hormone diffuses through the cell membrane into the extracellular fluid. Much of the cholesterol in steroid-producing cells is removed from the plasma, but there is also de novo synthesis of cholesterol from acetate.

Thyroid Hormones and Catecholamines Are Synthesized from Tyrosine. As with steroid hormones, there is no storage of thyroid hormones in discrete granules, and once thyroid hormones appear in the cytoplasm of the cell they leave the cell via diffusion through the cell membrane. In contrast to steroid hormones, there are large stores of thyroxine and triiodothyronine as part of a large iodinated protein *(thyroglobulin)* that is stored in the lumens of thyroid follicles.

In comparison, the other group of hormones derived from tyrosine, the adrenal medullary hormones *epinephrine* and *norepinephrine*, are taken up into preformed vesicles and stored until secreted. As with protein hormones stored in secretion granules, catecholamines are released from adrenal medullary cells through exocytosis.

Control of Hormonal Secretion and Negative Feedback

In most instances, the rate of hormonal secretion is controlled by negative feedback. In general, endocrine glands tend to oversecrete hormone, which in turn drives target cell function. When too much function of the target cell occurs, some factor about the function feeds back to the endocrine gland and causes a negative effect on the gland, decreasing its secretory rate.

Mechanisms of Hormonal Action *(p. 886)*

Hormonal Receptors and Their Activation

Hormones control cellular processes by interacting with receptors on target cells. These receptors are (1) either on or within the cell membrane, as in the case of peptide/protein and catecholamine hormones, and (2) within the cell, in either the cytoplasm or nucleus, as is the case for steroid and thyroid hormones. Receptors are usually specific for a single hormone. The hormone-receptor interaction is coupled to a signal-generating mechanism that then causes a change in intracellular processes by altering the activity or concentration of enzymes, carrier proteins, and so forth.

Mediating Hormonal Responses

Cell Responses to Protein/Peptide and Catecholamine Hormones Are Mediated by Second Messengers. In the case of peptide/protein and catecholamine hormones that do not readily pass the cell membrane, interaction with the receptor on or within the cell membrane often results in generation of a second messenger, which in turn mediates the hormonal response. Often, coupling *G-proteins* in the cell membrane link hormone receptors to the second messenger mechanisms. Second messenger mechanisms include the following:

- *Adenylyl cyclase–cyclic adenosine monophosphate* (cAMP). Hormone-receptor interaction may stimulate (or inhibit) the membrane-bound enzyme adenylyl cyclase. Stimulation of this enzyme results in synthesis of the second messenger cAMP. The cAMP activates protein kinase A, leading to phosphorylation that either activates or inactivates target enzymes.

- *Plasma membrane phospholipids.* Hormone-receptor interaction activates the membrane-bound enzyme *phospholipase C,* which in turn causes phospholipids in the cell membrane (especially those derived from *phosphatidylinositol*) to split into the second messengers *diacylglycerol* and *inositol triphosphate.* Inositol triphosphate mobilizes calcium from internal stores, such as the endoplasmic reticulum, and the calcium in turn activates *protein kinase C.* Phosphorylation of enzymes by protein kinase C activates and deactivates enzymes mediating the hormone responses. In addition, the activity of protein kinase C is further enhanced by the second messenger diacylglycerol. Finally, diacylglycerol is hydrolyzed to *arachidonic acid,* which is the precursor for prostaglandins, which also influence hormonal responses.

- *Calcium-calmodulin.* Hormone-receptor interaction activates calcium channels in the plasma membrane, permitting calcium to enter cells. Calcium may also be mobilized from intercellular stores such as the endoplasmic reticulum. The calcium ions bind with the protein calmodulin, and this complex alters the activity of calcium-dependent enzymes and thus intercellular reactions.

Protein/peptide hormones may exert actions independent of G-protein-linked second messenger events, and other second messenger mechanisms may transduce hormonal responses. For example, the second messenger cyclic GMP mediates the effects of atrial natriuretic peptide. Furthermore, in the case of the peptide hormone insulin, hormone binding to the cell surface receptor results in phosphorylation of an intracellular site of the receptor, which in turn alters enzymatic activity by phosphorylating (or dephosphorylating) other proteins in the cell.

Cell Responses to Steroid and Thyroid Hormones Are Mediated by Stimulating Protein Synthesis. In contrast to protein/peptide hormones and catecholamines, steroid and thyroid hormones enter the cell and bind to intracellular receptors located in the cytoplasm or nucleus of the cell. The hormone-receptor interaction results in a conformational change in the receptor. This permits binding of the hormone-receptor complex to specific points on DNA strands in the chromosomes, which results in activation of specific genes, transcription, and translation of proteins that are essential for mediating the hormonal response. Because the transcription mechanism is involved in mediating the hormonal response, hours may be required for the biologic effects to become evident.

Measurement of Hormone Concentrations in Blood *(p. 891)*

Most hormones are present in the blood in minute concentrations (often in nanograms per liter or even picograms per liter). These low concentrations of hormones can be measured by the following methods.

Radioimmunoassay. The principle of the radioimmunoassay is based on the combined incubation of the following substances:

- A fixed amount of antibody specific for the hormone
- A fixed amount of radioactive-labeled hormone
- The plasma sample

Because the amount of antibody present is limiting, the radioactive and unlabeled native hormones compete for the binding sites on the antibody. High concentrations of native hormone displace more of the labeled hormone from the antibody. At the end of the incubation period, bound and free hormones are separated, and the amount of radioactivity is determined. The greater the amount of native hormone in the plasma sample, the lower is the amount of radioactivity in the bound fraction. The amount of native hormone in the sample is calculated by comparison with a standard curve generated by incubation of different amounts of unlabeled hormone (rather than the plasma sample), with antibody and radioactively labeled hormone as described.

Other competitive binding procedures can be used to measure hormone levels in the plasma. For example, tissue receptor or plasma binding proteins can be used instead of antibody as the binding protein.

Enzyme-Linked Immunosorbent Assay (ELISA). The ELISA is a cost-effective enzyme based colorimetric or fluorometric assay that does not use radioactive isotopes. A typical ELISA is performed in a plastic plate containing 96 wells. Each well is coated with antibody (AB_1) that is specific for the hormone being measured. Unknown samples or standards are added to the wells, followed by a second hormone-specific antibody (AB_2). A third antibody (AB_3) is added that recognizes AB_2 and is coupled to an enzyme that converts an appropriate substrate into a colored or fluorescent product that can be detected by colorimetric or fluorescent optical methods. The amount of colored product is proportional to the amount of hormone present in the standard or unknown sample.

CHAPTER 75

Pituitary Hormones and Their Control by the Hypothalamus

Pituitary Gland and Its Relation to the Hypothalamus *(p. 895)*

The hypothalamus and pituitary gland have intimate anatomical and functional relationships; in turn, these structures regulate the function of a number of endocrine glands, including the thyroid, adrenal, and gonads. They play an important role in the regulation of growth, metabolism, lactation, and water balance.

The pituitary gland is composed of two distinct components: (1) the *anterior pituitary gland,* or *adenohypophysis,* which is derived embryologically from an upward invagination of cells from the oral cavity (Rathke's pouch) and (2) the *posterior pituitary gland,* or *neurohypophysis,* which is derived from a downgrowth of cells from the third ventricle of the brain. The pituitary gland is connected to the hypothalamus by the hypothalamic or pituitary stalk.

Neurohypophysis—Axons and Nerve Terminals for Storage of Neurohypophysial Hormones

Magnocellular neurons whose cell bodies are located in the *supraoptic* and *paraventricular nuclei* of the hypothalamus synthesize the *neurohypophysial hormones antidiuretic hormone* (ADH) and *oxytocin.* Secretion granules containing these neurohormones are transported from the cell bodies in the hypothalamus down axons in the pituitary stalk to storage sites in nerve terminals located in the posterior pituitary gland. ADH and oxytocin are released from secretion granules into the capillary plexus of the inferior hypophysial artery, the primary blood supply to the neurohypophysis.

Adenohypophysis—Cells That Synthesize, Store, and Secrete Adenohypophysial Hormones

There are five cell types in the anterior pituitary gland that synthesize, store, and secrete six polypeptide or peptide *adenohypophysial* hormones. One hormone, prolactin, acts on the breast; the other five are *tropic hormones* that stimulate secretion of hormones by other endocrine glands or, in the case of growth hormone (GH), the liver and other tissues. One cell type, the gonadotrope, secretes two hormones, folliclestimulating hormone (FSH) and luteinizing hormone

(LH). The cells that secrete the anterior pituitary hormones and the chemical structure and physiological actions of the adenohypophysial hormones are listed in Table 75–1.

There is considerable similarity in the chemical structures of the *glycoprotein hormones thyroid-stimulating hormone* (TSH), *FSH,* and *LH,* all of which are secreted from *basophilic cells.* Similarly, there is structural homology between *prolactin* and *GH,* both of which are secreted from *acidophilic cells.* The corticotropes synthesize a preprohormone containing the amino acid sequences for *adrenocorticotropic hormone* (ACTH) and *melanocyte-stimulating hormones* (MSHs). In humans, ACTH is generated in the anterior pituitary, but no appreciable amount of MSHs is secreted. Although the administration of MSHs in humans causes darkening of the skin by increasing synthesis of the black pigment *melanin,* it is likely that the pigmentary changes in endocrinological diseases are due to changes in circulating ACTH because ACTH has MSH activity.

Hypothalamus Controls Pituitary Secretion (p. 897)

Blood Supply to the Anterior Pituitary Gland— Hypothalamic-Hypophysial Portal Vessels

There is an extensive network of capillary sinuses surrounding the anterior pituitary cells; most of the blood entering these sinuses has first passed through another capillary plexus in the lower hypothalamus or *median eminence.* The blood from the latter capillary plexus comes from the superior hypophysial artery and flows through the *hypothalamic-hypophysial portal vessels* of the pituitary stalk to bathe the adenohypophysial cells.

Hypophysiotropic Hormones (Releasing and Inhibiting Hormones)—Secretion of Anterior Pituitary Hormones

In addition to the hypothalamic neuroendocrine cells, which synthesize neurohypophysial hormones, other neurons in discrete areas of the hypothalamus synthesize the *hypophysiotropic neurohormones (releasing and inhibiting hormones),* which control secretion of the anterior pituitary hormones. Although the axons from the magnocellular neurons of the supraoptic and paraventricular nuclei terminate in the posterior pituitary gland, the

Table 75–1. Adenohypophysial Cells and Hormones

Cell	Hormone	Chemistry	Physiological Actions
Corticotropes	Adrenocorticotropic hormone (corticotropin; ACTH)	Single chain of 39 amino acids	Stimulates production of glucocorticoids and androgens by the adrenal cortex; maintains size of the zona fasciculata and zona reticularis of cortex
Thyrotropes	Thyroid-stimulating hormone (thyrotropin; TSH)	Glycoprotein of two subunits, α (89 amino acids) and β (112 amino acids)	Stimulates production of thyroid hormones by thyroid follicular cells; maintains size of the follicular cells
Gonadotropes	Follicle-stimulating hormone (FSH)	Glycoprotein of two subunits, α (89 amino acids) and β (112 amino acids)	Stimulates development of ovarian follicles; regulates spermatogenesis in the testis
	Luteinizing hormone (LH)	Glycoprotein of two subunits, α (89 amino acids) and β (115 amino acids)	Causes ovulation and formation of the corpus luteum in the ovary; stimulates production of estrogen and progesterone by the ovary; stimulates testosterone production by the testis
Mammotropes, lactotropes	Prolactin (PRL)	Single chain of 198 amino acids	Stimulates milk secretion and production
Somatotropes	Growth hormone (somatotropin; GH)	Single chain of 191 amino acids	Stimulates body growth; stimulates secretion of insulin-like growth factor-1 (IGF-1); stimulates lipolysis; inhibits actions of insulin on carbohydrate and lipid metabolism

nerve fibers from the hypothalamic cell bodies that synthesize the hypophysiotropic hormones lead to the *median eminence*. Here, the releasing and inhibiting hormones are stored in secretion granules in the nerve terminals. On stimulation of these hypothalamic neuroendocrine cells, their neurohormones are released into the capillary plexus of the median eminence, flow through the hypothalamic-hypophysial portal vessels, and reach the sinusoids around the adenohypophysial cells. The anterior pituitary cells respond to the hypophysiotropic hormones by either increasing or decreasing the synthesis and secretion of adenohypophysial hormones.

The six established hypophysiotropic hormones are listed in Table 75–2. Releasing hormones are most important for secretion of most adenohypophysial hormones, whereas an inhibitory hormone is most dominant in the control of prolactin secretion. Note that GH secretion is influenced by both a releasing and an inhibiting hormone, and a single hypophysiotropic hormone, gonadotropin-releasing hormone (GnRH),

Table 75–2. Hypophysiotropic Hormones

Hormone	Structure	Primary Action on Anterior Pituitary
Thyrotropin-releasing hormone (TRH)	Peptide of 3 amino acids	Stimulates secretion of TSH by thyrotropes
Gonadotropin-releasing hormone (GnRH)	Single chain of 10 amino acids	Stimulates secretion of FSH and LH by gonadotropes
Corticotropin-releasing hormone (CRH)	Single chain of 41 amino acids	Stimulates secretion of ACTH by corticotropes
Growth hormone–releasing hormone (GHRH)	Single chain of 44 amino acids	Stimulates secretion of GH by somatotropes
Growth hormone–inhibiting hormone (somatostatin)	Single chain of 14 amino acids	Inhibits secretion of GH by somatotropes
Prolactin-inhibiting hormone (PIH)	Dopamine	Inhibits secretion of PRL by lactotropes

stimulates the gonadotropes to secrete both FSH and LH. All hypophysiotropic hormones are peptides, polypeptides, or derivatives of the amino acid tyrosine (see Table 75–2).

The hypothalamus receives neural inputs from many areas of the brain. This information, related to the well-being of the body, is integrated in the hypothalamus and has an impact on endocrine function in large part by the influence of the hypophysiotropic hormones on secretion of the anterior pituitary hormones. In turn, the trophic hormones from the anterior pituitary gland stimulate target endocrine glands and tissues. The resultant changes in target gland hormones and metabolic substrates in the peripheral blood exert negative feedback control on secretion of anterior pituitary hormones through a direct effect on the adenohypophysial cells and through an indirect action at the level of the hypothalamus to alter the release of hypophysiotropic hormones.

Physiological Functions of GH *(p. 898)*

GH—Multiple Physiological Effects

In contrast to the other pituitary hormones, which stimulate specific target glands, GH has multiple effects throughout the body.

- *Promotion of linear growth.* GH stimulates the *epiphyseal cartilage* or growth plates of the long bones. Under the influence of GH, the chondrocytes in the growth plate are stimulated, leading to proliferation of these cells and deposition of new cartilage, followed by conversion of this cartilage to bone. This process elongates the shaft of the long bones. By late adolescence, when there is no remaining epiphyseal cartilage and the shafts have fused with the epiphyses (epiphyseal closure), GH can no longer cause lengthening of the long bones. Because GH also increases osteoblastic activity, total bone mass is increased by GH even after epiphyseal closure.
- *Promotion of protein deposition in tissues.* GH is a protein *anabolic* hormone and produces a positive nitrogen balance. It increases amino acid uptake in most cells and the synthesis of amino acids into proteins.
- *Promotion of fat utilization for energy.* GH causes the mobilization of fatty acids from adipose tissue and the preferential utilization of free fatty acids for

energy. This action of GH, together with its protein anabolic effects, produces an increase in lean body mass. The lipolytic effects of GH require several hours to occur. At least part of this effect is due to the actions of GH to impair glucose uptake into adipose cells. Because GH increases plasma levels of free fatty acids and ketoacids, it is *ketogenic*.

- *Impairment of carbohydrate utilization for energy.* GH decreases the uptake and utilization of glucose by many insulin-sensitive cells, such as muscle and adipose tissue. As a result, blood glucose concentration tends to rise and insulin secretion increases to compensate for the GH-induced insulin resistance; thus GH is *diabetogenic*.

Somatomedins and Anabolic Effects of GH

The effects of GH on linear growth and protein metabolism are not direct, but they are indirectly mediated via the generation of polypeptides called *somatomedins* or *insulin-like growth factors* (IGFs). Somatomedins are secreted by the liver and other tissues. *Somatomedin C,* or *IGF-1,* is a circulating 70-amino-acid peptide produced by the liver that reflects plasma GH levels. The growth-promoting effects of GH, however, are due to locally produced as well as circulating somatomedins; in cartilage and muscle, locally produced somatomedins act in an autocrine or paracrine fashion to stimulate growth.

GH Secretion—Metabolic Stimuli

GH secretion is under the influence of both a hypothalamic releasing (GHRH) hormone and a hypothalamic-inhibiting hormone (somatostatin). Feedback regulation of GH secretion is mediated primarily by circulating IGF-I via actions at both the hypothalamus and pituitary. High plasma levels of somatomedin C decrease GH release by increasing secretion of somatostatin from the hypothalamus and acting directly on the pituitary to decrease responsiveness to GHRH.

GH secretion is highest during puberty and decreases in adult life. This may be partially responsible for the decline in lean body mass and increase in adipose mass that are characteristic of senescence. There are three general categories of stimuli that increase GH secretion:

- *Fasting, chronic protein deprivation,* or other conditions in which there is an acute fall in plasma levels of metabolic substrates such as glucose and free fatty acids

• *Increased plasma levels of amino acids,* such as occur after a protein meal

• *Exercise and stressful stimuli,* such as pain and fever.

Clearly, the increase in GH during fasting would be beneficial because GH enhances lipolysis and decreases peripheral utilization of glucose. After a protein meal, increased plasma levels of GH would favor the utilization of amino acids for protein synthesis.

Abnormalities of GH Secretion and Their Impact on the Skeletal System

The importance of GH in linear growth is reflected by the clinical states associated with a deficiency or excess secretion of GH before epiphyseal closure. Short stature *(dwarfism)* occurs when pituitary secretion of GH is deficient. In comparison, children grow tall *(gigantism)* when tumors of the somatotropes of the anterior pituitary secrete large amounts of GH. If a pituitary tumor secreting GH appears after epiphyseal closure, the adult form of the disease occurs. With *acromegaly,* linear growth is normal, but there is enlargement of the hands and feet, protrusion of the lower jaw (prognathism), and overgrowth of facial bones. In addition, virtually all internal organs are of increased size. The anti-insulin effects of GH may ultimately lead to diabetes mellitus in states of chronic GH excess.

Posterior Pituitary Gland and Its Relation to the Hypothalamus *(p. 904)*

The *neurohypophysial hormones ADH* and *oxytocin* are synthesized as preprohormones in the cell bodies of *magnocellular neurons* located in the *supraoptic* and *paraventricular nuclei.* They are then transported in secretion granules down axons to nerve terminals in the posterior pituitary gland. ADH is synthesized largely in the supraoptic nucleus, and oxytocin is synthesized largely in the paraventricular nucleus, although each hormone is synthesized in the alternate site. The secretion granules containing either ADH or oxytocin also contain an additional protein, or *neurophysin,* that is part of the preprohormone. When a nerve impulse travels from the cell body of the magnocellular neurons down the axon to the nerve terminal, both the neurohormone and the corresponding neurophysin are released from secretion granules into the capillary blood as separate polypeptides. ADH and oxytocin are nonpeptides with a similar chemical structure; only the amino acids in positions 3 and 8 differ.

Physiological Functions of Antidiuretic Hormone

ADH Regulates the Osmolality of Body Fluids by Altering Renal Excretion of Water. ADH plays an important role in the regulation of plasma osmolality. As discussed in Chapter 28, in the absence of ADH the collecting tubules and collecting ducts are largely impermeable to water, which prevents significant reabsorption of water in this portion of the nephron. This results in a large volume of dilute urine and a net loss of water; consequently, the osmolality of body fluids rises. In comparison, when increased ADH activates V_2-receptors on the basolateral side of the tubules via a cAMP second messenger system, cytoplasmic vesicles containing water channels (aquaphorin) are inserted in the apical membrane. This increases the permeability of the tubules to water; therefore water moves by osmosis from the tubular to the peritubular capillary fluid. In the collecting ducts, the urine becomes concentrated, and its volume decreases. As a result, there is retention of water in excess of solute, and the osmolality of body fluids decreases.

In accordance with its role in the regulation of the osmotic pressure of plasma, ADH secretion is sensitive to small changes in plasma osmolality (approximately 1%). When plasma osmolality increases above normal, the rate of discharge of ADH-secreting neurons in the supraoptic and paraventricular nuclei increases, and ADH is secreted from the posterior pituitary gland into the systemic circulation. Circulating ADH increases the permeability of the collecting ducts to water, which ultimately decreases plasma osmolality to normal levels. The opposite changes in neuronal discharge and ADH secretion occur when plasma osmolality declines. ADH secretion is regulated by *osmoreceptors* in the anterior hypothalamus that send nervous signals to the supraoptic and paraventricular nuclei. Osmoreceptors are outside the blood-brain barrier and appear to be located in the *circumventricular organs,* primarily the organum vasculosum of the lateral terminalis. These same osmoreceptors may also mediate the thirst response to increased plasma osmolality.

ADH Secretion Is Influenced by Multiple Factors.
Other than increased plasma osmolality, stimuli that
increase ADH secretion include hypovolemia, hypotension, nausea, pain, stress, and a number of drugs,
including morphine, nicotine, and barbiturates. Factors
that decrease ADH secretion include hypervolemia,
hypertension, and alcohol. The influence of these factors on the neurons in the supraoptic and paraventricular nuclei that secrete ADH may have an impact on the
regulation of body fluid osmolality. For example, in
hypovolemic states, elevated plasma levels of ADH
may decrease plasma osmolality.

**ADH Contributes to the Maintenance of Blood Pres-
sure During Hypovolemia.** Stimulation of ADH secretion by hypovolemia and/or hypotension is achieved
by reflexes initiated from receptors in both the high-
and low-pressure regions of the circulation. The high-
pressure receptors are those in the carotid sinus and
aortic arch; the low-pressure receptors are those in
the cardiopulmonary circulation, especially in the atria.
At least a 5% decrease in blood volume is necessary
to increase ADH secretion appreciably by this reflex
mechanism. Greater degrees of hypovolemia and hypotension can result in very large increases in plasma
ADH concentration to levels much higher than those
required to achieve maximal antidiuresis. When these
unusually high plasma levels of ADH occur, such as
during hypotensive hemorrhage, ADH constricts vascular smooth muscle and helps restore blood pressure
to normal levels. This action of ADH is a result of the
peptide binding to vascular V_1-receptors on arteriolar
smooth muscle. The vasoconstriction induced by
ADH is mediated by *calcium-* and *phospholipase C-*
generated second messengers.

Physiological Functions of Oxytocin Hormone

**Oxytocin Plays an Important Role in Lactation by Caus-
ing Milk Ejection.** Oxytocin causes contraction of the
myoepithelial cells of the alveoli of the mammary
glands; this forces milk from the alveoli into the
ducts so the baby can obtain it by suckling. The *milk
ejection* reflex is initiated by receptors on the nipples
of the breast. Suckling causes reflex stimulation of
oxytocin-containing neuroendocrine cells in the supraoptic and paraventricular nuclei and secretion of oxytocin from the posterior pituitary gland. The circulating

oxytocin then causes the myoepithelial cells to contract, initiating milk ejection.

Oxytocin Contributes to Parturition. Oxytocin also causes contraction of the smooth muscle of the uterus; the sensitivity of this response is enhanced by plasma levels of estrogen, which increase during pregnancy. During labor, the descent of the fetus through the birth canal stimulates receptors on the cervix, which send signals to the supraoptic and paraventricular nuclei and cause secretion of oxytocin. Secretion of oxytocin in turn contributes to labor by causing contraction of the uterus.

CHAPTER 76

Thyroid Metabolic Hormones

Synthesis and Secretion of Thyroid Hormones (p. 907)

The thyroid gland is composed of a large number of *follicles*. Each follicle is surrounded by a single layer of cells and filled with a proteinaceous material called *colloid*. The primary constituent of colloid is the large glycoprotein *thyroglobulin*, which contains the thyroid hormones in its molecule. The following steps are required for the synthesis and secretion of thyroid hormones into the blood (Figs. 76–1 and 76–2):

- *Iodide trapping (iodide pump) or sodium-iodide symporter (NIS)*. Iodine is essential to thyroid hormone synthesis. Ingested iodine is converted to iodide and absorbed from the gut. Most circulating iodide is excreted by the kidneys; much of the remainder is taken up and concentrated by the thyroid gland. To achieve this, the thyroid follicular cells actively transport iodide from the circulation across their basal membrane into the cell by the NIS. In a normal thyroid gland, the NIS concentrates the iodide many times over the concentration in the blood. Several anions, such as thiocyanate and perchlorate, decrease iodide transport by competitive inhibition. In so doing, they decrease the synthesis of thyroid hormones and are used to treat hyperthyroidism.

- *Oxidation of iodide*. Once in the thyroid gland, iodide is rapidly oxidized to iodine by *thyroid peroxidase*; this occurs at the apical membrane of the follicular cells.

- *Synthesis of thyroglobulin*. This glycoprotein is synthesized by the follicular cells and secreted into the colloid through exocytosis of secretion granules that also contain *thyroid peroxidase*. Each thyroglobulin molecule contains many tyrosyl groups, but only a fraction become iodinated.

- *Iodination (organification) and coupling*. Once iodide is oxidized to iodine, it is rapidly attached to the 3 position of tyrosine molecules of thyroglobulin to generate *monoiodotyrosine* (MIT). MIT is next iodinated in the 5 position to give *diiodotyrosine* (DIT). Thereafter, two DIT molecules are coupled to form *thyroxine* (T_4), the major product of the coupling reaction; or one MIT and one DIT molecule are coupled to form *triiodothyronine* (T_3). A small amount of *reverse T_3* (RT_3) is formed by condensation of DIT

Figure 76–1. Thyroid cellular mechanisms for iodine transport, formation of thyroid hormones, thyroxine, triiodothyronine, and RT_3 release into the blood. DIT, diiodotyrosine; MIT, monoiodotyrosine; RT_3, reverse T_3; T_3, triiodothyronine; T_4, thyroxine; T_G, thyroglobulin.

with MIT. These reactions are catalyzed by thyroid peroxidase and blocked by antithyroid drugs such as propylthiouracil. Approximately two thirds of the iodinated compounds bound to thyroglobulin are MIT or DIT; most of the remainder are the active hormones T_3 and, especially, T_4. Thyroglobulin is stored in the lumen of the follicle as colloid until the gland is stimulated to secrete thyroid hormones.

• *Proteolysis, deiodination, and secretion.* The release of T_3, T_4 and RT_3 into the blood requires proteolysis of the thyroglobulin. At the apical surface of the follicular cells, colloid is taken up from the lumen of the follicles through endocytosis. Colloid vesicles then migrate from the apical to the basal cell membrane and fuse with *lysosomes*. Lysosomal *proteases* release free RT_3, T_3, and T_4, which then leave the cell. Free MIT and DIT are not secreted into the blood but, instead, deiodinated within the follicular cell by the enzyme *deiodinase*; the free iodine is reused in the gland for hormone synthesis. More than 90% of the thyroid hormone released from the gland is T_4. The remaining secretion products are T_3 and very small amounts of the inactive compound reverse T_3.

Figure 76–2. Chemistry of thyroxine and triiodothyronine formation.

Transport and Metabolism of Thyroid Hormones

Thyroid Hormones Are Highly Bound to Plasma Proteins. On entering the blood, both T_4 and T_3 are highly bound to plasma proteins, especially *thyroxine-binding globulin* (TBG), but also to other plasma proteins such as *albumin* and *thyroxine-binding prealbumin*. Approximately 99.9% of T_4 is bound to plasma proteins, and less than 0.1% is free hormone. The binding of T_3 to plasma proteins is slightly less than that of T_4, but still less than 1% is free hormone. In the case of the thyroid hormones, it is the free hormone that is taken up by tissues, in which it exerts biological effects and is metabolized. As a result of the high degree of binding to plasma proteins, the half-lives of T_4 and T_3 are very long (7 and 1 day, respectively).

Alterations in Plasma TBG Levels Do Not Influence Free Thyroid Hormone Concentration. Reductions (e.g., during liver and kidney disease) and elevations (e.g., during estrogen administration and pregnancy) in plasma TBG levels decrease and increase, respectively, the total amount of thyroid hormones in the plasma but produce no more than a transient change in the free hormone concentration. This is because of the negative feedback effect of free thyroid hormones on pituitary secretion of thyroid-stimulating hormone (TSH). For example, during pregnancy, a fall in free thyroid hormone concentration induced by increased TBG levels in the plasma causes a compensatory rise in TSH secretion, which in turn increases the production of free thyroid hormones. Increased thyroid hormone secretion continues until plasma levels of free hormone are normal. At this time TSH levels are normal due to feedback, but total thyroid hormone concentration is elevated.

Most of the T_4 Secreted by the Thyroid Gland Is Metabolized to T_3. Although T_4 is the dominant secreted and circulated thyroid hormone, large amounts of the hormone are deiodinated in either the 5′ or the 5 position in peripheral tissues to produce T_3 and RT_3. In fact, most of the T_3 and RT_3 in the plasma come from circulating T_4 that has been deiodinated in peripheral tissues rather than secreted from the thyroid gland. Because most of the T_4 that enters cells is converted to T_3 (and RT_3), and because the T_3 in cells has a greater affinity than does T_4 for thyroid hormone receptors in the nucleus, T_4 has been considered to be a prohormone for T_3.

Functions of Thyroid Hormones in the Tissues *(p. 910)*

Thyroid Hormones and Transcription of Many Genes

After thyroid hormones enter the cell and bind to nuclear receptors in the DNA. This interaction either stimulates or inhibits transcription of a large number of genes. This leads to alterations in numerous enzymes that alter cell function. The actions of T_3 occur more rapidly and are more potent than are those of T_4 because T_3 is bound less tightly to plasma proteins and has a greater affinity for nuclear receptors. Because thyroid hormones act in large part through influencing transcription, a delay of several hours occurs before most hormonal effects are evident; these effects may last several days.

Physiological Effect of Thyroid Hormones—Cellular Metabolic Rate

In most tissues of the body, thyroid hormones increase oxygen consumption and heat production. Mitochondria increase in size and number, the membrane surface areas of the mitochondria increase, and the activities of key respiratory enzymes increase. A complete accounting of the cellular mechanisms responsible for the higher oxygen consumption is not possible at present. Because thyroid hormones increase the activity of membrane-bound *Na, K-ATPase*, the greater ATP consumption associated with the greater sodium transport is believed to contribute to the greater metabolic rate induced by thyroid hormone.

Specific Physiological Effects of Thyroid Hormones

Many of the Effects of Thyroid Hormones are Secondary to Increased Metabolic Rate. Thyroid hormones are responsible for the following functions:

- *Increased thermogenesis and sweating.* Skin blood flow increases because of the need for heat elimination.
- *Increased rate and depth of respiration* resulting from the need for oxygen.
- *Increased cardiac output* because increased metabolism and utilization of oxygen in tissues cause local vasodilatation. Increased cardiac output is associated with elevations in both stroke volume and heart rate, in part because thyroid hormones have direct and indirect effects on the heart to increase the heart rate and force of contraction.
- *Increased pulse pressure but not mean arterial pressure.* Because of the increased cardiac output (stroke volume) and reduced peripheral vascular resistance, systolic arterial pressure is elevated and diastolic arterial pressure is reduced. This results in an increase in pulse pressure but usually no change in mean arterial pressure.
- *Increased utilization of substrates for energy.* An increased metabolic rate is dependent on oxidation

of metabolic substrates. Thyroid hormones increase the utilization of carbohydrates, fats, and proteins for energy. If food intake is not increased sufficiently, there is depletion of body fats and proteins and weight loss. Although thyroid hormones promote lipolysis of triglycerides and increments in plasma levels of free fatty acids, they also decrease the circulating levels of cholesterol; this action is due to increased formation of low-density lipoprotein receptors in the liver, resulting in increased removal of cholesterol from the circulation. Because thyroid hormones increase the rate of metabolic reactions, the need for vitamins is greater, and excess thyroid hormone can lead to vitamin deficiency.

Thyroid Hormones Are Essential for Normal Growth and Development. Thyroid hormones are essential for many aspects of growth and development; they play an important role in the development of the skeletal system, teeth, epidermis, and central nervous system. In hypothyroid children, the rate of growth is greatly reduced. An important effect of thyroid hormone is to promote growth and development of the central nervous system in utero and for the first few years of postnatal life. If thyroid hormone is deficient at this time, irreversible brain damage occurs.

Thyroid Hormones Have Excitatory Effects on the Nervous System. Thyroid hormones enhance wakefulness, alertness, and responsiveness to various stimuli; they also increase the speed and amplitude of peripheral nerve reflexes and improve memory and learning capacity.

Regulation of Thyroid Hormone Secretion (p. 914)

Thyroid-Stimulating Hormone—Primary Controller of Thyroid Hormone Secretion

To maintain normal levels of metabolic activity in the body, the free plasma levels of thyroid hormone must be regulated. Thyroid hormone secretion is primarily regulated by *thyroid-stimulating hormone (thyrotropin, TSH)*. TSH secretion from the pituitary gland is increased by the hypophysiotropic hormone *thyrotropin-releasing hormone* (TRH) and is inhibited in a negative feedback fashion by circulating T_4 and T_3. Although some feedback occurs at the hypothalamus by influencing TRH secretion, the predominant feedback occurs at the level of the pituitary. Because T_4 is deiodinated to T_3 in the pituitary gland, T_3 appears to be the final effector that mediates the negative feedback.

TSH Promotes the Synthesis and Secretion of Thyroid Hormones. Binding of TSH to its receptors on the cell membrane of the thyroid gland activates *adenylyl cyclase* so that *cyclic AMP* mediates at least some of the actions of TSH. An immediate effect of TSH is to promote endocytosis of colloid, proteolysis of thyroglobulin, and release of T_4 and T_3 into the circulation. In addition, TSH stimulates steps in the synthesis of thyroid hormones, including iodine trapping, iodination, and coupling to form thyroid hormones.

TSH Has Chronic Effects to Promote Growth of the Thyroid Gland. The chronic effects of TSH include increased blood flow to the thyroid gland and induction of hypertrophy and hyperplasia of the follicular cells. With prolonged TSH stimulation, the thyroid enlarges, and a *goiter* occurs. In the absence of TSH, there is marked atrophy of the gland.

Diseases of the Thyroid (p. 916)

Graves' Disease Is the Most Common Form of Hyperthyroidism. Graves' disease is an autoimmune disease in which antibodies, *thyroid-stimulating immunoglobulins* (TSIs), form against the TSH receptor of the thyroid, bind to it, and mimic the actions of TSH. This leads to goiter and secretion of large amounts of thyroid hormones. As a result, several predictable changes occur: (1) increased metabolic rate, (2) heat intolerance and sweating, (3) increased appetite but weight loss, (4) palpitations and tachycardia, (5) nervousness and emotional lability, (6) muscle weakness, and (7) tiredness but inability to sleep.

Many patients with Graves' disease have protrusion of the eyeballs, or *exophthalmos*. This is due to the degenerative changes in the extraocular muscles as a result of an autoimmune reaction. TSH secretion from the pituitary gland is depressed in Graves' disease because of the feedback exerted by the high plasma levels of thyroid hormones.

Many of the Effects of Hypothyroidism Are Opposite to Those of Hyperthyroidism. Although hypothyroidism may have several causes, it often results from autoimmune destruction of the thyroid gland (Hashimoto's disease). The symptoms are, in general, opposite to those of hyperthyroidism: (1) decreased metabolic rate;

(2) cold intolerance and decreased sweating; (3) weight gain without increased caloric intake; (4) bradycardia; (5) slowness of movement, speech, and thought; and (6) lethargy and sleepiness. There is accumulation of mucopolysaccharides in interstitial spaces, giving rise to nonpitting edema. The puffiness of the skin is referred to as *myxedema,* a term used synonymously for adult hypothyroidism. If severe hypothyroidism occurs in utero or during infancy, irreversible mental retardation results, and growth is impaired; this condition is referred to as *cretinism.* If the hypothalamic-pituitary axis is normal, hypothyroidism is associated with increased plasma levels of TSH resulting from feedback.

Hypothyroidism can also be associated with *goiter.* In certain areas of the world, dietary iodine is deficient, so thyroid hormone secretion is depressed. Many individuals in these regions have enlarged thyroids, or *endemic goiter,* because high plasma levels of TSH stimulate the gland. The practice of adding iodine to table salt has decreased the incidence of endemic goiter in many areas of the world.

CHAPTER 77

Adrenocortical Hormones

The adrenal gland is composed of two distinct parts: (1) an inner *adrenal medulla,* which is functionally related to the sympathetic nervous system and secretes mainly *epinephrine* but some *norepinephrine* and (2) an outer *adrenal cortex,* which forms the bulk of the gland and secretes *corticosteroids.* The primary corticosteroids secreted by the adrenal cortex are as follows:

- *Mineralocorticoids.* C_{21} steroids that have important effects on sodium and potassium balance
- *Glucocorticoids.* C_{21} steroids that influence carbohydrate, fat, and protein metabolism
- *Sex hormones.* C_{19} steroids that are mostly *weak androgens* and contribute to secondary sex characteristics.

The secretion of mineralocorticoids and glucocorticoids is essential to life. Only small amounts of sex hormones are normally secreted by the adrenal cortex, and they have little effect on reproductive function.

Chemistry of Adrenocortical Secretion
(p. 921)

The Adrenal Cortex Is Composed of Three Distinct Layers or Cell Types: Zona Glomerulosa, Zona Fasciculata, and Zona Reticularis

- The *zona glomerulosa,* or outer zone, is relatively thin; it is the exclusive site of the enzyme *aldosterone synthase* (Fig. 77–1). Its major secretion product is the principal mineralocorticoid *aldosterone.* The primary controllers of aldosterone secretion are *angiotensin II* and *potassium.* Chronic increases in plasma angiotensin II concentration, such as occur during sodium depletion, cause hypertrophy and hyperplasia of zona glomerulosa cells only. Because the zona glomerulosa lacks the enzyme *17-hydroxylase* (see Fig. 77–1), it cannot synthesize cortisol or sex hormones.
- The *zona fasciculata,* or middle zone, is the widest zone; it secretes the glucocorticoids *cortisol* (the principal glucocorticoid) and *corticosterone.* This zone also secretes small amounts of sex hormones. The major controller of cortisol secretion is *adrenocorticotropic hormone* (corticotropin, ACTH).
- The *zona reticularis,* or inner zone, secretes sex hormones and some glucocorticoids; like the zona fasciculata, it is stimulated by ACTH. Chronic ACTH

Figure 77–1. Hormone biosynthesis in the adrenal cortex.

excess causes hypertrophy and hyperplasia of the inner two zones of the adrenal cortex. The most prevalent adrenal androgens are *dehydroepiandrosterone* (DHEA) and *androstenedione.*

Adrenocortical Hormones Are Synthesized from Cholesterol. Most of the cholesterol in adrenocortical cells is taken up from the circulation and then esterified and stored in lipid droplets. The rate-limiting step in the synthesis of adrenocortical hormones is the side-chain cleavage of cholesterol to form *pregnenolone* (see Fig. 77–1). This step includes the delivery of cholesterol to the inner mitochondrial membrane and the enzymatic cleavage (through *cholesterol desmolase*) of a six-carbon unit from cholesterol to yield pregnenolone. In all three zones of the adrenal cortex, this initial step in steroid biosynthesis is stimulated by the controllers of the major hormone products (aldosterone and cortisol). The conversion of cholesterol to pregnenolone and all the subsequent steps in the synthesis of adrenocortical hormones occur either in the *endoplasmic reticulum* or *mitochondria*. Not all of the compounds shown in Figure 77–1 are produced in all three zones of the adrenal cortex.

Adrenocortical Hormones Are Bound to Plasma Proteins. Approximately 90% to 95% of the cortisol in the plasma is bound to plasma proteins, especially *transcortin* or *corticosteroid-binding globulin* (CBG). As a result of this high degree of binding to plasma proteins, cortisol has a long half-life (about 60 to 90 minutes). Corticosterone is bound to plasma proteins to a lesser degree than cortisol and has a half-life of approximately 50 minutes. Even smaller amounts of aldosterone are bound to plasma proteins; consequently, aldosterone has a half-life of only approximately 20 minutes.

Adrenocortical Hormones Are Metabolized in the Liver. Cortisol and aldosterone are metabolized to various compounds in the liver and then conjugated to *glucuronic acid.* These inactive conjugates are freely soluble in plasma and are not bound to plasma proteins. Once released into the circulation, they are readily excreted in urine. The rate of inactivation of adrenocortical hormones is depressed in liver disease.

Functions of the Mineralocorticoids— Aldosterone *(p. 924)*

Aldosterone Is the Primary Mineralocorticoid Secreted by the Adrenal Cortex. Aldosterone accounts for approximately 90% of the mineralocorticoid activity of adrenocortical hormones. Most of the remainder of the mineralocorticoid activity can be attributed to (1) *deoxycorticosterone,* which has approximately 3% of the mineralocorticoid activity of aldosterone and is secreted at a comparable rate, and (2) *cortisol,* a glucocorticoid with weak mineralocorticoid activity that is normally present at plasma concentrations of more than 1000 times that of aldosterone. In vitro studies have shown that *cortisol* binds with high affinity to mineralocorticoid receptors. Because the kidneys have the enzyme *11β-hydroxysteroid dehydrogenase type 2,* cortisol is converted to cortisone, which does not avidly bind mineralocorticoid receptors. Consequently, cortisol does not normally exert significant mineralocorticoid effects in vivo. Under conditions in which 11β-hydroxysteroid dehydrogenase is either congenitally absent or inhibited (e.g., during excessive licorice ingestion), cortisol may have substantial mineralocorticoid effects.

Aldosterone Increases Sodium Reabsorption and Potassium Secretion. Aldosterone and other mineralocorticoids act on the distal nephron, especially the principal cells of the collecting duct, to increase sodium reabsorption and potassium secretion. These effects occur after the binding of aldosterone to intracellular receptors and the subsequent synthesis of proteins, including *Na,K-ATPase* in the *basolateral membrane* and sodium and potassium *channel proteins* in the *apical membrane.* As a result of increased Na,K-ATPase activity, sodium is pumped out of the tubular cells into the blood and exchanged for potassium. Potassium then diffuses into the tubular urine. As sodium is reabsorbed under the influence of aldosterone, there is enhanced tubular secretion of potassium ions. Aldosterone also causes secretion of hydrogen ions in exchange for sodium in the intercalated cells of the cortical collecting tubules. Because protein synthesis is required to mediate the tubular actions of aldosterone, a lag time of about 60 minutes occurs between exposure to aldosterone and its onset of action.

Aldosterone Affects Electrolyte Transport in Organs Other Than the Kidneys. Aldosterone binds to mineralocorticoid receptors in epithelial cells other than those of the kidney. Aldosterone increases sodium reabsorption from the colon and promotes potassium excretion in the feces. Similarly, aldosterone has an effect on sweat and salivary glands, decreasing the sodium/potassium ratio in their respective secretions.

Controllers of Aldosterone Secretion—Angiotensin II and Potassium

Angiotensin II Stimulates Aldosterone Secretion. *Angiotensin II* directly stimulates the cells of the *zona glomerulosa* to secrete aldosterone. This effect of angiotensin II is mediated via increments in intracellular levels of *calcium* and the *phosphatidylinositol* products, diacylglycerol and inosital triphosphate. These second messengers activate *protein kinase C,* which in turn stimulates both early *(cholesterol desmolase)* and late *(aldosterone synthase)* steps in the biosynthesis of aldosterone.

The control of aldosterone secretion by angiotensin II is closely linked to the regulation of extracellular fluid volume and arterial pressure (see Chapter 29). The renin-angiotensin system is activated in the presence of hypovolemia and hypotension; and high plasma levels of angiotensin II stimulate aldosterone secretion. In turn, aldosterone increases sodium reabsorption in the distal nephron; as fluid retention returns body fluid volumes and arterial pressure to normal levels, the stimulus for activation of the renin-angiotensin system wanes, and aldosterone secretion falls to basal levels. Accordingly, the activity of the renin-angiotensin system is inversely related to dietary sodium intake.

Potassium Stimulates Aldosterone Secretion. The cells of the zona glomerulosa are sensitive to small changes in the plasma potassium concentration. Increments in plasma potassium concentration increase aldosterone secretion by depolarizing the cell membrane, opening *calcium channels,* thereby increasing the intracellular calcium concentration. In response to these events, aldosterone secretion increases as a result of stimulation of the same early and late biosynthetic steps affected by angiotensin II (see previous discussion).

Aldosterone plays a critical role in eliminating ingested potassium and in feedback regulation of the plasma potassium concentration (see Chapter 29). Increments in plasma potassium concentration increase aldosterone secretion, which in turn stimulates tubular secretion of potassium. As plasma potassium concentrations fall to normal levels, the stimulus for aldosterone secretion is removed. The opposite sequence of events occurs when plasma potassium concentration decreases. Increases in plasma potassium concentration depolarize the cell membrane, activating voltage-dependent calcium channels. The rise in cytoplasmic calcium stimulates aldosterone secretion by the mechanism described above for angiotensin II.

ACTH Plays a Permissive Role in the Regulation of Aldosterone Secretion. So long as normal plasma levels of ACTH are present, the responsiveness of the zona glomerulosa to its major controllers, angiotensin II and potassium, is maintained. In contrast, if ACTH is chronically deficient, the aldosterone response to angiotensin II and potassium is diminished. High plasma levels of ACTH, which occur acutely during stress, stimulate aldosterone secretion; but in states of chronic ACTH excess (e.g., with Cushing's disease), hyperaldosteronism is not sustained.

Functions of the Glucocorticoids (p. 928)

Cortisol Is the Primary Glucocorticoid Secreted by the Adrenal Cortex. More than 95% of glucocorticoid activity exerted by the adrenocortical hormones can be attributed to cortisol; most of the remaining glucocorticoid activity is due to corticosterone. Cortisol mediates most of its effects by binding with intracellular receptors in target tissues and inducing or repressing gene transcription; this results in alterations in the synthesis of enzymes that alter cell function.

Cortisol Has Widespread Effects on Metabolism. There are pronounced disturbances in carbohydrate, fat, and protein metabolism in adrenal insufficiency. Some of the metabolic effects of cortisol are permissive in that cortisol does not initiate the changes, but its presence at normal plasma levels permits certain metabolic processes. Cortisol exerts the following effects on metabolism:

- *Decreases protein stores in extrahepatic tissues.* In muscle and other extrahepatic tissues, cortisol decreases amino acid uptake and inhibits protein synthesis; at the same time, it increases the degradation of proteins. As a result of these *catabolic* and *anti-anabolic effects* of cortisol, amino acids tend to increase in the blood and are taken up by the liver, where they are converted to glucose and proteins, including gluconeogenic enzymes.

- *Tends to increase the blood glucose concentration in two ways.* First, cortisol increases hepatic production of glucose by increasing *gluconeogenesis.* The proteins mobilized from peripheral tissues are converted to glucose and glycogen in the liver. By maintaining glycogen reserves, cortisol allows other glycolytic hormones, such as epinephrine and glucagon, to mobilize glucose in times of need, such as between meals. A second way in which cortisol tends to increase the blood glucose concentration is by impairing the utilization of glucose in peripheral tissues; cortisol has an *anti-insulin effect* in tissues such as muscle and adipose tissue and impairs the uptake and utilization of glucose for energy. Like growth hormone, cortisol is *diabetogenic* because it tends to increase the blood glucose concentration.

- *Plays an important role in the mobilization of fatty acids from adipose tissue.* Although weakly lipolytic itself, normal levels of cortisol exert a permissive effect on the mobilization of fatty acids during fasting. During fasting, cortisol allows other lipolytic hormones, such as epinephrine and growth hormone, to mobilize fatty acids from lipid stores.

Increased Cortisol Secretion Is Important for Resistance to Stress. Physical or mental stress increases ACTH secretion, which in turn stimulates the adrenal cortex to secrete cortisol. Although it is not clear how hypercortisolism mediates this response, the large rise in cortisol secretion in response to many stressors is essential to survival. Patients with adrenal dysfunction who are administered maintenance doses of steroids require extra glucocorticoid under stressful conditions.

Pharmacological Doses of Glucocorticoids Have Anti-Inflammatory and Antiallergic Effects and Suppress Immune Responses. Large doses of glucocorticoids decrease the *inflammatory response* to tissue trauma, foreign proteins, or infections through several effects, including the following:

- *Inhibition of phospholipase.* This decreases the synthesis of *arachidonic acid*, which is the precursor of *leukotrienes, prostaglandins,* and *thromboxanes,* mediators of the local inflammatory response that includes dilation of capillaries, increased capillary permeability, and migration of leukocytes into the area of tissue injury.
- *Stabilization of lysosomal membranes.* This decreases the release of proteolytic enzymes by damaged cells.
- *Suppression of the immune system.* Suppression is a result of decreased production of T cells and antibodies that contribute to the inflammatory process.
- *Inhibition of fibroblastic activity.*

Controller of Cortisol Secretion—ACTH *(p. 931)*

ACTH Stimulates Cortisol Secretion. The secretion of cortisol is under the control of the hypothalamic-pituitary, *corticotropin-releasing hormone* (CRH)-ACTH axis. The release of ACTH (corticotropin) from the pituitary is dependent on the hypophysiotropic hormone CRH. Once ACTH is secreted into the blood, it has a rapid effect on the inner two zones of the adrenal cortex, especially the *zona fasciculata,* to increase the secretion of *cortisol.* This effect of ACTH is achieved by increasing the conversion of cholesterol to pregnenolone and is mediated via the second messenger *cyclic*

AMP. Chronic stimulation of the adrenal cortex by ACTH causes hypertrophy and hyperplasia of the zona fasciculata and zona reticularis and increased synthesis of several enzymes that convert cholesterol into the final product cortisol. Under conditions of chronic ACTH excess, such as with Cushing's syndrome, there are sustained increases in the secretion of cortisol and adrenal androgens.

Blood levels of free (unbound) cortisol are controlled in a negative feedback fashion. Increased plasma levels of cortisol decrease ACTH secretion through a direct effect on the pituitary as well as indirect inhibition of CRH release from the hypothalamus. The secretion of cortisol is highest in the early morning and reaches its lowest in the late evening because there is a *diurnal* or *circadian rhythm* in ACTH secretion as a result of changes in the frequency and duration of CRH bursts from the hypothalamus. Because of the cyclic changes in cortisol secretion, plasma levels of cortisol are meaningful only when expressed in terms of the time of day when blood sampling occurred.

Stress Increases ACTH Secretion. Several physical and mental stressors stimulate the neuroendocrine cells of the hypothalamus to secrete CRH; as a result, there is increased ACTH secretion, which stimulates release of cortisol. Under conditions of stress, the inhibitory effect of cortisol on ACTH secretion is insufficient to counteract the extra neural input to the neuroendocrine cells secreting CRH. Consequently, plasma levels of ACTH are increased.

Adrenal Androgens (p. 934)

The *adrenal androgens DHEA* and *androstenedione* are secreted in appreciable amounts, but they have only weak androgenic effects. Consequently, the normal plasma concentrations of these hormones exert little effect on secondary sex characteristics, especially in males, in whom large amounts of testosterone, the most potent androgen, are secreted by the testes. In females, adrenal androgens are responsible for pubic and axillary hair. Most of the androgenic activity of adrenal hormones may be due to the conversion of adrenal androgens to testosterone in peripheral tissues. In contrast to the normal state, when adrenal androgens are secreted in excessive amounts, as with Cushing's syndrome, appreciable masculinization may be produced in both males and females. The secretion of adrenal androgens is stimulated by ACTH.

Abnormalities of Adrenocortical Secretion (p. 934)

Increased Plasma Levels of Glucocorticoids (Cortisol) Produce *Cushing's Syndrome.* Excess cortisol secretion can be caused by an adrenal tumor, a pituitary tumor that is secreting large amounts of ACTH and causing bilateral adrenal hyperplasia *(Cushing's disease),* or a tumor of the lungs or other tissues *(ectopic tumors)* that is secreting large amounts of ACTH and causing bilateral adrenal hyperplasia. Cushing's syndrome may also be produced by the administration of large amounts of exogenous glucocorticoids.

Symptoms of Cushing's syndrome include the following:

- Mobilization of fat from the extremities to the abdomen, face, and supraclavicular areas
- Hypertension and hypokalemia resulting from high plasma levels of cortisol and 11-deoxycorticosterone (when secreted in excess)
- Protein depletion resulting in muscle weakness, loss of connective tissue and thinning of the skin (leading to purple striae), and impaired growth in children
- Osteoporosis and vertebral fractures resulting from their direct effect on bone, decreased calcium absorption from the gut (antivitamin D action), and increased glomerular filtration rate and renal excretion of calcium
- Impaired response to infections resulting from a suppressed immune system
- Impaired carbohydrate metabolism, hyperglycemia, and even insulin-resistant diabetes mellitus
- Masculinizing effects when adrenal androgens are secreted in excess

Conn's syndrome (primary aldosteronism) is caused by a tumor in the zona glomerulosa. When a tumor is present in the zona glomerulosa that produces large amounts of aldosterone, the most notable features are hypertension and hypokalemia; usually hypertension is relatively mild because there is only a small increase in extracellular fluid volume resulting from "sodium escape" (see Chapter 29). The hypertension and hypokalemia are exacerbated by increased sodium intake.

Because of expansion of the extracellular fluid volume and the rise in arterial pressure, plasma renin activity is suppressed. The potassium depletion in Conn's syndrome decreases the concentrating ability of the kidneys, leading to polyuria, and causes muscle weakness and metabolic alkalosis.

Impaired secretion of adrenocortical hormones occurs in *Addison's disease*. Destruction of the adrenal cortex can result from autoimmune disease, tuberculosis, or cancer. These processes usually are gradual, leading to a progressive reduction in glucocorticoid and mineralocorticoid function. As a result of the decreased cortisol secretion, there is a compensatory increase in ACTH secretion, which produces *hyperpigmentation*. Symptoms of Addison's disease include the following.

Mineralocorticoid Deficiency

- Excessive loss of sodium, hypovolemia, hypotension, and increased plasma renin activity
- Excessive potassium retention and hyperkalemia
- Mild acidosis

Glucocorticoid Deficiency

- Abnormal carbohydrate, fat, and protein metabolism resulting in muscle weakness, fasting hypoglycemia, and impaired utilization of fats for energy.
- Loss of appetite and weight loss.
- Poor tolerance to stress. The inability to secrete increased amounts of cortisol during stress leads to an *Addisonian crisis* that may culminate in death if supplemental doses of adrenocortical hormones are not administered.

CHAPTER 78

Insulin, Glucagon, and Diabetes Mellitus

Chemistry, Synthesis, and Metabolism of Pancreatic Hormones *(p. 939)*

Insulin and Glucagon Are Synthesized in the Islets of Langerhans. The pancreas is composed of two types of tissue: (1) *acini*, which secrete digestive juices via the pancreatic duct into the duodenum (exocrine function) and (2) the *islets of Langerhans*, which do not secrete into ducts but, instead, empty their secretions into the blood (endocrine function). In humans, there are 1 million to 2 million islets of Langerhans, which contain at least four distinct cell types.

- *Beta cells* account for approximately 60% of the cells and secrete *insulin and amylin.*
- *Alpha cells* make up about 25% of the cells and are the source of *glucagon.*
- *Delta cells* secrete *somatostatin.*
- *PP cells* secrete *pancreatic polypeptide.*

Secretion of pancreatic hormones into the portal vein via the pancreatic vein provides a much higher concentration of pancreatic hormones in the liver than in the peripheral tissues. This is in keeping with the important metabolic effects of insulin and glucagon in the liver. The physiologic functions of *somatostatin* and *pancreatic polypeptide* have not been established.

Insulin and Glucagon Are Synthesized and Metabolized Like Most Peptide Hormones. Both insulin and glucagon are synthesized as large *preprohormones.* In the Golgi apparatus, the *prohormones* are packaged in granules and then largely cleaved into free hormone plus peptide fragments. In the case of the *beta cells, insulin* and *connecting (C) peptide* (which connects the two peptide chains of insulin) are released into the circulating blood in equimolar amounts. C peptide levels can be measured with a radioimmunoassay and is a measure of beta cell function in insulin-treated diabetic patients. Insulin is a polypeptide containing two amino acid chains (21 and 30 amino acids, respectively) connected by disulfide bridges. Glucagon is a straight-chain polypeptide of 29 amino acid residues. Both insulin and glucagon circulate unbound to carrier proteins and have short half-lives of 5 to 10 minutes. Approximately 50% of the insulin and glucagon in the portal vein is metabolized on the first pass in the liver; most of the remaining hormone is metabolized by the kidneys.

Insulin and Its Metabolic Effects (p. 941)

Insulin Is a Hormone Associated with Energy Abundance. In response to an influx of nutrients into the blood, insulin is secreted and permits these nutrients to be used by tissues for energy and anabolic processes; it also induces the storage of excess nutrients for later use when energy supplies are deficient. In the presence of insulin, stores of carbohydrates, fats, and proteins increase. Insulin has rapid (e.g., increased glucose, amino acid, and potassium uptake into cells), intermediate (e.g., stimulation of protein synthesis, inhibition of protein degradation, activation and inactivation of enzymes), and delayed (e.g., increased transcription) actions on carbohydrate, fat, and protein metabolism that occur within seconds, minutes, and hours, respectively.

Most of the Actions of Insulin Are Achieved through Autophosphorylation of Receptors. Insulin does not mediate its physiological effects through generation of second messengers as do most protein hormones; instead, signal transduction is achieved through *autophosphorylation* of the intracellular domains of its own receptor. The insulin receptor is a tetramer made up of *two α-subunits* that lie outside the cell membrane and *two β-subunits* that penetrate the cell membrane and protrude into the cytoplasm. Binding of insulin to the α-subunit of the receptor triggers *tyrosine kinase* activity of the β-subunits, producing autophosphorylation of the β-subunits on tyrosine residues. This results in phosphorylation of other intracellular proteins and enzymes, which mediates a multitude of responses.

Effects of Insulin on Carbohydrate Metabolism

In Muscle, Insulin Promotes the Uptake and Metabolism of Glucose. An important effect of insulin in muscle is that it facilitates glucose diffusion down its concentration gradient from the blood into cells. This is achieved by increasing the number of *glucose transporters* in the cell membrane. These transporters are recruited from a cytoplasmic pool of vesicles to the cell membrane. The increased glucose transported into muscle cells undergoes glycolysis and oxidation and is stored as glycogen. Because glucose entry into muscle cells is usually highly dependent on insulin, glucose uptake by these cells is restricted to the postprandial period when insulin is secreted or periods of exercise when glucose transport is non–insulin-dependent. During exercise the insertion of glucose transporters into the cell membrane is insulin independent.

In the Liver, Insulin Promotes Glucose Uptake and Storage, and Inhibits Glucose Production. It also has the following actions in the liver:

- *Increases the flux of glucose into cells.* This is achieved not by increasing the number of glucose transporters in the cell membranes but by inducing *glucokinase,* which increases the phosphorylation of glucose to glucose-6-phosphate.
- *Increases glycogen synthesis by activating glycogen synthase* (as well as by increasing glucose uptake).
- *Directs the flow of glucose through glycolysis by increasing the activity of key glycolytic enzymes* (e.g., phosphofructokinase and pyruvate kinase).
- *Decreases the hepatic output of glucose* in several ways. First, insulin impairs *glycogenolysis* by inhibiting *glycogen phosphorylase.* Second, insulin decreases the exit of glucose from the liver by inhibiting *glucose-6-phosphatase.* Third, insulin inhibits *gluconeogenesis* by decreasing the amino acid uptake into the liver (see discussion on effects on protein metabolism) and by decreasing the activity or levels of key *gluconeogenic enzymes* (e.g., pyruvate carboxylase and fructose-1,6-diphosphatase).
- *Enhances synthesis of fatty acids* in two ways. First, insulin increases the flow of glucose to pyruvate (glycolysis) and the subsequent conversion to *acetylcoenzyme A (acetyl-CoA).* Second, insulin stimulates *acetyl-CoA carboxylase,* which converts acetyl-CoA to malonyl-CoA. This is the rate-limiting step in the synthesis of fatty acids.

In Adipose Tissue, Insulin Facilitates Glucose Entry into Cells. This is achieved in much the same way that insulin promotes glucose uptake into muscle cells—by increasing glucose transporters in the cell membrane. Subsequently, the metabolism of glucose to α-*glycerol phosphate* provides the glycerol that is needed for esterification of fatty acids for storage as triglycerides (see discussion of effects on fat metabolsim).

Insulin Has Little Effect on Glucose Uptake and Use by the Brain. In the brain, insulin has little effect on glucose transport into cells. Because brain cells are quite permeable to glucose and highly dependent on this substrate for energy, it is essential that the blood glucose concentration is maintained at normal levels. If the blood glucose concentration falls too low, symptoms of hypoglycemic shock appear, including fainting, seizure, and even coma.

Effects of Insulin on Fat Metabolism

In Adipose Tissue, Insulin Enhances Storage and Inhibits Mobilization of Fatty Acids. This effect of insulin is accomplished in several ways:

- *Insulin inhibits hormone-sensitive lipase.* This decreases the rate of lipolysis of triglycerides and the release of stored fatty acids into the circulation.
- *Insulin increases glucose transport.* The subsequent metabolism of glucose to *α-glycerol phosphate increases the rate of esterification* of fatty acids for storage as *triglycerides.*
- *Insulin induces lipoprotein lipase.* This enzyme is present in the capillary wall and splits circulating triglycerides into fatty acids, which is necessary for their transport into fat cells.

In the Liver, Insulin Promotes the Synthesis and Inhibits the Oxidation of Fatty Acids. As discussed previously, insulin promotes the synthesis of fatty acids from glucose in the liver. Because of the increased availability of α-glycerol phosphate from glycolysis, fatty acids are esterified to form triglycerides. Oxidation of fatty acids is impaired because of the increased conversion of acetyl-CoA to malonyl-CoA by acetyl-CoA carboxylase, as discussed. Malonyl-CoA inhibits *carnitine acyltransferase,* which is responsible for shuttling fatty acids from the cytoplasm into the mitochondria for *β-oxidation* and *conversion to ketoacids;* insulin is *antiketogenic.*

Effects of Insulin on Protein Metabolism

Insulin is an *anabolic hormone.* It increases the uptake of several amino acids from the blood into cells by stimulating transport across the cell membrane; this limits the rise in plasma levels of certain amino acids after a protein meal. In addition, insulin increases protein synthesis by stimulating both gene transcription and translation of mRNA. Finally, insulin inhibits catabolism of proteins and therefore decreases the release of amino acids from muscle.

Insulin, like growth hormone, is essential to growth. Diabetic animals fail to grow. The anabolic effects of insulin and growth hormone are synergistic.

Control of Insulin Secretion

Glucose Is the Most Important Controller of Insulin Secretion. Although several factors can increase or decrease insulin secretion, the major control of insulin secretion is exerted by a feedback effect of blood glucose on the beta cells of the pancreas. When blood glucose concentration rises above fasting levels, insulin secretion increases. As a result of the subsequent effects of insulin to stimulate glucose uptake by the liver and peripheral tissues, the blood glucose concentration returns to normal levels. This provides an important negative feedback mechanism for controlling the blood glucose concentration.

Multiple Stimuli Other Than Hyperglycemia Increase Insulin Secretion. These stimuli include the following:

- *Amino acids*, especially arginine, lysine, leucine, and alanine. As a result, dietary amino acids are removed from the blood and used by cells to synthesize proteins. Amino acids have a synergistic effect with glucose in stimulating insulin secretion.
- *Gastrointestinal hormones*, especially *gastric inhibitory polypeptide* and *glucagon like polypeptide 1*. These hormones are released from the gastrointestinal tract after a meal is eaten and account for the greater increase in insulin secretion when glucose is administered orally than when comparable amounts are administered intravenously.
- Other hormones, including *cortisol* and *growth hormone*. These hormones increase insulin secretion in large part because they antagonize the effects of insulin on glucose uptake in peripheral tissues, leading to increased blood glucose concentration. Indeed, chronic increments in cortisol (with Cushing's syndrome) and growth hormone (with acromegaly) lead to hypertrophy and exhaustion of the beta cells of the pancreas and thereby cause *diabetes mellitus*.
- Autonomic nervous system, including both the sympathetic and parasympathetic nervous system. β-adrenergic stimulation increases insulin secretion, whereas α-adrenergic stimulation inhibits it. Activation of sympathetic nerves to the pancreas inhibits insulin secretion. Parasympathetic stimulation of the pancreas increases insulin secretion.

Glucagon and Its Functions *(p. 947)*

Most of the Actions of Glucagon Are Achieved by Activation of Adenylyl Cyclase. At physiological doses, the primary effects of glucagon occur in the liver and are opposite those of insulin. The binding of glucagon to hepatic receptors results in activation of *adenylyl cyclase* and generation of the second messenger *cyclic AMP*, which in turn activates *protein kinase A*, leading to phosphorylation that results in the activation or deactivation of a number of enzymes.

Glucagon Promotes Hyperglycemia in Several Ways

- *Glucagon stimulates glycogenolysis.* Glucagon has immediate and pronounced effects on the liver to increase glycogenolysis and the release of glucose into the blood. This effect is achieved through activation of *glycogen phosphorylase* and simultaneous inhibition of *glycogen synthase.*
- *Glucagon inhibits glycolysis.* Glucagon inhibits several key steps in glycolysis, including phosphofructokinase and pyruvate kinase. Consequently, *glucose-6-phosphate* levels tend to rise, leading to increased glucose release from the liver.
- *Glucagon stimulates gluconeogenesis.* Glucagon increases the hepatic extraction of amino acids from the plasma and increases the activities of key *gluconeogenic enzymes*, including pyruvate carboxylase and fructose-1,6-diphosphatase. Consequently, glucagon has delayed and protracted actions to promote glucose output by the liver.

Glucagon Is Ketogenic. Because glucagon inhibits *acetyl-CoA carboxylase*, there is decreased production of malonyl-CoA, an inhibitor of *carnitine acyltransferase.* Consequently, fatty acids are directed into the mitochondria for *β-oxidation* and *ketogenesis.*

Control of Glucagon Secretion

Glucose Is the Most Important Controller of Glucagon Secretion. Glucose is the most important controller of both glucagon and insulin secretion; however, glucose has opposing effects on the secretion of these two hormones. Hypoglycemia increases glucagon secretion; as a result of the hyperglycemic actions of glucagon, blood glucose concentration returns toward normal. Conversely, increases in blood glucose concentration decrease glucagon secretion; glucagon and insulin provide important, but opposing, mechanisms for the regulation of blood glucose concentration.

Amino Acids, **Especially Arginine and Alanine, Stimulate Glucagon Secretion.** After a protein meal, both insulin and glucagon secretion are stimulated, but the glucagon response is depressed if glucose is ingested simultaneously. The glucagon response to a protein meal is valuable because without the hyperglycemic effects of glucagon, increased insulin secretion would cause hypoglycemia.

Fasting **and** *Exercise* **Stimulate Glucagon Secretion.** Under these conditions, the stimulation of glucagon secretion helps prevent large decreases in blood glucose concentration. β-adrenergic stimulation increases glucagon secretion, whereas α-adrenergic stimulation inhibits it. However, in contrast to the inhibitory effects of the sympathetic nervous system on insulin secretion, glucagon secretion increases during sympathetic activation.

Somatostatin—Its Ability to Inhibit Glucagon and Insulin Secretion (p. 949)

Somatostatin is synthesized by the *delta cells* in the pancreas, as well as in the gut and hypothalamus, where it is a hypophysiotropic hormone (see Chapter 75). In the pancreas, the major product of the somatostatin prohormone is a 14-amino-acid peptide. Pancreatic somatostatin secretion is stimulated by factors related to the ingestion of food, including increased blood levels of glucose, amino acids, and fatty acids and a number of gastrointestinal hormones. Somatostatin inhibits gastrointestinal motility, secretion, and absorption and is a potent inhibitor of insulin and glucagon secretion; it delays the assimilation of nutrients from the gastrointestinal tract and the utilization of absorbed nutrients by the liver and peripheral tissues.

Diabetes Mellitus (p. 950)

With diabetes mellitus, carbohydrate, fat, and protein metabolism are impaired because of a deficient response to insulin. There are two forms of *diabetes mellitus*:

- *Type I diabetes mellitus,* also called *insulin-dependent diabetes mellitus* (IDDM), is caused by impaired secretion of insulin.

• *Type II diabetes mellitus*, also called *non–insulin-dependent diabetes mellitus* (NIDDM), is caused by resistance to the metabolic effects of insulin in target tissues.

Type I Diabetes Is Caused by Impaired Secretion of Insulin by the Beta Cells of the Pancreas. Often, type I diabetes is a result of autoimmune destruction of beta cells, but it can also arise from the loss of beta cells resulting from viral infections. Because the usual onset of type I diabetes occurs during childhood, it is referred to as *juvenile diabetes*.

Most of the pathophysiological features of type I diabetes can be attributed to the following major effects of insulin deficiency:

• *Hyperglycemia* as a result of impaired glucose uptake into tissues and increased glucose production by the liver (increased gluconeogenesis)
• *Depletion of proteins* resulting from decreased synthesis and increased catabolism
• *Depletion of fat stores and increased ketogenesis*

As a result of these fundamental derangements, the following occur:

• Glucosuria, osmotic diuresis, hypovolemia, and hypotension
• Hyperosmolality of the blood, dehydration, and polydipsia
• Hyperphagia but weight loss; lack of energy
• Acidosis progressing to diabetic coma; rapid and deep breathing
• Hypercholesterolemia and atherosclerotic vascular disease

Insulin Resistance Is the Hallmark of Type II Diabetes Mellitus. Type II diabetes is far more common than type I diabetes (accounting for approximately 90% of all cases of diabetes) and is usually associated with obesity. This form of diabetes is characterized by impaired ability of target tissues to respond to the metabolic effects of insulin, which is referred to as *insulin resistance*. In contrast to type I diabetes, pancreatic beta cell morphology is normal throughout much of the disease, and there is an elevated rate of insulin secretion. Type II diabetes usually develops in adults and therefore is also called *adult-onset diabetes*.

Although hyperglycemia is a prominent feature of type II diabetes, accelerated lipolysis and ketogenesis usually do not occur. Caloric restriction and weight reduction usually improve insulin resistance in target tissues; but in the late stages of the disease when insulin secretion is impaired, insulin administration is required.

CHAPTER 79

Parathyroid Hormone, Calcitonin, Calcium and Phosphate Metabolism, Vitamin D, Bone, and Teeth

The physiology of calcium and phosphate metabolism, the function of vitamin D, and the formation of bone and teeth are all tied together in a common system with the two main regulatory hormones parathyroid hormone (PTH) and calcitonin.

Calcium and Phosphate in the Extracellular Fluid and Plasma—Function of Vitamin D (p. 960)

Control of Vitamin D Formation

The active form of vitamin D, *1,25-dihydroxycholecalciferol,* is carefully regulated via the following steps:

- *In the skin,* 7-dehydrocholesterol is converted by ultraviolet light to vitamin D_3.
- *In the liver,* vitamin D_3 is converted to 25-hydroxycholecalciferol.
- *In the cortex of the kidney,* 25-hydroxycholecalciferol is converted to 1,25-dihydroxycholecalciferol in a reaction *stimulated and tightly controlled by PTH.*

Because PTH formation is stimulated by reduction in the extracellular fluid (ECF) concentration of calcium, formation of 1,25-dihydroxycholecalciferol also increases when the calcium concentration in the ECF falls.

Gastrointestinal Calcium Absorption— 1,25-Dihydroxycholecalciferol

In the epithelial cells of the small intestine, 1,25-dihydroxycholecalciferol stimulates formation of *calcium binding protein, calcium-stimulated ATPase,* and *alkaline phosphatase,* all of which promote absorption of calcium ions out of the lumen of the intestine.

Being a divalent cation, Ca^{2+} cannot cross the cell membrane of the epithelial cells without the mechanisms activated by 1,25-dihydroxycholecalciferol; *therefore, calcium absorption will occur at a rate determined specifically by the activity of the mechanisms regulated by 1,25-dihydroxycholecalciferol.*

Phosphate ions are absorbed in a relatively unregulated manner, although the rate of absorption is increased by administration of 1,25-dihydroxycholecalciferol.

Calcium and Phosphate in the Extracellular Fluid and Plasma (p. 955)

Accurate Regulation of Calcium Ion Concentration Is Essential to Normal Function of the Neuromuscular System and the Skeletal System. If the concentration of calcium in the ECF falls to less than 50% of normal for even brief periods, neuromuscular dysfunction of the skeletal muscles results, initially in the form of hyper-reflexivity and finally as tetanic contractions. If calcium ion concentration increases to 50% greater than normal, central nervous system depression occurs, along with slowing of the contractions of the smooth muscle of the gastrointestinal tract.

Calcium is found normally in the ECF in a total concentration of 2.4 mmol/L, or 9.4 mg/dL. In the ECF, 50% of the calcium is in the free divalent cation form, 40% is loosely bound to proteins, and 10% is in the nonionized form.

Phosphate ion concentration in the ECF can vary rather widely without physiologic impact. Phosphate in the ECF can be either monobasic ($H_2PO_4^-$) or dibasic (HPO_4^{2-}). The normal concentration of $H_2PO_4^-$ is 0.26 mmol/L, whereas HPO_4^{2-} is found at a concentration of 1.05 mmol/L. The relative concentrations of the two are affected by the pH of the ECF, with a reduction in pH increasing the amount of $H_2PO_4^-$ and decreasing the concentration of HPO_4^{2-}. Clinically, total phosphate concentration is usually expressed in milligrams per deciliter and is normally 3 to 4 mg/dL.

Bone and Its Relation to Extracellular Calcium and Phosphates (p. 957)

Bone Is Composed Mostly of Calcium and Phosphate Salts along with Organic Matrix. Approximately 70% of bone is calcium salts; most is in the form of large crystals of *hydroxyapatite*, $Ca_{10}(PO4)_6(OH)_2$. Bone is about 30% organic matrix, made up of collagen fibers and cells. Some calcium in bone is not in crystalline form and therefore is rapidly exchangeable with calcium in the ECF.

Bone Calcification. Bone formation begins with secretion of *collagen fibers* by *osteoblast cells;* the uncalcified collagen structure is referred to as *osteoid*. Calcification of the osteoid takes place over a period of weeks.

Bone Is Continually Deposited by *Osteoblasts* and Absorbed by *Osteoclasts*, a Dynamic Process Referred to as *Remodeling*. Bone has the capacity to undergo remodeling throughout life, although the process takes place much more rapidly in children and young adults than in the elderly. Osteoclast cells digest bone, after which *osteoblasts* deposit new bone. The balance between the two processes is affected by the following:

- *Mechanical stress* on the bone, which stimulates remodeling and formation of stronger bone at points of stress
- *PTH* and *1,25-dihydroxycholecalciferol*, which stimulate osteoclast activity and formation of new osteoclasts
- *Calcitonin*, which decreases the absorptive capacity of osteoclasts and decreases the rate of formation of new osteoclasts

The Calcium and Phosphate Present in Bone Serve as Reservoirs for the Ions in the ECF. About 99% of the total body calcium is in bone, whereas less than 1% is in the ECF. If the calcium ion concentration in the ECF falls below normal, calcium ions move from bone into the ECF. The calcium and phosphate distribution in bone and ECF is affected by PTH and 1,25-dihydroxycholecalciferol, which stimulate movement of calcium and phosphate from bone to the ECF, and by calcitonin, which has the opposite effect. Conversely, when the calcium concentration in the ECF increases above normal, calcium can be deposited in the bone.

Parathyroid Hormone (p. 962)

Parathyroid Hormone Secretion Increases in Response to Reduction in Extracellular Calcium Concentration. The hormone is formed in the *chief cells* of the parathyroid glands located immediately behind the thyroid gland. The rate of formation of PTH is strongly regulated by the ECF calcium ion concentration; small decreases in the concentration of the ion result in large increases in the rate of PTH formation. If the reduction below the normal level of calcium concentration persists, the parathyroid glands hypertrophy, as occurs with pregnancy and disease states such as rickets that are characterized by inadequate calcium absorption from the gastrointestinal tract.

Increases in PTH Concentration Decrease Renal Calcium Excretion. Normally, more than 99% of calcium filtered at the glomerulus is reabsorbed along the tubule. Approximately 5% of the filtered calcium is reabsorbed in the collecting tubules, and it is calcium transport in this segment that is stimulated by PTH. Other factors that affect calcium excretion include the following.

Increase Calcium Excretion	Decrease Calcium Excretion
Decreased [PTH]	Increased [PTH]
Increased ECFV	Decreased ECFV
Decreased [HPO_4^{2-}]	Increased [HPO_4^{2-}]
Metabolic acidosis	Metabolic alkalosis

Increases in PTH Concentration Elevate Phosphate Excretion. Phosphate excretion is regulated as a tubular maximum (T_m) system (see Chapter 29). Approximately 80% is reabsorbed in the proximal tubule, with additional absorption taking place at more distal sites in the nephron. PTH inhibits phosphate reabsorption in the proximal tubule; other factors that affect phosphate excretion include the following.

Increase HPO_4^{2-} Excretion	Decrease HPO_4^{2-} Excretion
Increased [PTH]	Decreased [PTH]
Increased ECF volume	Decreased ECF volume
Increased [HPO_4^{2-}]	Decreased [HPO_4^{2-}]
Metabolic acidosis	Metabolic alkalosis

Calcitonin (p. 966)

Calcitonin Secretion Increases in Response to Elevation of the Extracellular Calcium Concentration. The hormone is a polypeptide with 32 amino acids secreted from the *parafollicular cells* found in the interstitial tissue of the thyroid gland. In general, its effects are opposite those of PTH in the bone and renal tubule, and the magnitude of its effects is much less than that of PTH.

Overall Control of Calcium Ion Concentration (p. 966)

Calcium concentration in the ECF is controlled by a system that affects the distribution between the calcium stored in bone and the ECF, the rate of intake from the gastrointestinal tract, and the rate of excretion by the kidneys (Fig. 79–1).

Figure 79–1. Overview of calcium exchange between different tissue compartments in a person ingesting 1000 mg of calcium per day. Note that most of the ingested calcium is normally eliminated in the feces, although the kidneys have the capacity to excrete large amounts by reducing tabular reabsorption of calcium

Regulation of Calcium Distribution between Bone and Extracellular Fluid

When ECF calcium concentration falls, the following changes take place:

• Readily exchangeable calcium ions diffuse into the ECF.
• PTH formation increases, stimulating the activity of osteoclasts and causing movement of calcium from bone to ECF.

Regulation of Absorption from the Gastrointestinal Tract

When calcium concentration in the ECF falls, the following changes take place:

• PTH formation increases, causing a higher rate of formation of 1,25-dihydroxycholecalciferol.
• Elevated concentration of 1,25-dihydroxycholecalciferol stimulates the formation of calcium-binding protein and other factors in the epithelium of the small intestine, which increase the rate of absorption of calcium from the lumen of the gut.

Regulation of Renal Calcium and Phosphate Excretion

When calcium concentration in the ECF falls, PTH formation increases and the following changes occur:

1. Calcium absorption from the late distal tubules, collecting tubules, and collecting ducts increases, and excretion of calcium decreases.
2. Phosphate reabsorption from the proximal tubule decreases, and phosphate excretion increases.

In humans, the most important feedback control mechanism is the effect of a reduction in ECF calcium concentration to increase the PTH formation. The involvement of calcitonin in the control system is of minor importance in adults.

Pathophysiology of Parathyroid and Bone Diseases (p. 967)

Hypoparathyroidism Decreases Extracellular Calcium Concentration. With inadequate formation of PTH, osteoclasts become inactive and the formation of 1,25-dihydroxycholecalciferol declines to low levels. Transfer of calcium from bone to the ECF decreases, calcium absorption from the gut decreases to low levels, and calcium excretion by the kidneys is greater than the rate of absorption from the gut. As a result, the calcium concentration in the ECF falls below normal levels, and the phosphate concentration remains normal or is elevated. The condition can be treated with very large doses of vitamin D, which have the effect of stimulating gastrointestinal calcium absorption, or by the administration of 1,25-dihydroxycholecalciferol.

Excessive Formation of PTH by the Parathyroid Gland (Hyperparathyroidism) Causes Loss of Calcium from Bone and Increased Extracellular Calcium Concentration. Excessive PTH levels stimulate osteoclastic activity, renal retention of calcium and excretion of phosphate, and increased formation of 1,25-dihydroxycholecalciferol. Calcium concentration in the ECF is greater than normal, and phosphate levels are below normal. The most serious consequences are related to the damage done by excessive osteoclastic absorption of bone, which results in weakening of the bone.

Rickets Is Caused by Inadequate Absorption of Calcium from the Gastrointestinal Tract. This can be due to inadequate calcium in the diet or failure to form adequate amounts of 1,25-dihydroxycholecalciferol. If the kidneys are damaged or absent, 1,25-dihydroxycholecalciferol cannot be formed. Because of inadequate absorption of calcium, PTH levels are elevated, which stimulates osteoclastic resorption of bone and release of calcium to the ECF. In addition, the elevated PTH levels exert renal effects, causing retention of calcium and excretion of phosphate. The net results of these effects are weakening of the bones, a below-normal phosphate concentration, and for periods of months an only slightly below normal calcium concentration resulting from the transfer of calcium from bone to the ECF.

Osteoporosis Is Caused by Depressed Deposition of New Bone by the Osteoblasts. As a result, the rate of osteoclastic resorption of bone exceeds the rate of deposition of new bone.

The most common causes of the condition are (1) lack of physical stress on the bones because of insufficient physical activity; (2) postmenopausal lack of estrogen, because estrogen normally decreases the number and activity of osteoclasts; and (3) old age, in which growth hormone and other factors that contribute to bone formation diminish greatly.

In men, testosterone levels decline gradually but continue to provide a significant anabolic effect into the seventh and eighth decades of life. In women, estrogen formation falls to near zero at menopause, usually at about 50 years of age. The decline in estrogen concentration shifts the balance between deposition and resorption of bone, although no symptoms are apparent for many years. Starting even before menopause, calcium is continually lost from the skeleton. After years of the gradual wasting of calcium, the bones become weakened to the point that symptoms appear, such as vertebral compression and brittleness of the long bones and pelvis. The condition can be prevented with estrogen replacement therapy beginning at menopause. Calcium supplements after menopause are not effective because the condition is not characterized by inadequate calcium in the ECF.

Physiology of the Teeth (p. 969)

Teeth are composed of four parts: *enamel, dentine, cementum,* and *pulp.*

Enamel Makes Up the Outer Layer of the Crown of the Tooth. It is composed of very large, dense crystals of hydroxyapatite embedded in a tight meshwork of protein fibers similar to keratin in hair. The crystalline structure makes the enamel extremely hard, whereas the protein, which is completely insoluble, provides resistance to enzymes, acids, and other corrosive substances.

Dentine Makes Up the Main Body of the Tooth. It is composed of hydroxyapatite crystals embedded in a strong meshwork of collagen fibers, a structure similar to bone. Dentine has no cellular components; all of the nourishment of the structure is provided from *odontoblast cells,* which line the inner surface of the dentine along the wall of the pulp cavity.

Cementum Is a Bony Substance That Lines the Tooth Socket. It is secreted by the cells of the periodontal membrane. Collagen fibers pass from the bone of the jaw, through the periodontal membrane, and into the cementum. This arrangement provides the firm attachment between the teeth and jaw.

Pulp Is the Tissue that Fills the Pulp Cavity of the Tooth. It is composed of odontoblasts, nerves, blood vessels, and lymphatic vessels. During formation of the tooth, the odontoblasts lay down new dentine along the lining of the pulp cavity, making it progressively smaller.

CHAPTER 80

Reproductive and Hormonal Functions of the Male (and Function of the Pineal Gland)

The three major reproductive functions of the male are (1) spermatogenesis—the formation of sperm, (2) performance of the male sexual act, and (3) regulation of male reproductive functions by the various hormones. Associated with these reproductive functions are the effects of the male sex hormones on the accessory sexual organs, cellular metabolism, growth, and other functions of the body.

Spermatogenesis (p. 973)

Spermatogenesis Is the Process of Formation of Spermatocytes from Spermatogonia. It is initiated at puberty, continues throughout the remainder of a man's life, and takes place in the walls of the *seminiferous tubules.*

The walls of the tubules are composed of two compartments separated by tight junctions between the *Sertoli cells*:

- The *basal layer,* which consists of the *Leydig cells* and the *spermatogonia*
- The *adluminal layer,* which is made up of Sertoli cells and *spermatocytes*

The initial step in the process is transformation of *type A spermatogonia,* which are epithelioid in nature, to *type B spermatogonia,* a process involving four divisions. The type B cells embed in the Sertoli cells. In association with the Sertoli cells, the type B cells are transformed to *primary spermatocytes* and then, in a step involving the first meiotic division, to *secondary spermatocytes.* The secondary spermatocytes undergo a second meiotic division, yielding *spermatids,* each of which has 23 unpaired chromosomes. *The steps described are stimulated by testosterone and follicle-stimulating hormone (FSH).*

Spermiogenesis Is the Process of Transformation of the Spermatids, Which Are Still Epithelioid, to Sperm Cells. The process takes place with the cells embedded in the Sertoli cells; *it requires estrogen and FSH.*

Once the sperm cells are formed, they are extruded into the lumen of the tubule in a process stimulated by luteinizing hormone (LH). The first division of the type A spermatogonia to extrusion of the sperm cells requires a period of approximately 64 days.

The newly formed sperm cells are not functional and require a *maturation process*, which takes place in the *epididymis* over a period of 12 days. Maturation *requires both testosterone and estrogen*. The mature sperm are *stored in the vas deferens*.

Male Sexual Act (p. 978)

The male sexual act is the process that culminates in deposition of several hundred million viable sperm cells at the cervix of the man's sexual partner. The sperm cells are contained in a mixture of fluids produced by the male reproductive organs that is called *semen* and includes the following:

- *Seminal vesicle fluid,* which makes up 60% of the total volume of the semen. It contains mucoid, prostaglandin E_2, fructose, and fibrinogen.
- *Prostatic fluid,* which makes up 20% of the semen volume and contains $NaHCO_3$ (pH 7.5), clotting enzyme, calcium, and profibrinolysin.
- *Sperm cells.*

The average volume of semen ejaculated at each coitus is 3.5 mL, and each milliliter of semen contains approximately 120 million sperm cells. For normal fertility, the sperm count per milliliter must be greater than 20 million.

The *sexual act* takes place in three stages:

- *Erection and lubrication.* Erection is the process of filling the erectile tissue of the penis with blood at a pressure level near that of the arterial blood. The arteries leading to the erectile tissue dilate in response to parasympathetic impulses, which stimulate release of nitric oxide at the nerve endings on the arterial smooth muscle. Parasympathetic reflexes also stimulate secretion of mucus by the urethral glands and bulbourethral glands. The mucus aids in vaginal lubrication during coitus.
- *Emission.* This is the process of stimulating the smooth muscle surrounding the seminal vesicles, vas deferens, and prostate gland, causing the organs to empty their contents into the internal urethra, a process elicited by sympathetic reflexes from L1 and L2.
- *Ejaculation.* This is a skeletal muscle reflex elicited in response to distention of the internal urethra. The reflex results in contraction of the ischiocavernosus and bulbocavernosus muscles and the muscles of the pelvis, causing compression in the internal urethra and propulsion of the semen out of the urethra.

Male Sex Hormones (p. 979)

Testosterone Is an Anabolic Steroid Hormone Secreted by the Leydig Cells of the Testes. The hormone is formed from cholesterol in amounts ranging from 2 to 10 mg/day. In the blood, testosterone is carried in association with albumin or is tightly bound to *sex hormone-binding globulin.* The hormone is removed from the blood within 30 to 60 minutes of secretion by fixation to target tissue cells or degradation to inactive compounds. It is metabolized to dihydrotestosterone (the biologically active androgen) in target tissues and to estrogen in adipose tissue.

Testosterone has effects on reproductive and nonreproductive organs. The hormone is required for stimulation of prenatal differentiation and pubertal development of the testes, penis, epididymis, seminal vesicles, and prostate. Testosterone is required in adult men for maintenance and normal function of the primary sex organs. Testosterone also has effects on bone, stimulating growth and proliferation of bone cells, resulting in increased density of the bones. It also has effects on hair distribution and causes the skin to thicken. Testosterone affects the liver, causing synthesis of clotting factors and hepatic lipases. Under the influence of testosterone, blood high density lipoprotein levels decrease, and low density lipoprotein levels increase. Hematocrit and hemoglobin concentrations are elevated because of the effect of testosterone to stimulate production of erythropoietin. The hormone has a generalized effect in many tissues to enhance the rate of protein synthesis.

Being a steroid hormone, testosterone readily enters the cytoplasm of target tissue cells by diffusion through the cell membrane. The enzyme *5α-ketoreductase converts it to dihydrotestosterone,* which then binds with a cytoplasmic receptor protein. This combination migrates to the nucleus, where it binds with a nuclear protein that induces DNA-RNA transcription.

Gonadotropin-Releasing Hormone Increases Release of LH and FSH from the Anterior Pituitary Gland. The polypeptide hormone, which is also referred to as gonadotropin-releasing hormone (GnRH), is secreted from the hypothalamus into the hypothalamic-hypophysial portal system. Its formation is inhibited by testosterone and estrogen (Fig. 80–1).

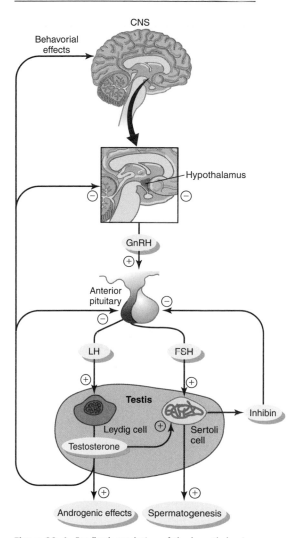

Figure 80–1. Feedback regulation of the hypothalamic-pituitary-testicular axis in males. Stimulatory effects are shown by ⊕ and negative feedback's inhibitory effects are shown by ⊖. FSH, follicle-stimulating hormone; GnRH, gonadotropin-releasing hormone; LH, luteinizing hormone.

LH Stimulates Testosterone Formation by the Leydig Cells, and FSH Stimulates Spermatogenesis and Spermiogenesis. They are secreted from the basophilic cells of the anterior pituitary. Their release is stimulated by GnRH.

Inhibin Is Formed by Sertoli Cells and Inhibits FSH Secretion. Inhibin formation increases as the rate of sperm cell production increases.

Male Infertility *(p. 985)*

Approximately 15% of couples in the United States are infertile, and approximately 50% of the dysfunction is in the male partner; 5% of men in the United States are believed to be infertile. The causes of male infertility include the following:

- *Androgen dysfunction with normal sperm cell production,* caused by hypothalamic-pituitary defects, Leydig cell defects, or androgen resistance
- *Isolated dysfunction of sperm cell production with normal androgen levels,* resulting from infection or trauma, congenital deformation of passages, or formation of nonmotile or otherwise abnormal sperm
- *Combined androgen and sperm cell production defects* resulting from (1) developmental defects, such as Klinefelter's syndrome or abnormal testicular descent, or (2) acquired testicular defects, such as infections, autoimmune reactions, or systemic diseases such as chronic liver and kidney diseases

In 50% of infertile males, no cause can be identified.

CHAPTER 81

Female Physiology Before Pregnancy and Female Hormones

Female Hormonal System (p. 987)

Reproductive function in the female is regulated by interactions of hormones from the hypothalamus, anterior pituitary, and ovaries. Several of the hormones important for female reproductive functions are also found in males.

- *Gonadotropin-releasing hormone (GnRH)* is the releasing factor from the hypothalamus that stimulates secretion of follicle-stimulating hormone (FSH) and luteinizing hormone (LH) from the anterior pituitary. The release of GnRH is inhibited by estrogen and progesterone.
- *LH* is secreted from basophilic cells of the anterior pituitary gland and stimulates development of the corpus luteum in the ovaries.
- *FSH* is secreted from the basophilic cells of the anterior pituitary gland in response to GnRH and stimulates development of the follicles in the ovaries.
- *Estrogen* and *progesterone* are the steroid hormones secreted by the follicle and corpus luteum of the ovary.

The 28-day period of the female sexual cycle is determined by the time required for the development of the follicles and corpus luteum after menstruation and the feedback effect on the hypothalamus of the hormones they secrete.

Monthly Ovarian Cycle (p. 988)

One mature ovum is released from the ovary during each monthly cycle, and the endometrium of the uterus is prepared for implantation of the fertilized ovum at the appropriate time. To achieve these results, all of the hormones of the female reproductive system must interact. The changes of the blood concentrations of the most important hormones of the system over the course of the 28-day cycle are illustrated in Figure 81–1.

Ovarian Follicle Development—The "Follicular" Phase

At the Beginning of the Monthly Cycle, No Mature Follicles or Corpus Lutea Are Present. Estrogen and progesterone concentrations in the blood are at their

Figure 81–1. Appropriate plasma concentrations of the gonadotropins and ovarian hormones during the normal female sexual cycle.

lowest levels (see Fig. 81–1). As a result, the hypothalamus receives no inhibitory signals to block secretion of GnRH. The GnRH that is secreted stimulates FSH and LH secretion from the pituitary, and the FSH stimulates development of 12 to 14 primary ovarian follicles. The follicles are surrounded by *granulosa cells,* which begin to secrete fluid into the center of the structure; this in turn expands to form a fluid-filled antrum that surrounds the oocyte. At this stage, the structure is referred to as an *antral follicle.* The fluid is rich in estrogen, which diffuses into the blood and results in a progressive rise in its concentration. The follicles continue to develop, stimulated by FSH, LH, and the estrogen secreted by the follicles. Proliferation of the granulosa cells proceeds, accompanied by growth of surrounding layers of *thecal cells* derived from the stroma of the ovary. With accumulation of additional fluid and continued development, the follicle is referred to as a *vesicular follicle.*

After approximately 1 week of development, one follicle begins to outgrow the others. The remaining follicles, which developed to the follicular stage, undergo *atresia* and degenerate; the cause of this process is unknown. The remaining dominant follicle continues to develop rapidly, with proliferation of granulosa and thecal cells stimulated by FSH and estrogen. The estrogen promotes development of additional FSH and LH receptors on the granulosa and thecal cells, which provides a positive feedback cycle for rapid development of the maturing follicle.

Because of the rapidly rising concentration of estrogen in the blood (see Fig. 81–1), the hypothalamus receives an inhibitory signal to depress GnRH secretion. This results in suppression of FSH and LH secretion from the pituitary; the reduction in the secretion of FSH prevents the development of additional follicles. The dominant follicle continues to develop because of its intrinsic positive feedback cycle, whereas the other vesicular follicles involute, and no additional primary follicles begin to develop.

Ovulation

Ovulation in a woman who has a normal 28-day female sexual cycle occurs 14 days after the onset of menstruation. About two days before ovulation, a *surge of LH secretion*, 6- to 10-fold above normal, occurs. This LH surge is necessary for ovulation to occur.

Associated with the LH surge, the thecal cells begin to secrete progesterone for the first time. The blood flow in the thecal layers increases at this time, as does the rate of transudation of fluid into the vesicle. The thecal cells also secrete a proteolytic enzyme into the follicular fluid.

At a point of weakness in the wall of the follicle on the surface of the ovary, a protrusion, or *stigma*, develops. The wall ruptures at the stigma within 30 minutes of its formation; and within minutes of the rupture, the follicle evaginates, and the *oocyte* and surrounding layers of granulosa cells, referred to as the *corona radiata*, leave the vesicle and enter the abdominal cavity at the opening to the fallopian tube.

Corpus Luteum—"Luteal Phase of the Ovarian Cycle"

The structure of the follicle remaining on the surface of the ovary after ovulation contains layers of granulosa and thecal cells. The high concentration of LH before ovulation converts these cells to *lutein cells*, which enlarge after ovulation and become yellowish; this structure is referred to as the *corpus luteum*. The granulosa cells secrete large amounts of progesterone and smaller amounts of estrogen, and the thecal cells produce androgenic hormones, testosterone, and androstenedione, most of which are converted by the granulosa cells to the female hormones.

The cells of the corpus luteum require stimulation by the preovulatory surge of LH to undergo transformation and proliferation. The corpus luteum secretes large amounts of progesterone and estrogen for approximately 12 days under the continuing stimulatory influence of the declining concentration of LH. After 12 days, when LH levels are minimal due to feedback inhibition of the hypothalamus by estrogen and progesterone (see Fig. 81–1), the corpus luteum degenerates and ceases to secrete hormones. Within 2 days of failure of the corpus luteum, menstruation begins (see subsequent discussion). At the same time, FSH and LH secretion from the pituitary begins to increase owing to the absence of inhibition of the hypothalamus by estrogen and progesterone. As the concentration rises in the blood of the stimulatory hormones from the pituitary, a new group of primary follicles begins to develop, initiating another cycle.

Summary of Ovarian Cycle

About every 28 days, gonadotropic hormones from the anterior pituitary gland cause about 8 to 12 new follicles to begin to grow in the ovaries. One of these follicles finally becomes "mature" and ovulates on the 14th day of the cycle. During growth of the follicles, mainly estrogen is secreted.

After ovulation, the secretory cells of the ovulating follicle develop into a corpus luteum that secretes large quantities of both major female hormones, progesterone and estrogen. After another 2 weeks, the corpus luteum degenerates, whereupon the ovarian hormones estrogen and progesterone decrease greatly, and menstruation begins. A new ovarian cycle then follows.

Functions of the Ovarian Hormones— Estradiol and Progesterone (p. 991)

The ovaries secrete two classes of hormones: *estrogens* and *progestins; estradiol* is the most important of the estrogens, and *progesterone* is the dominant progestin. In the nonpregnant female, essentially all of the estrogen compounds are secreted from the ovaries, with only minute amounts being synthesized in the adrenal cortex. Nearly all of the progesterone in nonpregnant females is produced in the corpus luteum; only small amounts are formed in the mature follicle during the day immediately before ovulation.

Functions of Estrogen

Estrogens cause growth and proliferation of the cells of the female sex organs and other tissues associated with reproduction.

Estrogen Stimulates the Growth and Development of the Uterus and External Female Sex Organs. At puberty, the levels of estrogen rise rapidly, causing rapid growth in the ovaries, fallopian tubes, uterus, vagina, and external genitalia. The lining of the uterus, the *endometrium,* becomes thickened under the effect of estrogen, as discussed later.

Estrogens Stimulate Development of Stroma Tissue of the Breasts, Growth of an Extensive Ductile System, and Deposition of Fat in the Breasts. Estrogens initiate growth of the breasts and of the milk-producing apparatus. They are also responsible for the characteristic growth and external appearance of the mature female breast. However, they do not complete the job of converting the breasts into milk-producing organs.

Estrogen Causes Growth of the Skeleton by Stimulating Osteoblastic Activity. At puberty, the effect on the osteoblast causes a period of rapid growth in the long bones, although this "growth spurt" lasts only a few years because of the effect of estrogen to cause closure of the epiphyses of the bones. Longitudinal growth occurs only at the epiphyses, so once they are closed additional lengthening of the bones cannot take place.

Estrogen Has a Weak Effect to Increase Total Body Protein and Metabolic Rate. It promotes deposition of fat in the subcutaneous tissue, particularly in the breasts, hips, and thighs.

Functions of Progesterone

The Most Important Function of Progesterone Is to Promote Secretory Changes in the Uterine Endometrium During the Latter Half of the Monthly Sexual Cycle. This prepares the uterus for implantation of the zygote. Progesterone has a similar effect on the lining of the fallopian tubes, causing secretion of the fluid that provides nutrition for the fertilized ovum during its passage to the uterus. The hormone also reduces the excitability and motility of the uterine smooth muscle.

Progesterone Stimulates Development of the Lobules and Alveoli of the Breasts. This effect causes the alveolar cells to enlarge, proliferate, and become secretory in nature, although the cells do not produce milk in response to progesterone.

Progesterone Causes an Upward Resetting of the Body Temperature Control System by About 0.5° F. This effect can be used to determine the time of ovulation because progesterone is not produced until the preovulatory LH surge, which takes place a few hours before ovulation.

Monthly Endometrial Cycle and Menstruation

Driven by the cyclic production of ovarian hormones, the endometrium goes through a monthly cycle characterized by three phases: (1) proliferation, (2) development of secretory changes, and (3) menstruation.

The Proliferative Phase Is Initiated by Secretion of Estrogen from the Developing Follicles. At the beginning of each cycle, most of the endometrium has been lost during menstruation, and only a thin layer of basal endometrial stroma remains. The only remaining epithelial cells are located in the crypts of the endometrium and in the deep portions of the endometrial glands. Estrogen secreted from the developing follicles during the early portion of the cycle stimulates rapid proliferation of the stromal and epithelial cells. The entire endometrial surface is re-epithelialized within 4 to 7 days of the beginning of menstruation. During the next 10 days, the stimulatory effects of estrogen cause development and thickening of the endometrium of up to 4 mm.

The Secretory Phase Results from Changes Brought About by Progesterone. After ovulation, the corpus luteum secretes large amounts of progesterone and estrogen. The effect of the progesterone is to cause swelling and secretory development of the endometrium. The glands secrete fluid, and the endometrial cells accumulate lipids and glycogen in their cytoplasm. The vascularity of the endometrium continues to develop in response to the requirements of the developing tissue. At the peak of the secretory phase, at 1 week after ovulation, the endometrium is approximately 6 mm thick.

Menstruation Follows within 2 Days of Involution of the Corpus Luteum. Without the stimulation of the estrogen and progesterone secreted by the corpus luteum, the endometrium rapidly involutes, to about 65% of its previous thickness. Then, starting approximately 24 hours before menstruation, the blood vessels supplying the endometrium become vasospastic, resulting in ischemia and finally necrosis of the tissue. Hemorrhagic areas develop in the necrotic tissue, and gradually the outer layers separate from the uterine wall. At about 48 hours after the start of menstruation, all the superficial layers of the endometrium are desquamified. Distention of the uterine cavity, elevated levels of prostaglandin E2 released from the ischemic and necrotic tissue, and low levels of progesterone contribute to stimulation of uterine contractions, which expel the shed tissue and blood. The menstrual fluid is normally nonclotting resulting from the presence of *fibrinolysin* released from the endometrial tissue.

Regulation of the Female Monthly Rhythm—Interplay between the Ovarian and Hypothalamic-Pituitary Hormones *(p. 996)*

At the beginning of each monthly cycle, a new group of primary follicles begins to develop, secreting increasing levels of estrogen in response to the trophic hormones from the pituitary, FSH, and LH.

Estrogen in small amounts strongly inhibits secretion of LH and FSH through a direct pituitary effect, although estrogen also inhibits the hypothalamic secretion of GnRH. Progesterone acts synergistically with estrogen, but it has only a weak inhibitory effect by itself.

As the level of estrogen rises, the rate of secretion of the pituitary hormones begins to fall; however, for unknown reasons, the pituitary gland secretes a large amount of LH immediately before ovulation, when estrogen levels are elevated. This surge of LH at a time when LH secretion "should" be suppressed by the inhibitory influence of estrogen triggers ovulation and transformation of the granulosa and thecal cells to luteal cells.

After ovulation, the estrogen and progesterone secreted from the corpus luteum again exert an inhibitory effect on the secretion of LH and FSH.

Inhibin also is secreted from the corpus luteum. As in males, inhibin in females inhibits secretion of FSH and, to a lesser extent, LH.

Once the levels of LH fall to minimal values, because of the inhibitory influence of the hormones from the corpus luteum the corpus luteum involutes, and estrogen and progesterone secretion rates decline toward zero. Formation of LH and FSH increases in the absence of inhibition as menstruation begins, initiating the development of a new group of follicles.

Puberty, Menarche, and Menopause

Puberty Is the Onset of Adult Sexual Life. It is marked by a gradual increase in the secretion of estrogen from developing follicles driven by increasing concentrations of FSH and LH from the pituitary.

Menarche Is the Onset of Menstruation. It marks completion of the first cycle of the system, although the first several cycles usually do not include ovulation.

Menopause Is the Period during which the Cycles Cease and the Ovarian Hormone Levels Fall to Minimal Values. The cessation of the cycling is the result of the presence of an inadequate number of primary follicles in the ovary to respond to the stimulatory effect of FSH. As a result, the estrogen-secretory dynamics during the first portion of the cycle are inappropriate for triggering the LH surge, and ovulation does not occur. After several irregular anovulatory cycles, estrogen production declines to near zero. Without inhibition, the rate of LH and FSH secretion proceeds at very high levels for many years after menopause.

Female Sexual Act (p. 1000)

Both psychic and local sensory stimulation are important for satisfactory performance of the female sexual act. Sexual desire is affected to some extent by estrogen and testosterone levels in the female; consequently, desire may be greatest a few days before ovulation, when estrogen secretion from the follicle is greatest.

Erectile tissue analogous to that in the penis is located around the introitus and extending into the clitoris. Dilation of the arteries leading into the tissue is mediated by parasympathetic nerves that release nitric oxide from their nerve endings on the vascular smooth muscle of the arteries. Parasympathetic stimulation also causes secretion of mucus from Bartholin's gland, which is located underneath the labia minora.

With appropriate local sensory and psychic stimulation, reflexes are initiated that cause the female orgasm.

Female Fertility *(p. 1000)*

Female fertility depends on properly timed ovulation, ability of sperm to reach the ovum in the fallopian tube within 24 hours of ovulation, and the ability of the zygote to implant and survive in the endometrium. Several problems can make a woman infertile.

- *Failure to ovulate* can result from the following:
  1. Mechanical obstruction on the surface of the ovary resulting from (1) the presence of a thickened capsule; (2) scarring from infection; and (3) overgrowth of the surface by cells of endometrial origin, a condition referred to as *endometriosis.*
  2. Absence of an LH surge or other hormonal abnormalities.
- *Obstruction of the fallopian tubes* is often a result of infection or endometriosis.

CHAPTER 82

Pregnancy and Lactation

Transport, Fertilization, and Implantation of the Developing Ovum *(p. 1003)*

While still in the ovary, the *primary oocyte* undergoes meiotic division shortly before ovulation, giving rise to the first polar body, which is expelled from the nucleus. With this division, the oocyte is transformed to a *secondary oocyte* containing 23 unpaired chromosomes. A few hours after a sperm cell enters the oocyte, the nucleus divides again and a second polar body is expelled, forming the *mature ovum,* which still contains 23 unpaired chromosomes.

The Ovum Enters the Fallopian Tube (Oviduct) (*Fig. 82–1*). At ovulation, the ovum and surrounding layers of granulosa cells, referred to as the *corona radiata,* are expelled from the ovary into the peritoneal cavity at the ostium, or opening, of the fallopian tube. The ciliated epithelium lining the tubes creates a weak current that draws the ovum into the tube.

Fertilization Takes Place in the Fallopian Tube. Within 5 to 10 minutes of ejaculation, sperm cells reach the ampullae at the ovarian ends of the fallopian tubes aided by contractions of the uterus and fallopian tubes. Normally, approximately several hundred million sperm are deposited at the cervix during coitus, but only a few thousand reach the ampullae of the fallopian tubes where fertilization usually takes place.

Before fertilization can occur, the *corona radiata* must be removed through the successive actions of many sperm cells that release the proteolytic enzymes in the *acrosome* at the head of the sperm cell. Once the way is cleared, one sperm cell can bind to and penetrate the *zona pellucida* surrounding the ovum and enter the ovum. The 23 unpaired chromosomes from the sperm cell rapidly form the *male pronucleus,* which then align themselves with the 23 unpaired chromosomes of the *female pronucleus* to form the 23 pairs of chromosomes of the fertilized ovum or *zygote.*

The Zygote Is Transported in the Fallopian Tubes. Three to 5 days are required for passage of the zygote through the fallopian tube to the cavity of the uterus. During this time the survival of the organism is dependent on the secretions of the epithelium of the tube. The first series of cellular divisions take place while the ovum is in the fallopian tube, so by the time it enters the uterus the structure is referred to as a

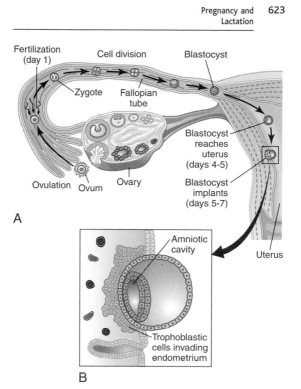

Figure 82–1. *A*, Ovulation, fertilization of the ovum in the fallopian tube, and implantation of the blastocyst in the uterus. *B*, Action of trophoblast cells during implantation of the blastocyst in the uterine endometrium.

blastocyst. Shortly after ovulation the *isthmus* of the fallopian tube (the last 2 cm before the tube enters the uterus) becomes tonically contracted, blocking movement between the tubes and uterus. The final entry into the uterus does not take place until the smooth muscle at the isthmus relaxes under the influence of rising levels of progesterone from the corpus luteum.

The Blastocyst Implants in the Endometrium. The developing blastocyst remains free in the cavity of the uterus for an additional 3 days before implantation begins. On about the seventh day after ovulation, the *trophoblast cells* on the surface of the blastocyst begin to secrete proteolytic enzymes that digest and liquefy the adjacent endometrium. Within a few days, the blastocyst has invaded the endometrium and is firmly attached to it. The contents of the digested cells, which contain large amounts of stored nutrients, are actively transported by the trophoblast cells for use as substrates to enable rapid growth of the blastocyst.

Function of the Placenta (p. 1005)

Development of the Placenta

The trophoblast cells form cords that grow into the endometrium. Blood capillaries grow into the cords from the vascular system of the embryo; about 21 days after fertilization, blood flow begins into the capillaries. Simultaneously, on the maternal side, sinuses develop that are perfused with blood from the uterine vessels, surrounding the trophoblast cords. The cords branch extensively as they continue to grow, forming the *placental villi* into which embryonic capillaries grow. The villi contain capillaries carrying fetal blood, and they are surrounded by sinuses filled with maternal blood. The two blood supplies remain separated by several cell layers, and no mixing occurs of the blood from the mother and fetus.

Blood enters the fetal side of the placenta from two umbilical arteries and returns to the fetus by way of a single umbilical vein. The paired uterine arteries of the mother give rise to branches that supply blood for the maternal sinuses, which are drained by branches of the uterine veins.

Placental Permeability and Transport

Oxygen Diffuses from the Maternal Blood through the Placental Membranes and into the Fetal Blood. The mean Po_2 for the blood in the maternal sinuses is about 50 mm Hg, whereas in the venous end of the fetal capillaries, the Po_2 averages 30 mm Hg; the 20-mm Hg pressure gradient is the driving force for the *diffusion* of oxygen from the maternal to the fetal blood.

Several factors assist in the diffusion of oxygen from the mother to the fetus:

- The fetal hemoglobin has a greater affinity for oxygen than does adult hemoglobin. At the partial pressures of O_2 present in the placenta, fetal hemoglobin can carry 20% to 50% more oxygen than maternal hemoglobin.
- The concentration of hemoglobin in the fetal blood is 50% greater than that in the maternal blood.

- The *Bohr effect* operates in favor of transfer of oxygen from the maternal blood to that of the fetus. The Bohr effect refers to the action of an increase in Pco_2 to decrease the affinity of hemoglobin for O_2. Fetal blood entering the placenta has a high Pco_2, but it rapidly diffuses into the maternal blood because of a favorable pressure gradient. As a result, the Pco_2 in the fetal blood decreases while that of the maternal blood increases, causing the affinity of the fetal hemoglobin for oxygen to increase and the affinity of the maternal hemoglobin to decrease.

Carbon Dioxide Diffuses Readily through the Membranes of the Placenta. Even though the pressure gradient driving the diffusion averages only about 2 to 3 mm Hg, the CO_2 molecule is extremely soluble in biologic membranes and can move easily across the layers of the placenta.

Movement of Metabolic Substrates Such as Glucose and Fatty Acids across the Placenta Occurs by the Same Mechanisms That Operate in Other Parts of the Body. Glucose diffusion is aided by a facilitated diffusion process, and fatty acids cross the membranes by simple diffusion. Electrolytes such as sodium and potassium move by both diffusion and active transport.

Removal of Waste Products from Fetal Blood to Maternal Blood. Metabolic waste products formed in the fetus also diffuse through the placental membrane into the maternal blood and are then excreted along with the excretory products of the mother. These include especially the *nonprotein nitrogens* such as *urea, uric acid,* and *creatinine.*

Hormonal Factors During Pregnancy (p. 1007)

In pregnancy, the placenta forms especially large quantities of *human chorionic gonadotropin, estrogens, progesterone,* and *human chorionic somatomammotropin,* the first three of which, and probably the fourth as well, are all essential to a normal pregnancy.

Human Chorionic Gonadotropin—Persistence of the Corpus Luteum and Prevention of Menstruation

Human chorionic gonadotropin (hCG) is a glycoprotein hormone produced by trophoblast cells beginning 8 to 9 days after fertilization. It reaches the maternal blood and binds to luteinizing hormone (LH) receptors in the cells of the corpus luteum. At about this time, LH levels begin to decline; if fertilization does not occur, the corpus luteum involutes and menstruation begins within a few days. The hCG effect on the corpus luteum is the same as that of LH: the hCG maintains the function of the corpus luteum and continues to stimulate its secretion of large amounts of progesterone and estrogen, so the endometrium can continue in a viable state that would support early development of the embryo. As a result of the hCG secretion, menstruation does not occur.

In addition, hCG binds to LH receptors in the Leydig cells of the testes of male embryos; this stimulates testosterone secretion, which is essential to differentiation of the male sex organs.

Estrogen and Progesterone

The *syncytial trophoblast* cells of the placenta secrete both estrogens and progesterone. Late in pregnancy, the estrogen secretory rate is approximately 30 times the normal rate. The high concentrations of estrogens cause the following conditions:

- Enlargement of the mother's uterus
- Enlargement of the mother's breasts, with growth of the ductile structure
- Enlargement of the mother's external genitalia

Progesterone is also necessary for pregnancy. The rate of secretion reaches 10 times the maximum level present during nonpregnant cycles. Its functions include the following:

- Promotion of storage of nutrients in the endometrial cells, transforming them into *decidual cells*
- Reduction of contractility of the uterine smooth muscle, *preventing contractions*
- Promotion of secretion of nutrient-rich fluids from the epithelium of the fallopian tubes that *sustain the zygote* before implantation
- Promotion of development of the *alveoli of the breasts*

Human Chorionic Somatomammotropin

Human chorionic somatomammotropin is a third placental hormone, and it is secreted by the placenta starting during the fifth week of pregnancy. The specific function of the hormone remains unknown, although it does have metabolic effects similar to those of growth hormone. It reduces insulin sensitivity of tissues and decreases glucose utilization. Human chorionic soma-tomammotropin also promotes releases of fatty acids from fat stores.

Parturition (p. 1011)

Increased Uterine Excitability Near Term

Parturition is the process by which the baby is born. Toward the end of pregnancy, the uterus becomes progressively more excitable until it begins strong rhythmical contractions that expel the baby. Changes in hormonal levels and mechanical properties of the uterus and its contents contribute to the increase in uterine contractility.

Hormones Increase Uterine Contractility. Beginning in the seventh month of pregnancy, the rate of progesterone secretion remains constant, whereas the rate of estrogen secretion continues to rise. Although progesterone reduces the contractility of uterine smooth muscle, estrogen has the opposite effect. *Because the estrogen-to-progesterone ratio increases during the final weeks of pregnancy, the excitability of the organ increases.*

Oxytocin, which is secreted from the posterior pituitary, can cause uterine contractions. During the final weeks of pregnancy the oxytocin receptors on the cells of the uterine smooth muscle increase, which increases the intensity of response for a given concentration of hormone. At the time of labor, the oxytocin concentration is elevated considerably above normal. There is reason to believe that oxytocin contributes to the mechanism of parturition.

Stretch of the Uterus and Cervix Increases Uterine Contractility. Stretch of smooth muscle increases its excitability. The size of the fetus near the end of pregnancy provides continual distention of the uterus, and the vigorous movements of the maturing fetus provide intermittent stretch of portions of the smooth muscle wall of the organ. The cervix becomes greatly distended as the end of pregnancy approaches. Contractions initiated by stretch of this part of the uterus can spread upward through the body of the uterus. In addition, stretch and distention of the cervix elicit reflexes that cause release of oxytocin from the posterior pituitary gland.

Onset of Labor—A Positive Feedback Mechanism for Its Initiation

Beginning in the sixth month of pregnancy, the uterus undergoes periodic slow rhythmical contractions called *Braxton-Hicks contractions*. As the duration of pregnancy increases, the frequency and intensity of these contractions increase. At some point, a contraction occurs that is sufficiently powerful, and the uterine muscle is sufficiently excitable that the effect of the contraction elevates the level of excitability still more; thus, after several minutes another contraction is initiated. If the second contraction is more powerful than the first, an even greater elevation of excitability results, followed by an even more powerful contraction. Such a *positive feedback cycle* appears to operate during parturition. The cycles continue to intensify the strength of contractions until delivery finally occurs.

Lactation *(p. 1014)*

High Levels of Estrogen and Progesterone During the Later Months of Pregnancy Promote the Final Developmental Changes in the Breasts that Prepare Them for Lactation. These hormones do not stimulate milk production by the alveolar cells. Milk formation is achieved through the effects of prolactin, an anterior pituitary hormone that is secreted in rising concentrations throughout pregnancy. The stimulatory effect of prolactin is blocked by the high concentrations of estrogen and progesterone secreted by the placenta, so no milk is formed until after delivery of the baby. When the levels of estrogen and progesterone fall, the stimulatory effect of prolactin causes the cells of the alveoli to synthesize milk, which accumulates in the alveoli and ducts of the breast.

The Mechanical Stimulation Associated with Suckling Elicits a Reflex to the Hypothalamus, Releasing Oxytocin from the Posterior Pituitary Gland. Oxytocin travels to the breast in the blood and causes contraction of the *myoepithelial cells* that surround the ducts of the breast. The contraction increases the pressure of the milk filling the ducts, causing milk to flow from the nipple to the baby. Milk is not usually ejected from the breast until the baby suckles the nipple.

After delivery, prolactin levels tend to fall toward nonpregnant levels. Stimulation of the nipples associated with suckling, however, increases the release of prolactin, which in turn stimulates milk production. The greater the duration of suckling, the greater is the response of prolactin and the greater is the amount of milk produced by the breast. This feedback control system regulated by the baby's desire for milk and duration of suckling provides for a well regulated supply of milk for the baby from the time it is born until as long as 1 year or more after birth, when its requirements for milk have increased greatly. When the baby discontinues breast-feeding, the signal for prolactin secretion stops, and milk production declines rapidly.

Prolactin is regulated by hypothalamic release of *prolactin-inhibitory factor (PIF)*, which is believed to be *dopamine.* Elevated dopamine release from the hypothalamus inhibits prolactin secretion from the pituitary gland.

During the period of breast-feeding, the mother's ovarian cycle is interrupted, so ovulation and menstruation do not occur for several months after delivery. The precise cause for this effect is not known.

Human milk is composed of 88.5% water, 3.3% fat, 6.8% lactose, 0.9% casein, and other proteins and minerals. When a woman is lactating heavily to supply the needs of a rapidly growing, large baby, she may secrete 2 to 3 g of calcium phosphate into the milk per day. This can lead to depletion of calcium from the bones if the mother does not carefully choose a diet that is rich in calcium.

CHAPTER 83

Fetal and Neonatal Physiology

Growth and Functional Development of the Fetus (p. 1019)

Circulatory System. The heart begins to beat during the fourth week after fertilization, which is about the same time that the first non-nucleated red blood cells form. During the first two thirds of gestation, red blood cells are formed outside the bone marrow; only during the final 3 months of gestation are most of the red blood cells formed in the bone marrow.

Respiratory System. Although some respiratory movements take place during the first and second trimesters, respiratory movements are inhibited during the final 3 months of gestation. This inhibition prevents filling of the lungs with debris from the amniotic fluid.

Nervous System. The organization of the central nervous system is completed during the first months of gestation, but full development and even complete myelination do not take place until after delivery.

Gastrointestinal Tract. By midpregnancy, the fetus ingests amniotic fluid and excretes *meconium* from the gastrointestinal tract. Meconium is composed of residue from amniotic fluid and waste products and debris from the epithelium of the gastrointestinal tract. By the final 2 to 3 months of gestation, gastrointestinal tract function approaches maturity.

Kidneys. The fetal kidneys can form urine beginning in the second trimester, and urination takes place during the latter half of gestation. Abnormal kidney development or severe impairment of kidney function in the fetus greatly reduces the formation of amniotic fluid *(oligohydramnios)* and can lead to fetal death The ability of the kidneys to regulate the composition of the extracellular fluid accurately is poorly developed until several months after birth.

Fetal Metabolism. The fetus uses mainly glucose for energy and has a high capability to store fat and protein, much if not most of the fat being synthesized from glucose rather than being absorbed directly from the mother's blood.

The average fetus accumulates about 22.5 g of calcium and 13.5 g of phosphorus during gestation. About half of this accumulation occurs in the last 4 weeks before birth, coincident with a period of rapid ossification of the fetal bones and rapid weight gain off the fetus.

Adjustments of the Infant to Extrauterine Life *(p. 1021)*

Onset of Breathing. Normally, a baby begins to breathe within seconds of delivery. The stimuli for the sudden activation of the respiratory system probably include hypoxia incurred during delivery and sudden cooling of the face on exposure to the air. A normal pattern of breathing develops within 1 minute of delivery, although in some cases the onset of breathing may be delayed. Newborn infants can tolerate 8 to 10 minutes without breathing before permanent damage occurs; in adults, death or severe damage takes place if breathing is interrupted for 4 to 5 minutes.

Expansion of the Lungs at Birth. The surface tension of the fluid-filled lungs at birth keeps the alveoli in a collapsed state. Approximately 25 mm Hg of negative inspiratory pressure is required to overcome the surface tension. At birth, the first inspirations are powerful and generate as much as 60 mm Hg negative intrapleural pressure.

Circulatory Readjustments at Birth *(p. 1022)*

Two primary changes occur in the fetal circulation at birth:

- A *doubling of systemic vascular resistance* resulting from loss of the placenta, which has very low vascular resistance. This increases aortic pressure and left ventricular and left atrial pressures.
- A *fivefold decrease in pulmonary vascular resistance* resulting from expansion of the lungs following the first inspiration. As a result, pulmonary arterial, right ventricular, and right atrial pressures decrease.

After these initial changes, several other alterations follow:

- The *foramen ovale, which is located between the right and left atria, closes* owing to the pressure in the left side being greater than the pressure in the right.
- The *ductus arteriosus between the pulmonary artery and descending aorta closes.*
- The *ductus venosus closes.* During fetal life, it carries blood from the umbilical vein and the fetal portal bed directly to the inferior vena cava, bypassing the fetal liver.

With these adjustments, the fetal circulation is transformed within a matter of hours to the neonatal configuration.

Special Problems in the Neonate *(p. 1023)*

In the newborn, most of the cardiovascular, hormonal, and neural control systems are poorly developed and are often unstable.

Respiratory System. Because of the relatively small residual capacity (less than one half the volume per kilogram of body weight than that of adults), relatively high metabolic rate of the newborn, and immaturity of the neural components of the respiratory control system, blood gas values fluctuate widely during the first weeks of life.

Circulation. *Blood volume* at birth is normally about 300 mL. If the baby is left attached to the placenta for a few minutes after birth, approximately 75 mL of additional blood can enter the baby's circulatory system, which is equivalent to a transfusion of 25% of the blood volume. This overload could contribute to an elevation of left atrial pressure and a tendency to develop pulmonary edema.

Liver Function. *Bilirubin* formed from the breakdown of hemoglobin from red blood cells is normally excreted by the liver into the bile conjugated with glucuronic acid; however, the neonatal liver has inadequate ability to conjugate bilirubin at the rate it is formed. As a result, the blood concentration of bilirubin rises for the first 3 days after birth and then returns to normal as the capability of the liver increases. This condition is referred to as *physiologic hyperbilirubinemia* and can be seen in some cases as a slight jaundice or yellowish tint in the skin and sclera of the eyes.

In addition to the potential problems associated with bilirubin conjugation, the limited capability of the liver during the first few days of life can lead to difficulty synthesizing adequate quantities of protein for maintaining colloid osmotic pressure, adequate amounts of glucose, and necessary amounts of the factors required for coagulation. These potential limitations of hepatic function rapidly diminish during the first weeks of postnatal life.

Fluid Balance and Renal Function. On a per-kilogram of body weight basis, the neonate takes in seven times as much fluid as an adult. In addition, the metabolic rate per kilogram of body weight of the newborn is twice as great as that of the adult. These and other factors can contribute to problems in the newborn regarding the regulation of fluid balance, electrolyte concentrations, pH, and colloid osmotic pressure.

Digestion and Metabolism. The gastrointestinal absorptive capacity and hepatic digestive function of neonates are limited to some extent in the following ways:

- *Absorption of starches* is limited by a deficient rate of secretion of pancreatic amylase, which breaks down complex carbohydrates such as starches.
- *Absorption of fat* is not as great in neonates as it is in older children.
- *Gluconeogenic capacity* of the liver is not sufficient in many newborns to maintain the blood glucose concentration in the normal range for long periods after feeding. It is important to maintain the newborn on a schedule of frequent feedings.

All of these gastrointestinal limitations are exacerbated in preterm infants. The limited capacities for absorption of starches and fats are worsened by feeding cow's milk-based formulas to preterm and newborn infants. The carbohydrates and fats in human milk are digested and absorbed more readily than those in non-human milk and formula preparations.

The *basal metabolic rate* of the newborn is twice as high per kilogram of body weight as that of an adult, and the surface area to body rate ratio is much greater in the neonate than in the adult. As a result, body temperature control is relatively unstable, especially in preterm infants.

XV

Sports Physiology

CHAPTER 84

Sports Physiology

Few of the normal, day-to-day stresses to which the body is exposed even approach the extreme stresses of heavy exercise. For example, the metabolic rate increases about 100% in a person with a high fever, but the metabolism of a marathon runner may increase to 2000% of normal during a race.

Female and Male Athletes (p. 1031)

Total body muscle mass greatly influences muscle strength, pulmonary ventilation, and cardiac output, which in females are two thirds to three fourths of the values found in males. If measured in terms of strength per square centimeter of muscle cross-sectional area, however, a female can achieve the same maximum force of contraction as men: 3 to 4 kg/cm^2. Much of the difference in athletic performance of males and females is due to the smaller amount of muscle mass in females.

Testosterone is primarily responsible for the increased amount of muscle mass in males and has strong *anabolic effects* on protein deposition, especially in muscles. Even a nonathletic male may have 40% more muscle mass than his female counterpart. In comparison, *estrogen* in females causes increased fat deposition in the breasts and subcutaneous tissue. The nonathletic female may have about 27% body fat in contrast to 15% body fat in a nonathletic man. In addition, testosterone promotes some aggressiveness, which may play a role in some athletic events.

Muscles During Exercise (p. 1031)

The *Contractile Strength* of a Muscle Is Directly Related to Its Size. A person with large muscles is generally stronger than one with small muscles. The strongest muscle in the body is the quadriceps muscle, which has a cross-sectional area of up to 150 cm^2 has a maximum contractile strength of 525 kg (1155 pounds). When an athlete is using the quadriceps muscles for lifting, a tremendous amount of stress is applied to the patellar tendon. This or any other highly strenuous activity places much stress on joints, tendons, muscles, and ligaments. The *holding strength* of a muscle is approximately 40% greater than the maximal contractile strength and is the force required to stretch out a muscle after it has contracted.

The *Power* of a Muscle Is the Amount of Work That Can Be Performed Per Unit Time. The power is determined not only by muscle strength but also by the distance it contracts and number of times it contracts each minute; this is usually measured in kilogrammeters per minute. Table 84–1 shows that muscle power is very high during the first 8 to 10 seconds of exercise and then decreases.

A large power surge occurs in a race such as a 100-m dash (see Table 84–1), but in a longer-distance race much lower power levels are available—about one fourth as much. The velocity achieved in a 100-m dash, however, is only about 1.75 times as great as that achieved in a 10,000-m run.

***Endurance* Depends on Maintaining a Nutrition Supply for the Muscle.** As seen in Table 84–2, a person on a high-carbohydrate diet stores more glycogen in the muscles, which increases his or her endurance in races at marathon speeds. This is why marathon runners eat a large amount of carbohydrates, such as pasta, on the day before the race.

Table 84–1.   Muscle Power During Exercise

Time	Muscle Power (kg-m/min)
First 8–10 seconds	7000
Next 1 minute	4000
Next 30 minutes	1700

Table 84–2.   Effects of Glycogen Storage on Exercise Endurance

Diet	Glycogen Stored in Muscle (g/kg of muscle)	Endurance Time at Marathon Speed (min)
High carbohydrate	40	240
Mixed	20	120
High fat	6	85

Muscle Metabolic Systems During Exercise

The basic sources of energy for muscle contraction are the following:

• *Phosphagen system,* which consists of adenosine triphosphate (ATP) and phosphocreatine
• *Glycogen–lactic acid system*
• *Aerobic system*

ATP Is the Basic Source of Energy for Muscle Contraction. ATP, which consists of adenosine with three high-energy phosphate bonds attached, supplies the short-term energy needs of the muscle fibers. ATP is converted to adenosine diphosphate (ADP) by the removal of one high-energy phosphate radical; this releases 7300 calories per mole of ATP. This energy is used for muscle contraction as ATP combines with the myosin filaments. The removal of another phosphate radical converts ADP to adenosine monophosphate (AMP) and supplies an additional 7300 calories per mole of ADP.

The amount of ATP present in muscle sustains maximal muscle contraction for only 3 seconds, but the phosphocreatine system also supplies energy. The combination of the cellular ATP and phosphocreatine system is called the *phosphagen energy system.*

Phosphocreatine (or *creatine phosphate)* is the combination of creatine and a phosphate radical connected with a high-energy phosphate bond, which, when broken, provides 10,300 calories per mole. Adding to the importance of this system is the fact that muscle cells have twofold to fourfold more phosphocreatine than ATP.

Phosphocreatine reversibly combines with ADP to form ATP and creatine in the cell. This phosphagen energy system by itself, however, supplies only enough energy for 8 to 10 seconds of maximal muscle contraction, or nearly enough energy for a 100-m race.

The Glycogen–Lactic Acid System Supplies Energy through Anaerobic Metabolism. The glycogen stored in muscle rapidly splits into glucose molecules that can be used for energy. The initial stage of this process is called *glycolysis;* it occurs without the use of oxygen and is referred to as *anaerobic metabolism.* The glycogen in this process is mostly converted to lactic acid and supplies four ATP molecules for each molecule of glucose. An advantage of this glycogen–lactic acid system is that it forms ATP 2.5 times as fast as oxidative metabolism in the mitochondria. The system supplies enough energy for maximal muscle contraction for 1.3 to 1.6 minutes.

For longer periods of muscle use, energy for muscle contraction must be supplied through the aerobic system. In this system, glucose, fatty acids, and amino acids are oxidized in the mitochondria to form ATP.

Recovery of Energy Systems after Exercise Requires Oxygen. After exercise is completed, the energy sources of muscle must be reconstituted. Any lactic acid formed during exercise is converted to pyruvic acid and then metabolized oxidatively or reconverted to glucose (mainly in the liver). The extra liver glucose forms glycogen, which replenishes the glycogen stores in muscles.

The aerobic system is also replenished after exercise by two means:

- *The increased respiration that occurs after exercise replenishes the oxygen debt.* The oxygen debt is the deficit in the oxygen stored in the body as air in the lungs, dissolved in body fluids, and combined with hemoglobin and myoglobin.

- *The glycogen is replaced in the muscle.* This process can take days to complete after extreme long-lasting exercise, with the recovery time highly dependent on the diet of the person. An individual on a high-carbohydrate diet replenishes muscle glycogen stores much faster than one on either a mixed diet or a high-fat diet.

Resistive Training Significantly Enhances Muscle Strength

If the muscles are exercised under no load, even for hours, little increase in strength occurs. However, if muscles are contracted with at least a 50% maximum force for a few times each day three times a week, an optimal increase in muscle strength occurs, and muscle mass increases through a process called *muscle hypertrophy.* Most of the hypertrophy is caused by an increase in the size of the muscle fibers, but the number of fibers increases moderately. Other changes occur in the muscle during training, including the following:

- Increase in number of myofibrils
- Up to 120% increase in mitochondrial enzymes
- A 60% to 80% increase in the components of the phosphagen energy system

- A 50% increase in stored glycogen
- A 75% to 100% increase in stored triglycerides

Fast-Twitch and Slow-Twitch Muscle Fibers and Various Types of Exercise

Fast-twitch muscle fibers give a person the ability to contract their muscles rapidly and forcefully. *Slow-twitch fibers* are used for prolonged lower leg muscle activity. The differences between fast-twitch and slow-twitch fibers include the following:

- Fast-twitch fibers are about twice as large in diameter.
- Enzymes that release energy from the phosphagen and glycogen–lactic acid energy systems are two to three times as active in the fast-twitch fibers.
- Slow-twitch fibers are used more for endurance exercise, using the aerobic system of energy; there are more mitochondria in slow-twitch fibers than in fast-twitch fibers.
- Slow-twitch fibers contain more myoglobin, which is a hemoglobin-like substance that combines with oxygen in muscle.
- Capillary density in slow-twitch fibers exceeds that of fast-twitch fibers.

Fast-twitch fibers generate a great amount of power in a short period of time, such as during a sprint. In contrast, slow-twitch fibers are used for endurance exercises, such as marathons.

Respiration During Exercise *(p. 1036)*

Maximum Oxygen Consumption Increases During Athletic Training. The maximum oxygen consumption of the average untrained male is 3600 mL/min; this increases to 4000 mL/min in the athletically trained male and to 5100 mL/min in the male marathon runner. The maximum oxygen consumption increases during training, but the high values in marathon runners may be partly genetically determined by factors such as large lung capacity in relation to body size and strength of respiratory muscles.

At maximal exercise, pulmonary ventilation is 100 to 110 L/min, but maximum breathing capacity exceeds this by 50%. The lungs have a built-in safety mechanism that can be helpful if exercise is attempted (1) at a high altitude, (2) under hot conditions, or (3) with some abnormality in the respiratory system.

Pulmonary Oxygen-Diffusing Capacity Increases in Athletes. The oxygen-diffusing capacity is the rate at which oxygen diffuses from the alveoli into the blood per millimeter of mercury oxygen pressure. During exercise, the diffusing capacity increases in a nonathlete from a resting value of 23 mL/min/mm Hg to 48 mL/min/mm Hg. The diffusing capacity increases during exercise mainly because of the opening of underperfused pulmonary capillaries, which provides more surface area for diffusion of oxygen.

Cardiovascular System During Exercise (p. 1038)

As discussed in Chapter 20, the blood flow through muscle increases up to 25 times that of normal during exercise. Most of the muscle blood flow occurs between contractions because the blood vessels are compressed during the contractile process. An increase in arterial pressure during exercise directly increases flow. Stretching of the arteriolar walls by the increase in pressure decreases vascular resistance and increases flow much more.

Athletic Training Increases Stroke Volume and Decreases Resting Heart Rate. If a normal person starts extensive athletic training of the aerobic type, both the heart size and maximum cardiac output increase. The *stroke volume* thus increases, and the resting heart rate decreases. Table 84–3 shows the results of training. Note that the stroke volume increases only 50% during maximum exercise in the marathoner, and the heart rate

Table 84–3. Comparison of Cardiac Output between Marathoners and Nonathletes

Condition	Stroke Volume (mL)	Heart Rate (beats/min)
Resting		
Nonathlete	75	75
Marathoner	105	50
Maximum		
Nonathlete	110	195
Marathoner	162	185

increases 270%. Cardiac output can be calculated from the data in Table 84–3 with the following formula:

$$\text{Cardiac Output} = \text{Stroke Volume} \times \text{Heart Rate}$$

The increase in heart rate provides a much greater proportion of the increase in cardiac output in the marathoner than does the increase in stroke volume.

The Heart Limits the Amount of Exercise One Can Perform. During maximum exercise cardiac output is at 90% of its maximum value, but pulmonary ventilation is only 65% of its maximum. The cardiovascular system usually limits the amount of exercise that can be performed.

During any type of cardiac disease, the maximum cardiac output decreases, which limits the amount of exercise that can be performed. Any type of respiratory disease that severely limits pulmonary ventilation or oxygen-diffusing capacity also limits exercise.

Body Heat During Exercise (p. 1039)

The body produces a large amount of heat during exercise, and problems with elimination of this heat from the body can limit exercise. Hot, humid conditions limit heat loss and can lead to *heat stroke*; symptoms include nausea, weakness, headache, profuse sweating, confusion, dizziness, collapse, and unconsciousness. The person is treated by decreasing his or her body temperature as quickly as possible.

Dehydration also occurs in hot, humid conditions during exercise and can lead to nausea, muscle cramps, and other effects. Therapy is provided by replacing the fluid, sodium, and potassium losses.

Note: Page numbers followed by *f* indicate figures and *t* indicate tables.